Short Notes for Dental PG Entrance Examinations

Second Edition

Including Review for UG Students

Clinical Sciences Volume 5

- Periodontics
- Prosthodontics
- Radiology

Volumes in the Series

Short Notes for **Dental PG Entrance Examinations**

Second Edition

Basic Sciences

- **Volume 1** BDS I
- **Volume 2** BDS II
- **Volume 3** BDS III

Clinical Sciences

- **Volume 4** Operative Dentistry, Endodontics, Oral Surgery, Local Anaesthesia, Orthodontics, Pedodontics
- **Volume 5** Periodontics, Prosthodontics, Basic Radiology Self-Assessment Paper, Model Test Papers

Short Notes for Dental PG Entrance Examinations

Second Edition

Including Review for UG Students

Clinical Sciences Volume 5

SANDEEP GOYAL MDS (Orthodontics)
Professor
Department of Orthodontics and Dentofacial Orthopedics
ITS College of Dental Sciences and Research
Murad Nagar, UP

Edited by
Sonia Goyal MDS (Oral and Maxillofacial Surgery)
Associate Professor, Department of Oral and Maxillofacial Surgery,
ITS College of Dental Sciences and Research, Murad Nagar, UP

CBS Publishers & Distributors Pvt Ltd

New Delhi • Bangalore • Pune • Cochin • Chennai

Second Edition

Short Notes for Dental PG Entrance Examinations Volume 5

First Edition : 2006
Second Edition : 2010

ISBN : 978-81-239-1802-0

Published by Satish Kumar Jain and produced by Vinod K. Jain for
CBS Publishers & Distributors Pvt Ltd
4819/XI Prahlad Street, 24 Ansari Road, Daryaganj,
New Delhi 110 002, India.
Fax: 011-23243014 e-mail: cbspubs@vsnl.com; delhi@cbspd.com
Website: www.cbspd.com

Branches

- **Bangalore:** Seema House 2975, 17th Cross, K.R. Road, Banasankari 2nd Stage, Bangalore 560 070
  Fax: 080-26771680 e-mail: cbsbng@gmail.com
- **Pune:** Shaan Brahmha Complex, Basement, Appa Balwant Chowk,
  Budhwar Peth, next to Ratan Talkies, Pune 411 002
  Fax: 020-24464059 e-mail: pune@cbspd.com
- **Cochin:** 36/14 Kalluvilakam, Lissie Hospital Road, Cochin-682018, Kerala
  e-mail: cochin@cbspd.com
- **Chennai:** 20, West Park Road, Shenoy Nagar, Chennai 600030.
  email: chennai@cbspd.com

Printed at Somya Printers, Delhi-110053

dedicated
to
Ma Vaishno Devi,
my parents
and
my teachers

Acknowledgments

At the very outset, I bow my head to the Almighty God and my Guruji for all the grace showered on me to compile the second edition of the book. I am also thankful to my parents for their unforgettable sacrifices and choicest blessings.

I acknowledge the words of advice given to me by Dr Prof. Hari Parkash, Director General, ITS College of Dental Sciences and Research, Murad Nagar.

I place on record my deep gratitude towards my mentors and guides, my respected teachers during my postgraduation, Dr D N Kapoor, the then Professor and Head; Dr V P Sharma, Professor; Dr Pradeep Tandon, Professor, Department of Orthodontics and Dentofacial Orthopedics, Faculty of Dental Sciences, KGMC, Lucknow, for all their blessings, ideas and inspiration.

Prof P B Sood, Principal, ITS College of Dental Sciences and Research, Murad Nagar, has always been a constant source of insipiration and advice.

Dr Sanjay Tiwari, Professor and Head, Department of Endodontics, and Principal, GDC, PGIMS, Rohtak, for all his good wishes, the support, stimulating criticism and magnanimous help during my UG/PG days and afterwards.

My wife Dr Sonia Goyal MDS (oral and maxillofacial surgery), for her support, constant advice, contribution and editing the text, and all the pains she took during the compilation of the project.

Mr S K Jain and Mr Y N Arjuna of CBS Publishers & Distributors Pvt Ltd and their team of professionals for their best suggestions and help in getting this work published in the present form.

Last but not the least, I acknowledge all my family members and friends for their best wishes to boost my morale.

Sandeep Goyal MDS

Preface to the Second Edition

We thank all our readers for their overwhelming support and inputs for the first edition of our series **Short Notes for PG Dental Entrance Examinations**. However, with the increasing competition and increasing base of knowledge, a strong requirement for the improvement has been felt.

In the second edition, we have tried to incorporate a few new topics which will be helpful to postgraduate aspirants. We have now compiled the basic subjects and clinical subjects separately. This will help those undergraduate students also who aspire to compete for postgraduate entrance examination in the future. This edition will help and guide them to build their knowledge base from the very beginning of their dental career and will be helpful in their regular BDS examinations and also *viva voce* examinations.

We have included MCQs in this new edition for the side-by-side exercise and testing the skills and growth of their knowledge base. The book in the second edition has now been split into five volumes, considering the valuable additions made in the text as well new sections of MCQs which have been selectively added to strengthen the inherent appeal of this title amongst the potential readers. Basic Sciences are covered in Vols 1–3 and Clinical Sciences in Vols 4 and 5.

We request our readers to continue sending their suggestions to us for future improvements for the benefit of their friends, juniors and other future dental surgeons.

In the end, we again emphasize that all the aspirants should synergize their knowledge by reading standard theory books to smoothly sail through the ocean of entrance examination, since our volumes may not be complete in every aspect.

Sandeep Goyal MDS
Sonia Goyal MDS
goyalsandeep2000@rediffmail.com
goyalsandeep2000@gmail.com

Preface to the First Edition

There has been a marked increase in competition in dental PG entrance examinations, which have become tougher in recent times. A proper guidance to the aspirants is, therefore, necessary for making their preparations.

The trend of today being MCQ-based, the aspirants just memorise the MCQs from the books available in the market without going into the depth of the statement, leading to errors during the examination. Also, a series of MCQs currently available in the market unfortunately contain 50 to 60% repetition of the questions, and the answers to many questions given in the answer key are also misleading and confusing for the students.

Most of the students do not want to undertake a detailed study of the subjects for their preparation and hence look for the easiest method to get through in the examinations which they consider to be present in the MCQ books.

In my view, MCQ books are for practice only. Your basic knowledge is tested through MCQs and they help to churn your mind, but you should not read them blindly thinking that they will be repeated in the examinations as such. The paper setters change the statements and options of the MCQs for better judgement of the student, therefore, only those students who have a strong basic knowledge can easily analyze and correlate the statement and the option. Also, for some of those students who read the textbooks and do not make notes but rather underline the text or write in the textbooks only, revision becomes very confusing and time-consuming.

This book has been compiled with an idea in mind to provide handy information in the form of a ready-reckoner to the aspirants. This volume covers eight important subjects, and other subjects will be included in the latter volume(s). The motive of compiling information in this manner is to bring important points of each topic together so that a student while reading the topics can revise all the key points immediately and at one stretch.

I have tried with the best possible efforts to tabulate and alphabetically arrange most of the important information so as to make it easy for the students to search for the required topic. The book speaks about the points to be stressed in the form of lists, like the most common terms, syndromes, synonyms, etc.

This book gives the students the guidelines and information about the topics most often asked in the examinations. However, they are advised to go for **further detailed reading from standard textbooks to supplement and reinforce their knowledge.**

I have attempted my best to include almost 80 to 90% of the important information on the covered subjects. However, the readers must study additionally and add their own points on the topics for their benefit.

No project can be completed and improved upon without **feedback**, constructive criticism and healthy suggestions. It is my humble request to all the readers and students to send me their suggestions and points/topics to be added in further editions of the book, to make it more informative and useful for their younger friends and students. It is promised that these suggestions will be suitably incorporated in the future editions and all the contributors will be suitably acknowledged. My e–mail address is goyalsandeep2000@sify.com. Wishing you all the success in your examinations.

Sandeep Goyal MDS

Suggested Readings

Since we do not claim this book to be complete in all the respects, we advise the students to further supplement their information by going through other standard textbooks on particular topics. We are providing below a list of some books for reference for the students.

	Author	*Textbook on*
1.	Monheim's	Local anesthesia
2.	Malamed's	Local anesthesia
3.	Graber's	Orthodontics – an art or science
4.	Profitt's	Orthodontics
5.	Grossman's	Endodontics
6.	Cohen's	Endodontics, i.e. pathways to the pulp
7.	Ingle's	Endodontics
8.	Gupta	Removable Partial Prosthodontics
9.	Orban's	Dental and oral histology
10.	Ten cate's	Oral histology
11.	Shafer's	Oral pathology
12.	Stone's	Oral pathology
13.	Burkitt's	Oral medicine
14.	Sikri	Dental Radiology, 4/e
15.	Sikri	Conservative Dentistry
16.	Goaz /White	Radiology
17.	Singh	Embryology
18.	Garg	Histology, 4/e

Standard books of MCQs which should be read definitely:

- ❑ Series of NDBs, i.e. national dental board papers, available upto L – series in I and II volumes.
- ❑ Rudman's
- ❑ Boucher's
- ❑ Steele's
- ❑ Gardiner's
- ❑ Cawson's
- ❑ Reed's Vols I & II
- ❑ Arco's Vols I & II

Besides these books, the students should always refer to the MCQ books available in the market for practice but they should not get confused.

Contents of Volume 5

Contents of Volume 4

CLINICAL SCIENCES
Volume 4

Abbreviations Used in the Book

AD	autosomal dominant
A.	artery
Ag/Ab/	antigen/antibody
Aka	also known as
Alv.	alveolar
Ant./post.	anterior/posterior
As	arsenic
Ass.	associated
B/W	between
Bact.	bacteria
BCC	basal cell ca.
C/E	clinical exam.
Ca.	carcinoma
Ch.	chronic/characteristics
Chr.	chromosomes
Cp.	compared
CT	connective tissue
Def.	deficiency
Dev.	develop/developmental
Dis	disease/distance as per the case
D/D	differential diagnosis
Enz.	enzyme
Epith.	epithelium/-al
ECA/ICA	external/internal carotid A
H/E	histology examination
IU	intrauterine
LAP	lymphadenopathy
LN	lymph nodes
LO	lateral oblique
M.	muscles
Mm	mucous membrane
MO/m.o.	malocclusion
Md/mand	mandibular
Memb.	membrane
MNGC	multinucleated giant cells
MNP/LNP	median/lateral nasal process
Mo.	months

Mx/max	maxillary
n.m.	neuromuscular
O/F	oral features
Org./orgs	organism/organisms
OTM	orthodontic tooth movement
OMV	occipito-mental view
OFD	object–film distance
PO	presence of
PA	periapical/posteroanterior
PNS	para nasal sinus
Pt.	patient
PDL	periodontal ligament
R/G	radiograph
R/L	radiolucent
R/O	radiopaque
REE	reduced enamel epith
Reqd.	required
SCC	squamous cell ca.
SG	salivary gland
S/S	signs and symptoms
SMV	submento-vertex view
Synd	syndrome
TFD	target–film distance
TOD	target–object distance
Vit.	vitamin

How to Prepare for the Entrance Examinations

This is my personal experience for PG entrance preparation and a time-tested method as many of my friends who have followed this method have been successful in the exams.

1. You have to believe in that hard work and luck go side by side.
2. Keep at least 6–8 months for preparation, which should be free from any sort of disturbance and forget about your surroundings.
3. Devote at least 8–10 hrs/day for the studies.
4. Divide your time and make a time bound schedule.
5. Pick important subjects first depending on the numbers of questions asked in the examinations. The subjects to be studied and stressed during entrance preparation are : general anatomy; dental materials; dental histology; pharmacology; oral pathology; fluorides; endodontics; periodontology; local anaesthesia; pedodontics; basics of all the clinical subjects.
6. Make your daily routine and diligently follow it.
7. Read MCQs two times from NDBs and any other standard book available on a particular subject. This will give you an idea about the style of MCQs and the part of the topic from which the question has been picked from the text, e.g. many MCQs are taken from the legends written below the figures in the book especially dental histology, periodontology, orthodontics.
8. Pick up a standard textbook which you have read during UG days. Read the topics and make notes separately and underline the important points. This will help you to strengthen your knowledge on that topic. Then take other subjects and follow the same pattern.
9. Read only relevant parts of the non-clinical subjects. Stress on anatomy, embryology, dental histology, pharmacology and physiology during the preparation.

10. All the topics and subjects should be covered in the time that at least two months are left for revision before the examination which you are preparing for.
11. When you have finished all the subjects, pick the MCQs books and read the 2–3 times. Any problem can be referred to your notes/textbooks.
12. Mark difficult MCQs in the book with different colors and read them carefully everytime.
13. 15 days before exams, read the notes on all the subjects, followed by one more revision of MCQs.
14. Discussion with your friends is a very important part of preparation. It gives an insight into the topics and more informations.
15. Take all the exams as far as possible; it tells you the trend; your standing and reshuffles your knowledge.

If you follow these rules, I can guarantee you 100% success in the examinations.

Syllabus

Given below is brief outline of the syllabus and topics the students should follow during preparation which should be supplemented by other topics for better knowledge.

Subjects	**Topics**	**Books advised**
Anatomy	◆ Head and neck — complete ◆ Brain — basics	Chaurasia's
Embryology	◆ Basics ◆ Pharyngeal arches ◆ Fetal circulation ◆ Fate of germ layers ◆ Development of oral cavity and face	I B Singh
Histology	◆ Basics ◆ Cell structure, cell division ◆ All glands and appendages, spleen, liver, etc. ◆ Skin, epithelium, A, V, N, M, CT	I B Singh
Dental materials	Complete	Skinners
Physiology	◆ Basics ◆ Blood, GIT, CVS, respiration, endocrinology	Chatterjee
Biochemistry	Basic concepts, enzymes, DNA/RNA, Krebs's cycle, HMP, etc. cycles carbohydrate/ lipid/ protein structure and metabolism, vitamins, minerals, energy requirements, etc.	Rama Rao, Harper's

Subjects	Topics	Books advised
Dental histology	Complete	Orbans
Dental anatomy	Basics, difference in morphology of molars, premolars, canines, mand lateral incisors, etc., occlusion, TMJ, alveolar bone	Wheeler's
Microbiology	Basics, sterilisation, structure of bacteria and virus, immunity, Ag–Ab reactions, *Strept.*, *Staph.*, *Clostridia*, *Mycobacterium,* HIV, Hepatitis virus	Ananthnarayan
Pathology	Basics only, neoplasia definitions, blood pathology (Do not waste much time on it.)	Robins
Pharmacology	Basic concepts, pharmacokinetics and dynamics, dental pharmacology, antibiotics, analgesics, LA/GA, sympathomimetic/lytic drugs, cholinergics/adrenergic, etc., briefly about CVS, CNS, antiepileptic, etc. Mechanism of action of all the drugs, MCQs	K D Tripathi
Oral pathology	Complete	Shafer's
Surgery/ medicine	Basics only, HT, TB, DM, infections, etc.	Any book
PCD	Fluorides, epidemiology, definitions, indices;	
Orthodontics	Basics, growth, ceph, diagnosis, appliances, wire properties, tissue reactions, forces, anchorage, tooth movements	Graber's, Proffit's

Subjects	**Topics**	**Books advised**
Local anesthesia	Complete	Monheim's, Malamed
Oral surgery	Basics; sterilisation, sutures, grafts, fascial infections, maxillary sinus, TMJ, salivary glands, fractures and x-rays	Kruger's, Killey's
Operative	Basics, cavity preparation, classification, cariolgy, instruments, cements and restorative materials, differences between cavity of silver, gold, porcelain, etc.	Sturdevant, Marzouk
Endodontics	Complete book	Grossman, Weine
Pedodontics	Complete book	Mcdonald's, Finn's
Periodontics	Complete book	Glickmann's
Radiography	Brief, basics	Any standard book
Prosthodontics	Basics of CD/impressions; materials, occlusions, jaw relations, implants, TMJ, movements, immediate dentures, etc.	Boucher's Fenn Winkler's
	Basics of FPD preparations, finish lines, crown preparations, principles, gingival retraction, impression, casting, etc.	Shillinburg Dykema
	Basics of RPD, DR, IR, connectors, classification of RPDs, diagnosis and Rx plan, surveyor, etc.	McCracken's Steward

Clinical Sciences

Volume 5

- Periodontics
- Prosthodontics
- Basic Radiology
- *Self-Assessment Paper*
- *Model Test Papers*

10

Periodontics

Important points

- **Mean thickness** of PDL is 0.2 mm (0.15–0.38 mm).
- **2 days** old supragingival plaque has = streptococci.
- **Plaque in** caries is = acidic.
- Plaque in PD diseases = is basic.
- **Keye's technique** = i.e. applying hypertonic salts in an oxidative antiseptic for controlling plaque.
- Subgingival plaque is more tenacious than supragingival plaque.
- **Supragingival** contains = 10^{11} bact./gm wet wt.
- Plaque cannot mineralise in = acid environment.
- LJP is usually severe in patients with = defective neutrophils.
- Alveolar bone/ID septum = 1.5 mm below CEJ.
- In plaque, acid fermentation of carbohydrate occurs in = 2–5. minutes, or few seconds.
- Only oral microbes which produces collagenase = bacteroides melaninogenicus.
- Lactobacilli are prominent in caries, because they are secondary invaders and acid atmosphere is favourable for them.
- Bacteria dominant in root surface caries are—**Actinomyces**.
- Bacteria which decrease the damaging potential of lactic acid by using it as a metabolite are—**Neisseria and Veillonella**. So they are anti–caries bacteria. Veillonella acts as ***symboint of streptococci***.

- PH of normal plaque is 7.1; while pH of plaque in caries prone persons is 5.5, i.e. acidic due to lactic acid.
- Sucrose → glucose + fructose.
- Glucose → dextrans (alpha- 1, 3 linkage).
- Fructose → levans.
- Cyanoacrylate = is an adhesive, which can be used instead of sutures.
- Sounding = is know as transgingival probing.
- Free gingival groove is related to = arrangement of supra alveolar fibres.
- **Tartar controlling agents** used in tooth pastes are—triclosan; zinc citrate pyrophosphate.

Causative microbes

Root surface caries	Actinomyces viscosus
Bacteria which form intracellular apatite crystals	Veillonella
Green stain of plaque	Aspergillus and penicillin
Bacteria to colonise first after tooth surface is cleaned	*Strept. Sanguis* and *S mitis*
Early supragingival plaque	G + cocci and rods
Mature supragingival plaque	Spirochetes/G (–) rods, e.g. bacteroides, which causes gingivitis
Tooth ass. sub-gingival plaque	G + cocci and rods, e.g. actinomyces, which cause root caries
Epith ass. sub-gingival plaque	G (–) bacteria
Caries initiated by	*S mutans*
Bacteria prominent in dentinal caries/deep cavity	Lactobacilli
Bacteria prominent in pits and fissures	Lactobacilli

Causative microbes (*Contd.*)

Bact prominent in smooth surface caries	*S mutans*
Bacteria which decrease damagingpotential of lactic acid by using it as a metabolite	Veillonella and neisseria
Symbiont of streptococci	Veillonella

Bluish line of gingiva in plumbism = known as **Burtonian line.**

Immunoglobulins—are glycoproteins; source for preparation of human gamma globulins is placenta.

Ig for auto-immune reactions	IgM
Ig **maximum in saliva**	Salivary IgA
Ig **maximum in sulcular** fluid	IgG
Smallest Ig, **most abundant**	IgG
Ig that **crosses placenta**	IgG
Warm antibodies	IgG
Blocking antibodies	IgG
Largest immunoglobulins	IgM
Earliest antibody to be synthesised	IgM
Natural antibodies	IgM
Mainly **intravascular** immunoglobulins	IgM
Cold antibodies	IgM
Reaginic antibodies (allergies)	IgE
Heat labile Ig	IgE
Ig with **minimum half life**	IgE
Ig that **protects the surface**	Ig A
Commonest Ig **deficiency**	Ig A
Prevents adhesion of bacteria to mucosa	IgA
Ig present in **milk**	IgA and IgG
By G + bacteria	IgG
By G – bacteria	IgM

IgM	First to be formed after infection, i.e. has a role in early stages of infection. Also activates the complement system.
IgE	Responsible for severe acute allergic response. Attaches to mast cells and basophilic leucocytes.
IgD	Binds with B-cells. Triggers lymphocytic stimulation. Does not activate complements (unlike IgG, M).
IgA	Main Ig of exocrine secretions, i.e. tears, milk, saliva, etc. 2 types—serum IgA is monomer; found in GCF; secretory IgA is dimmer; resistant to digestion. Does not activate complements (unlike IgG, M).
IgG	Most abundant in serum; distributed equally b/w blood and extravascular fluids. Neutralizes the bacterial toxins and helps phagocytosis. Passes through placental barrier. Provides newborns with the humoral immunity of the mother.

Cells maximum in sulcular fluid = PMN.

Lymphocytes predominent in sulcular fluid = B-cells.

Lymphocytes predominent in blood = T-cells.

Stages of Gingivitis

Stages	**Lesion**	**Predominant cells**
I.	Initial lesion	Neutrophils
II.	Early lesion	Lymphocytes
III.	Established lesion	Plasma cells
IV.	Advanced lesion	—

Brushing:

Technique	**Directions of bristles**	**Comment**
Scrub tech	Horizontal	Most common to cause abrasion
Bass/	Pointing apically, at **sulcular**	Most common 45 to long axis of teeth recommended tech
Roll tech	Pointing apically, parallel to long axis of teeth	Least efficient
Mod. Stillman's	Pointing apically, at 45 to long axis of teeth	Recommended if gingival recession and root exposures
Charter's tech	Pointing occlusally, at 45 to long axis of teeth	Recommended after gingival surgeries
Fone's tech	Horizontal	Recommended in children
Stillman's	Pointing apically, at 45 to long axis of teeth	

Tooth brushing techniques

Technique	**Bristle position**	**Motion**	**Effects**
Horizontal scrub	90° to teeth	Horizontal strokes	Supraging cleaning Gingival stimulation
Fones	Do	Large circles over teeth and gingiva	Do
Leonard	Do	Vertical strokes	Do

Tooth brushing techniques (*Contd.*)

Technique	Bristle position	Motion	Effects
Smith-Bell	At occlusal surface	Sweep gingivally	Supragingival cleaning
Rolling strokes	Apically at attached gingiva	Sweep in arc occlusally	Supraging cleaning gingival stimulation
Stillman	45 to apex; part on gingival margin, part on cervix of tooth	Vibratory pulsing	Gingival stimulation
Modified charters	90° to teeth	Sweep occlusally, circular vibratory	Interdental cleaning Gingival stimulation
Modified bass	45 to apex; in sulcus	Sweep occlusally, vibratory, horizontal jiggle	Supraging cleaning Gingival stimulation

Important points about tooth brushing

- Most commonly used method which causes tooth abrasions–scrub technique.
- Most commonly recommended method, bass or sulcular method.
- Least efficient method is—roll technique.
- Method which is recommended in gingival recession and root exposures—modified stillman method.
- Method which is recommended after pd surgeries—charter's method.
- Recommended method in children—fones technique.

- Brushing efficiency depends on 3 factors—technique; frequency and duration; brush design.
- Modified Bass technique = only technique which **cleanses the sulcus** effectively; **best technique.**
- Modified Charters technique = useful for cleaning **fixed orthodontic appliances**.
- Horizontal scrub technique = worst; however it is most commonly used technique.
- Fones technique = for children; easy to learn and mastered by children.
- Powered tooth brushes are superior to manual tooth brushes; esp for removing interdental plaque.
- 3 minutes brushing time is ideal.
- Brush should be usually changed once in 90 days/3 months.
- Most widely used ***disclosing agent*** is **erythrosin**.

Differences between adult and child's tooth brush

Adult	Child
Has 4 rows	Has 3 rows
Has 10–14 vertical tufts	6 tufts
Size of head = larger	Is 2/3rd of that of adult brush

- Nylon bristles—flexible; non absorbent; rounded ends.
- Floss—unitufted–multitufted; waxed-unwaxed; twisted-unnon twisted.
- **Best floss**—unwaxed; multitufted; twisted.
- Each tuft of brush—has 18–20 bristles.
- Tooth pick is made of—**orange wood.**
- Tooth paste—its abrasive content should specify less than or equal to 100 rad, i.e. radioactive dentinal abrasion value.

Important points

- Instruments = best for root planing = curet.
- Most harmful premature occlusal contacts exist on—non-working side; facial incline of max. lingual cusps and lingual inclines of mand facial cusps.
- Most frequent osseus lesion in periodontitis = crater.
- Gingival clefts may be caused by = faulty tooth brushing.
- Main result of TFO = mobility.
- First fibre group destroyed to allow JE migration = dentogingival, i.e. G1 fibres.
- In gingivitis:
  - Earliest lesion = neutrophils collect.
  - Established lesions = lymphocytes.
  - Advanced lesions = plasma cells.
- Plaque irritates gingival tissue = **biochemically.**
- Gingivitis in a child is frequently related to each of the following except = SPIROCHETES.
- Treatment of hypersensitivity = in anterior teeth = $SrCl_2$ or $CaCl_2$, as they cause no staining; in posterior teeth = by $AgNO_3$.
- Treatment of hypersensitivity = pot. oxalate is most commonly used agent.
- Treatment of hypersensitivity = apply NaF paste (from NDB).
- Histoplasma = a fungus having both capabilities, i.e. dimorphism and produces gingivitis also.
- Histoplamosis microbes are also found in RE system.

Gingival index by Loe and Silness

- 0 = clinically healthy gingiva.
- 1 = no bleeding upon palpation.
- 2 = bleeding.
- 3 = spontaneous bleeding.

Plaque index by Silness and Loe

FUNCTIONS OF FOLLOWING

1. I_2 = iodine = antimicrobial, astringent.
2. H_2O_2 = kills anaerobes, removes debris by nascent oxygen, RC irrigant.
3. 0.2% chlorhexidine = antiseptic.
4. KNO_3 = desensitizer in tooth paste, cariostatic.
5. 0.2% NaF = remineralisation, antibacterial.

Types of embrasures

1. Type I = floss.
2. Type II = proxa brush.
3. Type III = unitufted brush.

- In periodontitis = an increased IgA would suggest the possibility of an increased response to oral Ag—stimulation.
- First stage of LJP = destruction of principal fibers of PDL; degeneration.
- First step in pathogenesis of PD pocket formation = is breakdown of sulcular epithelium.
- For epithelium to migrate apically = group A, i.e. (G1) fibers must be destroyed, as these are the fibers attached immediately apical to the epithelium attachment.
- Plasma cell gingivitis = is ass. with use of chewing gums.
- Sterile necrosis by TFO.
- Natural Abs = IgM.
- Hemiseptum = one walled bony defect.
- Intra-bony pockets = 3 walled defect.
- After PD surgery—epitheium attachment takes 8 weeks for healing and so floss is not recommended.
- Estrogen and progesterone act as growth factors for bacteroides by substituting for vitamin K, i.e. menadione.
- Epithelium of epithelium—attachment does not contain = rete-pegs, but which are acquired during apical migration.

HYPERSENSITIVITY

Type I, Anaphylaxis or immediate	IgG, i.e. blocking Ab, IgE, i.e. reaginic Ab	IgG + mast cell complex reacts with Ag	Histamine, SRS-A are released
Type II, Cytotoxic	IgG, IgM	(Cell with Ag) r.w. Ab	Cell lysis, e.g. RBCs, as in autoimmune diseases, e.g. pemphigus, pemphigoid, SLE, rheumatoid arthritis, mickulicz's dis
Type III, Arthus' reaction	Local tissue damage, vascular endothelium	Ag rw Ab	Lysosomal enzymes
Type IV, Delayed hypersen-sitivity	No Abs involved here	T-cells r.w. Ag	Lymphokines, OAF, etc. released

Schwartzman's reaction = is not an immune reaction, but an alteration in factors affecting intravascular coagulation. So first dose is intradermal; and second dose is I/V, which then causes necrotic lesion at the site of first dose.

e.g. in Waterhouse = Friderichsen syndrome, acute adrenal deficiency, here, endotoxins play a role in Schwartzman's reaction.

Systemic form of Arthus reaction = is serum sickness.

DISTANCES

1. Mean thickness of PDL is 0.2 mm (0.15–0.38 mm).
2. Marginal gingiva 1 mm.

3. Gingival sulcus 2–3 mm.
4. Attached gingiva max CI = 3.5–4.5 mm, maximum.

   M and CI 3.3–3.9 mm.

   Max First PM 1.9 mm.

   M and first PM 1.8 mm, minimum.
5. Junctional epithelium 0.25–1.35 mm.
6. JE-epithelium bone crest 1.07 mm (in young) 2.81 mm (in olds).
7. Physiologic mesial migration 1.0 cm on each side,
8. Radius of action of plaque 1.5–2.5 mm.
9. Bone loss/year in periodontitis.
10. Bone loss/year after full mouth extractions.
11. Cementum is thickest at apex, its thickness is 150–200 microns.
12. Cementum is thinnest at apex, its thickness is 20–50 microns.
13. Specific gravity of saliva 1.003.
14. Amount of GCF secreted per day by normal gingival 0.5–2.4 ml.
15. Concentration of tetracycline in GCF is 2–10 times that of plasma.
16. Probing depth of normal gingival sulcus is 2–3 mm.
17. Histologic depth of normal gingival sulcus is 1.5–1.8 mm.
18. Oxygen coefficient of normal gingival is 1.6 ± 0.37.
19. Diameter of standard probe tip is 0.35–0.55 mm.
20. Recommended probing force is 0.25 N or 2.5 gm, w.
21. Total no. of intra-oral films recommended for complete full mouth survey is = 18; (IOPA–14; bitewings–4).
22. Plaque contains bacteria as 1.7×10^{11} per gm wt (i.e. 1.7×10^{8} per mg wt).
23. Average daily increment in calculus former is 0.1–0.15%.
24. Minimum levels of cyclosporine in plasma above, which gingival hyperplasia occurs is 150 nanogm/ml.
25. Duration of each masticatory cycle is 0.6–1.0 sec.

26. Number of swallows per day in an individual is 600 times/24 hrs.
27. Total occlusal points in dentition are 138.
28. Normal Ca and P precipitate concentration is 35–40%.
29. Tooth brush abrasion of dentin is more than enamel by 15–25 times.
30. Cementum is abraded more than enamel by 35 times.
31. Conc. of chlorhexidine used in mouthwashes is 0.12–0.2%.

Furcation lesions can be graded as

Grade	Features
I.	Incipient early lesion; pocket is suprabony; bone loss is minimal; cannot be detected.
II.	Bone destroyed on one aspect of the furcation; a part of PDL and alveolar bone end is intact; partial penetration of probe possible.
III.	Interradicular bone is completely absent; probe can be passed through and through; but furcation not visible as it is covered by gingival tissue.
IV.	Same as grade III, but furcation is visible and denuded.

1. Grade 1 = bone loss upto 1/3rd of the tooth width, i.e. about 3 mm of horizontal attachment loss.
2. Grade 2 = bone loss b/w 1/3rd and 2/3rd of the tooth width.
3. Grade 3 = a through and through lesion.

- Extent of furcation is measured by Naber's probe.

Tooth mobility = according to Miller's index is:

1. Score 1 = mobility upto 1 mm.
2. Score 2 = mobility of 1–2 mm.
3. Score 3 = mobility over 2 mm and or rotation or depression in the socket.

Recession: According to Miller's classification.

Class I; prognosis is good to excellent	Marginal gingival recession does not extend to mucogingival line. No soft tissue and bone loss seen in I/D area.
Class II; prognosis is good to excellent	Marginal gingival recession extends to MGL or beyond; no soft tissue and bone loss seen in I/D area.
Class III; partial coverage can be seen	Marginal gingival recession extends to MGL or beyond; soft tissue and bone loss seen in I/D expected area and malpositioning of teeth.
Class IV; hopeless prognosis	Marginal gingival recession extends to MGL or beyond; severe soft tissue and bone loss seen in I/D area and severe malpositioning of teeth.

Periodontal indices

DEBRIS INDEX = by Green and Vermillion 1960.

0 no plaque.

1 plaque covering 1/3rd tooth.

2 plaque covering 2/3rd tooth.

3 plaque totally covering tooth.

Plaque index, Silness and Loe 1964.

0 no plaque detected.

1 looks clean but material can be removed from gingival 1/3rd with probe.

2 visible plaque.

3 tooth covered with abundant plaque.

Modified gingival index, Loe 1967.

0 healthy gingiva.

1 gingiva looks inflammed, but do not bleed on probing.

2 gingiva looks inflammed, and bleeds on probing.

3 ulceration and spontaneous bleeding.

Community periodontal index of Rx needs: CPITN.

CPITN probe = has a ball end of 0.5 mm in diameter; colour coded area extends from 3.5–5.5 mm; probing force of 20–25 gm is recommended.

Code 0	Healthy gingival tissues with no bleeding after probing.
Code 1	Bleeding on probing, plaque present, but no calculus or defective restoration margins, pockets < 3.5 mm.
Code 2	Bleeding on probing, calculus detected or defective restoration margins, but pockets < 3.5 mm.
Code 3	Pockets within colour coded area, i.e. pocket > 3.5 mm to < 5.5 mm.
Code 4	Colour coded area disappears indicating pocket > 5.5 mm.

False pocket = where increased probing depth is due to gingival enlargement without loss of attachment of the PDL.

True pocket = where increased probing depth results from destruction of PDL.

Recession = where the gingival margin lies apical to the CEJ.

ORAL HYGIENE AIDS

Tooth brushes	The mimp features are the size of head, texture of filaments, rounded ends of the bristles.
Electric tooth brush	Beneficial in patients with reduced manual dexterity.
Single tufted brushes	Cleans around lone-standing teeth; partially erupted M3, proximal spaces adj to saddle areas in partially dentate patients.
Floss **Tape**	Broader than floss; used in i/d areas.

ORAL HYGIENE AIDS (*Contd.*)

Superfloss	Used for cleaning under the bridges.
Floss threader	Used to pass floss below the FPD.
Interproximal/ bottle brushes	Method of choice for i/d cleansing when space permits.
Wooden sticks	Not so effective than interproximal brushes.

Root planning involves removal of subgingival plaque, calculus and infected cementum.

Scaling instruments

Instrument	**Description**	**Area of use**
Chisel/push scaler	Chisel head angled at 45.	Applied from labial to remove gross supragingival deposits from approximal surfaces of mand ant teeth.
Point scaler/ + sickle scalers and jacquettes	Are triangular in cross section and have 2 cutting edges, which converge to a sharp point.	All buccal and lingual embreasures, supragingival and 2–3 mm subgingival. Manipulated with wrist movements.
Hoes	Have a blade set at 100 angle to shank and cutting edge is bevelled at 45. A set of 4 is required to give access to all tooth surfaces.	Access to deep pockets; used in a series of pull strokes. Subgingival depostits.
Curettes	Curved spoon shaped blade with 2 cutting edges, which meet to form a rounded hoe.	Supra, and esp subgingivally throughout the mouth. Used after hoes in root planning.
Ultrasonic scalers		Avoid in patients fitted with a cardiac pacemaker.

Differences b/w periodontal abscess and periapical abscess

C/F	PD abscess	PA abscess
Pain	Acute onset	H/O tooth ache
Swelling	Usually localised, extra-oral swelling unlikely	Over tooth apex; more likely to be extensive
Pocket	Always present; more likely in p.o. PD disease	Pocket may/may not be present
Sinus	Frequently on attached gingiva	Tracks to the apex
Percussion	Tender to percussion; worse laterally	Tender to percussion; esp axially
Restoration status	More likely if tooth caries free/ unrestored	More likely in heavily filled tooth
Vitality	Tooth is vital	Non-vital
Radiograph	Little evidence in early stages; bone loss	Loss of lamina dura in PA areas; after 10 days or so.

Endo-perio lesions = when infection involves both pulp chamber and PDL space simultaneously.

Splint = a means of increasing tooth support by joining to an adjacent tooth or teeth.

A primary function of the PD tissues is to support the tooth when a load is applied.

Trauma from occlusion cannot induce periodontal tissue breakdown, but in p.o. pre-existing PD disease, excessive occlusal loading may increase the PD breakdown.

- Temporary splint for 2–6 mos.
- Provisional splint for 6–12 mos.
- Permanent splint for > 12 mos.

Important procedures

Procedure	Indications
Currettage	• Supra bony pockets. • New attachment attempts. • Maintenance Rx. • In patients with systemic conditions where surgery is C/I.
Gingivectomy	• Supra bony pockets. • Gingival hyperplasia. • Supra bony PD abscess.
Full thickness flaps	Osseous surgery.
Partial thickness flap	For apical repositioning of flap.
Osseous surgery	Infra bony pockets.
Flaps	• Furcation. • Infra bony pockets. • Osseous defects and gingival enlargement.
Mucogingival surgery	• Widening the zone of the attached gingiva. • Coverage of denuded roots. • Shallow vestibules.

Most common Pathogens causing various PD diseases

Disease	Pathogens
Early gingivitis	Actinomyces.
Long standing gingivitis	Fusobacterium and veillonella.
Adult periodontitis	B gingivalis.
Pregnancy gingivitis	Bacteroides intermedius; it can substitute progesterone/estradiole for vitamin K as growth factor.

Most common Pathogens causing various PD diseases (*Contd.*)

Disease	**Pathogens**
Rapidly progressing periodontitis	B gingivalis; B intermedius; small spirochetes, etc. Functional defects in neutrophils or monocytes.
Refractory periodontitis	B gingivalis, etc.
LJP	A. actinomyecetamcomitans (AA); capnocytophaga; Neutrophil chemotactic defect and decreased phagocytosis. Concentration of AA is 6 times greater than the normal sites; Increased Ab levels to AA esp IgG. Serotype B is the commonest.
GJP	B gingivalis is most common. C high IgG titers esp to serotype C.
Periodontitis in juvenile diabetes	Actinomyces and streptococci.
ANUG	• Principal bacteria = B intermedius; unnamed intermediate sized spirochetes; • Superficial bacteria = **Borrelia vincenti; fusiform bacilli.** • **Increased Ab titers IgG; IgM.**
AIDS	• Bacteroides melaninogenicus. • G + bacilli. • G – wet spreaders.
In IDDM; gingivitis	• Actinomyces. • Streptococci. • Veillonella. • Fusobacterium.

Most common Pathogens causing various PD diseases (*Contd.*)

Disease	Pathogens
In IDDM, periodontitis	• Capnocytophaga. • Anaerobes. • It is different than adult periodontitis in which B gingivalis is predominant.
PD abscess	• B gingivalis.
Prepubertal	• Decreased chemotaxis of PMN and periodontitis monocytes. • Main bacteria are fusobacterium, selemonas, etc.

Important values

- ♦ Force applied during brushing = < 500 gm.
- ♦ Dentin abraded = 25 times faster than enamel.
- ♦ Cementum abraded = 35 times faster than enamel.
- ♦ Dentrifrices contain F = 1100 ppm.
- ♦ Distance b/w apical edge of calculus and bottom of pocket = 0.2–1.0 mm.
- ♦ In gingivitis, ratio of T4–T8 cells = 2:1.
- ♦ In periodontitis, ratio of T4–T8 cells = 1:1.
- ♦ In AIDS, ratio of T4–T8 cells is << 1.
- ♦ In sulcular fluid, ratio of T cell : B cells = 1:3.
- ♦ In PBF, the ratio of T cell : B cells = 3:1.
- ♦ Zone of J E = 500 microns or 0.25–1035 mm.
- ♦ Rate of bone loss = 0.2 mm/yr on facial surfaces, 0.3 mm/yr on proximal surfaces.
- ♦ Radius of action required = 1.5–2.5 mm.
- ♦ Loss of attachment occurs 6–8 mos before the bone loss.

Tooth whitening systems

- ♦ It is the Rx of choice if the patient has realistic expectations; teeth are only moderately stained.

- Power bleaching = is an in office procedure; it uses 30–35% of H_2O_2 with heat or light.
- At home tray based system = has 10% H_2O_2 or 22% urea carbamide peroxide solution; used for more than 2 hrs daily.
- Paint on liquid gel = 6.5% H_2O_2.
- Whitening strips = 6.5% H_2O_2.
- Oral irritation is largely associated with tray whitening systems.
- Potassium nitrate is used to overcome dentinal hypersensitivity.

PERI-IMPLANTITIS

- It is an inflammatory process affecting tissues surrounding the osseo-integrated dental implant.
- In healthy peri-implant tissues = aerobic bacteria; high no. of coccoid cells; low no. of G +ve bacteria.
- In unhealthy peri-implant tissues = G –ve anaerobes; spirochetes; motile organisms.
- Pocket depth of more than 3 mm requires investigation.
- Cleaning of implants is done with = carbon fiber curettes; rubber cups and polishing paste.
- Daily rinsing with chlorhexidine digluconate 0.12–0.2%.
- Antibiotic given if pockets are more than 6 mm; amoxycillin + metronidazole is given.
- If pocket depth is more than 5 mm = surgical intervention is done.

FOR MEDICINE PART

- There is an association between low grade infections and cardiovascular diseases.
- CRP lipoprotein LPa; RAS activation, etc. are the non-traditional risk indicators for heart diseases.
- Viral and bacterial infections, e.g. CMV and chlamydia pneumoniae are associated with atherosclerosis.
- LDL is also know as **bad cholesterol**.

- LPS is a toxic component of G –ve cell wall bacteria, which initiates inflammatory responses and monocytic adhesion to walls of blood vessels.
- Activated monocytes also known as **macrophages**.
- Macrophages filled with LDL are know as **foam cells**.
- Plasma level of CRP, i.e. C–reactive protein indicates systemic inflammation.
- High levels of CRP are predictive of increased risk of heart attack years before they occur.
- NIMIT'S NOTES:

GINGIVA

NORMAL PERIODONTIUM

- It contains 2 hard tissues, i.e. cementum and alveolar bone; and 2 soft tissues, i.e. gingival and PDL.
- Origin of periodontium is dental follicle.
- Gingival has 3 parts, i.e. free gingiva (FG); attached gingiva (AG) and interdental papilla.
- FG demarcated from AG by free gingival groove (FGG).
- AG separated from alveolar mucosa by mucogingival junction (MGJ).
- **Colour** of the normal gingiva = coral pink; it depends on the vascularity; degreee of keratinization and pigmentation.
- Under absolute normal or ideal conditions, the depth of gingival sulcus is or about zero.
- Keratinized gingiva = includes marginal and attached gingival.
- Hard tissues of dento-gingival apparatus are cementum and bone; soft tissuc are PDL and gingiva.

Width of attached gingiva

- Is greatest in the incisor region = 3.5 to 4.5 in maxilla; 3.3 to 3.9 mm in mandible.
- Less in posterior segment.

- Least width in the first premolar area = 1.9 mm in maxilla and 1.8 mm in mandible.
- It increases with age and in supra-erupted teeth, although the position of MGJ remains stationary throughout life.

◆ Histology of gingival.

◆ Gingival epithelium may be orthokeratinized; parakeratinized and non-keratinized.

◆ **Orthokeratinized epithelium** has a well defined stratum granulosum with no nuclei in stratum corneum. It has 4 layers, i.e. basale; spinosum; granulosum and corneum.

◆ **Parakeratinized epithelia**, stratum corneum retains **pyknotic nuclei** and ***keratohyalin granules*** are dispersed, not giving rise to a stratum granulosum. It has basale; spinosum and corneum layers.

◆ **Non-keratinized epithelia** has neither stratum granulosum nor stratum corneum layers. It has only basale and spinosum.

◆ **Other cells** = e.g. Langhans cells are antigen presenting cells; Merkel cells are tactile preceptors.

◆ Interdental papilla = is pyramidal in shape in anterior segment and col-shaped in posterior segment.

◆ Col = facial and lingual papilla joined by a valley like depression.

◆ Col is covered by thin, stratified squamous non-keratinized epithelium.

◆ **Basal lamina** is seen under an electron microscope. It is 300–400 A thick. It has **2 layers,** viz. *lamina lucida (glycoprotein laminin) and lamina densa* (type IV collagen).

◆ **Basement membrane** is seen under light microscope. It consists of ***basal lamina and connective tissue elements***.

◆ ***Sulcular epithelium*** and ***non-keratinized stratified squamous*** epithelium are ***without rete pegs*** and extends from the coronal limit of the junctional epithelium JE to the crest of the gingival margins.

◆ JE is stratified squamous non-keratinizing epithelium formed by confluence of oral epithelium and reduced enamel epithelium/ REE during tooth eruption.

- JE and the gingival fibers form a functional unit know as **dento-gingival unit**.
- Gingival connective tissue is mainly **collagen fibers type–I**.
- **Gingival sulcus and probing depth**:
  - Under absolutely ideal conditions; the depth is zero or about zero.
  - Histologic depth = 0–6 mm.
  - Clinically normal gingival sulcus = 2–3 mm.
- **Collagen**:
  - Most abundant protein in the animal kingdom.
  - Polypeptide of 3 alpha–chains, i.e. alpha–1, 2, 3.
  - Collagen molecule may be a homotrimer or hetertrimers.
  - Characterized by repeating Glycine amino acid sequence.
  - In vertebrate collagen = the amino acid at gamma position are hydroxyproline or hydroxylysine.
  - Size of collagen molecue is 300 A × 15 Å. (Å = angstrom unit)
  - Collagen fibers are characterized by a special banding of pattern at 64 nm interval.
  - Collagen biosynthesis involve hydroxylation of proline and lysine, which require oxygen; ferrous ions and vitamin C as cofactors.
- **Stippling** = it is orange-peel like appearance of the surface; gingival has a textured surface know as stippling. It is due to the elevations. Only attached gingival and centre of inter-dental papilla is stippled. Effect of age not in infants and in edentulous patients.
- **Active eruption** is the actual movement of the tooth towards the occlusal plane. **Passive eruption** is the exposure of the tooth by apical migration of gingival.
- **Theories of eruption Supra-eruption.**

PERIODONTAL LIGAMENT/ DETAILS (Also refer to section of dental histology in Vol. I.)

- PDL fibers are known as principal fibers.

- Fibers are mainly formed ***by fibroblasts***.
- Terminal parts of principal fibers which is embedded in the bone and cementum is known as Sharpey's fibers.
- PDL fibers are composed of amino acids, the most prominent of these being the ***collagen type I***.
- Types of collagen fibers ____ locations ____.
- Terminal ends of PDL fibers are embedded in the cementum and bone, and are know as **Sharpey's fibers**.
- Epithelial rests of Malassez are remnants of Hertwig's epithelial root sheath ____ details ____ depth ____ function.
- It has the ***shape of hourglass***, being narrowest in the region of the axis of rotation.
- **Types of principal fibers**

Trans-septal	• Also know as supracrestal fibers ____. • Extend inter-proximally over the alveolar crests and are inserted in the cementum of adjacent tooth. • These fibers are reconstructed even after the destruction of bone has occurred in PD disease. • Are responsible for relapse of rotations after orthodontic Rx.
Alveolar	Run from cementum to bone in the ____ apical direction ____.
Horizontal oblique	• Are largest group of the fibers, i.e. maximum in no. • Run from cementum in a coronal direction to the bone. • Bear most of the masticatory load.
Apical	Not seen in teeth with incompletely formed roots, run almost in a vertical direction from the apex of tooth to bone.
Inter-radicular	Seen only in multi-rooted teeth.

- Calcified masses in PDL are know as cementicles.
- **Sensory receptors in the PDL**:

Free nerve endings	Carry pain sensations.
Ruffini like organs	Mechanoreceptors; located in apical areas.
Meissner's corpuscles	Mechanoreceptors; located in midroot regions.
Spindle like endings	Pressure and irritations sensations.

CEMENTUM (Also refer to section of dental histology in Vol. I.)

- It is formed by the cells know as cementoblasts.
- It is an avascular, mesenchymal tissue.
- 2 sources of collagen fibers in cementum.
  - **Extrinsic fibers** = i.e. **Sharpey's fibers**; are basically PDL fibers embedded in cementum.
  - **Intrinsic fibers** = which belong to cemental matrix. Are formed by cementoblasts.
- It is of 2 types.
- Acellular cementum—is the ***first formed cementum***. It covers the cervical 3rd or half of the root. It does not contain cells. It is formed before the tooth reaches the occlusal plane.
- Cellular cementum = formed after the tooth reaches the occlusal plane; it contains cells and is ***less calcified than acellular*** type. It covers apical part _____ Its thickness _____ , etc.
- Junction between cementum and enamel is of 3 types:

Type of junction	**% age**
Cementum overlaps the enamel	60–65%
Edge to edge butt joint	30%
Cementum and enamel fail to meet	5–10%

- Thickness of cementum varies from 16–60 microns in the coronal half to 150–200 microns in the apical areas.
- Cementum is thickest in apical third and in furcation areas of the tooth.
- Both cementum and PDL are thicker on distal surfaces of roots than on the mesial surface.
- Cementum repair is not affected by the vitality of the tooth.
- Cellular and acellular cementum are differentiated under light microscope.

ALVEOLAR BONE

- Alveolar process is that part of the maxilla and mandible that forms and supports the tooth sockets.
- It is formed by intramembranous ossification.
- **Basal bone** = that part of the jaw located apically to teeth.
- **Alveolar bone proper** is the inner wall of the tooth socket; it is seen as **lamina dura** in R/G; on H/E, it contains small holes through, which neurovascular bundles link PDL with cancellous bone, i.e. ***cribriform plate***.
- **Lamina dura** = the cribriform plate of socket is seen in R/G as thin radiopaque line.
- **Bundle bone** = i.e. bone adjacent to PDL which contains a large no. of Sharpey's fibers. It is localized within alveolar bone proper.
- **Woven bone** = is the first formed bone/immature bone.
- **Lamellar bone**—mature bone made up of layers or lamellae.
- **Cancellous bone/spongy bone/trabecular bone**—it is structurally similar to compact bone, except for the presence of trabecular spaces. More cancellous bone is found in maxilla than the mandible.
- **Bone marrow**—in the embryo and newborns, all bone cavities are occupied by red marrow; in adults, the red marrow changes to yellow/fatty marrow. But red marrow may still be found in ribs, sternum, vertebrae, skull and humerus.

- **Even in jaws,** the foci of red bone marrow may be seen in maxillary tuberosity; maxillary and mandibular molar and premolar areas; and the mandibular symphysis and ramus angle.
- **Periosteum** has 2 layers:
  - Inner layer is composed of osteoblasts surrounded by osteoprogenitor cells.
  - Outer layer is composed of collagen fibers and fibroblasts.
- **Endosteum** is single layered—it is composed of osteoblasts and a small amount of connective tissues.
- Osteoblasts originate from pluripotent stem cells of bone marrow while osteroclasts originate form hematopoietic system.
- Osteoclasts are characterized by their size (50–100 microns); multiple nuclei (2–10); and its presence within resorption lamina at the calcified matrixbone marrow interface.
- Parathormone/PTH acts on bone to produce resorption, thereby increasing the serum calcium levels; but the receptors of PTH in bone are located on osteoblasts (AIPG–99) and not on the osteoclasts.
- Osteoblasts are characterized by the presence of enzyme alkaline phosphatase, while osteoclasts have enzyme acid phosphatase.
- The mesio-distal angulation of the crest of the interdental septum usually parallels a line drawn between the CEJ of the approximating teeth.
- **Fenestrations** are isolated areas, in which the root is denuded of the bone, but the marginal bone is intact. Root is covered only by the periosteum and overlying gingiva.
- **Dehiscence,** i.e. when the denuded areas extend through the marginal bone, it is know as dehiscence.
- Typical feature which distinguishes the gingivitis from periodontitis is the presence of clinically detectable attachment loss.
- Incidence = probability that a person will become a case. It is the ratio of no. of new cases to the no. of persons at risk.
- Prevalence = proportions of persons in a population, who have the disease at a given period of time. It is the ratio of no. of persons with the disease to the no. of persons in the population.

- Sensitivity of a test = is the proportion of subjects with the disease who test positive. It is the ratio of no. of subjects who test positive to the no. of subjects with the disease.
- Specificity of the test = proportion of subjects without the disease who test negative. It is the ratio of subjects who test negative to the no. of subjects without disease.

PLAQUE

- It is a host–associated biofilm. It is defined as soft deposits that form the biofilm adhering to tooth surface or other hard surfaces in the oral cavity.
- Acquired pellicle _____.
- Most common sites are near the orifices of salivary glands.
- More than 500 distinct bacterial species are found in plaque.
- Inorganic component is mainly Ca and P.
- Initial bacteria colonizing the pellicle coated tooth surface are predominantly gram positive facultative microbes, e.g. actinomyces viscosus and streptococcus sanguis.
- Pregnancy associated gingivitis is associated with dramatic increase in the level of P. intermedia/which uses steroids as their growth factors.
- Scurvy diabetes mellitus _____.
- Bismuth pigmentation/Burtonian line is linear, steel grey in colour _____. Other lines of pigmentations lead arsenic, etc. silver, etc. _____.
- Main Ig in saliva = IgA.
- Main Ig in GCF = IgG.

PERIODONTAL MICROBIOLOGY

Plaque = soft deposits that form the biofilm adhering to the tooth surface or other hard surfaces in the oral cavity including removable and fixed restorations.

Materia alba = soft accumulations of bacteria and tissue cells that lack the organized structure of dental plaque and are easily displaced by water spray.

Calculus = is the mineralized plaque.

Plaque = 3 types, i.e. supragingival; marginal; subgingival.

Supragingival plaque causes root caries; calculus formation.

Marginal plaque causes gingivitis.

Subgingival plaque is of 2 types = tooth associated (which causes root caries and calculus) and tissue associated (which causes periodontitis).

More than 500 distinct microbial species are found in dental plaque.

During plaque formation, the initial bacteria colonizing the pellicle coated tooth surface are gram-positive facultative micro-organisms, e.g. actinomyces viscosus and streptococcus sanguis.

The composition of plaque formed on all types of restorative materials is similar with the exception of that formed on silicate.

Pregnancy gingivitis is associated with increases levels of Provetella intermedia, which uses steroids as growth factors in place of vitamin K.

Viruses associated with chronic periodontitis are EBV–1; HCMV.

Localized aggressive periodontitis = actinobacillus actinomycetamcomitans serotype–B (gram negative rods).

Necrotizing periodontal diseases = by P. intermedia and spirochetes.

Calculus = 2 types, i.e. supragingival and subgingival.

Supragingival calculus—most common locations are buccal surfaces of maxillary molars and the lingual surfaces of mandibular anterior teeth. It is because of the presence of the openings of major salivary glands in these vicinity.

Location and extent of subgingival calculus may be evaluated by careful tactile perception with an explorer.

Saliva is the source of mineralization for supragingival calculus, while GCF provides the minerals for subgingival calculus.

Differences b/w supragingival and subgingival calculus:

Properties	**supragingival**	**subgingival calculus**
Colour	Yellow	Black
Consistency	Soft	Hard
Source	Saliva	GCF

Inorganic component of calculus is crystalline in nature. The four main crystal forms are:

1. Hydroxyapatite = 58%.
2. Magnesium whitlockite = 21%.
3. Octacalcium phosphate = 12%.
4. Brushite = 9%.
5. Brushite is more common in ***mandibular anterior region***.
6. Hydroxyapatite and octacalcium phosphate are detected most frequently.
7. Magnesium whitlockite is common in the posterior region.

BACTERIOLOGY

Bacteria	**Features**	**Importance**
Neisseria	G negative cocci, anaerobe	
Veillonella	G negative cocci, anaerobe	
Peptostreptococcus	G positive cocci, anaerobe	
Bacteroides	G negative bacilli	
Eubacterium	G positive bacilli	
Actinobacillus actinomycetam comitans	Gram negative rods	
Provetella	G negative bacilli	
Campylobacter	Gram negative vibrio	
Porphyromonas	G negative bacilli	
Fusobacterium	G negative bacilli	

- Interproximal attachment loss is generally a consequence of bacteria induced periodontitis. While buccal and lingual attachment loss is frequently the result of tooth brush abrasion.

DIABETES

- There is an alteration of oral flora with greater preponderance of Candida albicans; hemolytic strept; staphylococci.
- There is an increased collagenase activity and decreased collagen synthesis render the periodontal tissues more susceptible to destruction.

PREGNANCY

- Pregnancy itself does not cause gingivitis.
- Gingival disease during pregnancy is caused by bacterial plaque, but hormonal change during pregnancy accentuates the gingival response to plaque and modifies the resultant clinical picture.
- Bacteria which increase significantly during pregnancy is = Prevotella intermedia.
- Gingival has "rasp-berry like" appearance.

GINGIVAL ENLARGEMENT

- Hyperplasia vs hypertrophy—No. of cells increase in former.
- Drugs causing gingival enlargement are phenytoin; cyclosporin; nifedipine.
- Idiopathic gingival enlargement involves/affects gingival margin; attached gingival and interdental papillae.
- Capnocytophaga species is implicated in the initiation of pubertal gingivitis.
- Epulis are inflammatory (non-neoplastic) masses of the gingiva.

ACUTE GINGIVAL INFECTIONS

- ANUG; primary herpetic gingivo-stomatitis and pericoronitis are acute gingival infections.

- ANUG is caused by spirochetes Treponema intermedia and fusiform bacilli.
- ANUG is also know as trench mouth.
- Primary infection of AHG is asymptomatic.

PERIODONTAL POCKETS

- It is the pathologically deepened gingival sulcus.
- The only reliable method of locating pocket and determining their extent is CAREFUL PROBING.
- ***Pseudopocket/gingival/false/relative pocket***: Are caused by gingival enlargement without destruction of the underlying periodontal tissues.
- ***True pockets/periodontal/absolute pockets***: It is formed by the destruction of supporting periodontal tissues. It is of suprabony and infrabony types.
- ***Suprabony pockets***: Also known as supracrestal or supraalveolar pocket; bottom of the pocket is coronal to the underlying alveolar bone.
- ***Infrabony pocket:*** Also known as infrabony, subcrestal or intra-alveolar pocket; bottom of the pocket is apical to the level of the adjacent alveolar bone.

Difference between suprabony and infrabony pockets

Suprabony	Infrabony
Base of pocket is cornonal to alveolar crest.	Apical to crest of alveolar bone.
Pattern of destruction of underlying bone is horizontal.	Vertical/angular.
Interproximally, the transseptal fibers restored during PD disease are arranged horizontally.	Obliquely arranged.
PDL fibers below the PD pocket follow normal horizontal-oblique course.	Follow angular pattern.

- ***Simple pocket*** = involves one-tooth surface.
- ***Compound pocket*** involves 2 or more tooth surfaces.
- ***Complex pocket*** = it originates from one tooth surface and twisting around the tooth to involve one or more additional surfaces. Involves more than 2 tooth surfaces. These are spiral type of pockets. These are most common in furcation areas.
- The only reliable method of locating the periodontal pocket is by probing of the gingival margin along each tooth surface.
- Periodontitis is always preceded by gingivitis, but not all gingivitis proceed to periodontitis. Most important cause of gingivitis is plaque.
- The distance b/w the apical extent of calculus and the alveolar crest in human periodontal pockets is most constant, having a mean length of 1.97 mm ± 33.16%.
- The distance b/w JE and alveolar bone is relatively constant.
- Distance b/w attached plaque and bone is 0.5 mm–2.7 mm.
- Intrabony pockets most often occur interproximally, but may be located on facial and lingual tooth surfaces.
- Horizontal bone loss vs vertical bone loss.
- ***Angular bony defects/vertical bony defects*** are classified on thc basis of the no. of osseous wall remaining, i.e.1-walled, 2-walled; 3-walled defects, combined, 1½ walled, circumferential defects.
- 3-walled defects are also known as ***intrabony defects***; they mostly occur on mesial aspect of 2nd and 3rd molars.
- 1–walled defects is also known as ***hemiseptum***.
- Prognosis of 3 walled defects is better than the 2-walled defects; worst prognosis is of 1-walled defects.
- ***Combined osseous defect*** = i.e. the number of walls in the apical portion of the defect are greater than its occlusal part.
- **Other angular defects** can be shallow and narrow; shallow and wide; deep and narrow; deep and wide. Surgical exposure is the only sure way to determine the presence and configuration of vertical osseous defect.
- **Most common** location of vertical defects is on distal surfaces of molars.

- **Most common bony lesion** = crater.
- ***Craters*** = concavities in the crest of interdental bone confined within the facial and lingual walls.
- ***Reverse architecture*** = bony defects produced by loss of interdental bone including the facial and lingual plates or both, *without concomitant loss of radicular bone* thereby reversing the normal architecture. These are more common in maxilla.
- Radiological evaluation of bone changes in periodontal disease is based mainly on the appearance of the I/D septa, because the relatively dense root structure obscures the facial and lingual bony plates.
- Crest of the I/D septa is parallel to the line b/w the CEJs of the adjacent teeth.
- Healthy gingiva is associated with coccoid cells and straight rods; while diseased gingival is associated with increased numbers of spirochetes and motile rods.
- ***Histopathology*** = pocket formation starts as an inflammatory change in CT wall of gingival sulcus.
- ***Many zones*** are present: junctional epithelium; zone of destroyed collagen; zone of partial destruction; area of normal attachment;
- Collagen destruction may be due to enz collagenase; and increased numbers of **PMN cells**. If volume of PMN cells reaches approx 60% of JE, it detaches from the tooth surface and migrates apically. PMN increase in number, which migrate through the gaps b/w epithelial cells.
- Discoloration is due to circulatory stagnation; bleeding is due to engorged vessels and pain is due to ulceration of inner aspect of the pocket wall.
- **Plasma cells** increased in CT; JE is reduced to 50–100 microns (normal width of JE is 500 microns); migration of JE along the root requires the presence of healthy epithelial cells. So degeneration of JE retards the pocket formation. Degenerative changes at the base of pocket, i.e. in JE are less severe than those in the epithelium of lateral wall of the pocket.
- Pockets are said to be healing lesions, but the rate of destructive changes are more than the rate of healing/constructive changes.

- **Root caries** = here, proteolysis of Sharpey's fibers occurs and cementum gets softened; this caries tends to progress around rather than into the tooth. Main cause is **Actinomyces viscosus**.
- Main bacteria in PD abscess are G (–) anaerobic rods.

TRAUMA FROM OCCLUSION

It refers to the tissue injury but not the occlusal forces. It is the tissue injury that results when occlusal forces exceed the adaptive capacity of the tissues. It occurs in supporting tissues and does not affect the gingival. It does not cause pockets formation.

- **Traumatic occlusion**—i.e. an occlusion producing such injury. Any occlusion which produces periodontal injury is traumatic.
- **Acute TFO** i.e. which occurs from an abrupt change in occlusal forces.
- **Chronic TFO**—more common; develops from gradual changes in the occlusion produced by tooth wear, drifting movements; bruxism, etc.
- **Primary TFO**—i.e. if TFO is the main cause of periodontal destruction. More than normal occlusal forces are the cause. It does not alter the level of CT attachment an do not initiate pocket formation, because supracrestal fibers are not affected and so JE does not migrate.
- **Secondary TFO**—i.e. when the adaptive capacity of the tissues to withstand normal occlusal forces is impaired. Alveolar bone loss is the most common cause of secondary TFO. The periodontium becomes vulnerable to injury, e.g. decrease in PD area due to marginal inflammation.
- **Capillary** pulse pressure is 20–26 gm/sq. cm; width of PDL is 0.2–0.25 mm.
- Bifurcation and trifurcation are the areas most susceptible to injury from increased occlusal forces.
- Most common sign of TFO is mobility of teeth and R/G there is widened PDL; thickened lamina dura; vertical bone loss; root resorption, etc.
- **Pathologic migration**—occurs mostly in anterior region; mobility and rotation of the affected teeth occur. It occurs under

conditions that weaken the PD support and/or increase or modify the forces exerted on the teeth.

- **Drifting**—it is different from pathologic migration, in that it does not result from destruction of PD tissues. It usually occurs mesially with tilting or extrusion. Premolars drift distally.

Oral manifestations of AIDS

Manifestations	**Clinical features**
Oral hairy leukoplakia	• Primarily occurs in persons with HIV infections, esp due to **Epstein Barr** virus. • Found esp on the **lateral borders of tongue**; frequently has a bilateral distribution. • Lesion does not rub-off. • Lesion has hyperparakeratosis and acanthosis and balloon cells, which contain Ebviruses. • Microscopically, it contains some characterisitic koilocytes/**balloon cells,** which contain virus particles of herpes group. • Lesions also reveal surface colonization by candida, but it is a secondary invader.
Candidiasis	• Most common oral lesion in HIV esp on hard and soft palate. • Is due to diminished host resistance. • Seen in approx 90% of AIDS patients. • Diagnosis of candidiasis is made by H/E of a tissue sample or smear of material scraped from the lesion.
Kaposi sarcoma	• Is a rare, vascular neoplasm. • Closely associated with **human herpes virus-8**.

Oral manifestations of AIDS (*Contd.*)

Manifestations	Clinical features
	• In its classical form, it is a localized and slow growing lesion; but in AIDS patient it is a much more aggressive lesion. • Contains mononuclear inflammatory cells esp of **plasma cells**.
Bilateral epithelioid angiomatosis	• Infectious vascular proliferative diseases. • Caused by rickettessia like organism, bartonellaciac henselia; quintana or others.
Atypical ulcers	• Patients have a higher incidence of ***recurrent herpetic lesions and aphthous stomatitis***. • In non-HIV patients, herpes presents on the keratinizing mucosa and aphtae on non-keratinizing surfaces. But in HIV patients, herpes may involve all mucosal surfaces and extend to the skin.
Linear gingival erythema	• It may be limited to marginal tissue or may extend into AG in a punctate or a diffuse erythema or extend into alveolar mucosa. • Candida dubliniensis has been implicated in some cases of LGE.
Atypical periodontal disease	• Severe soft tissue necrosis; like ANUG. • Rapid PD destruction. • Deep interdental craters. • Exposure of alveolar bone and sequestration. • Severe pain .

- Is caused by HIV/HTLV–3 and is characterized by destruction of lymphocytes.
- It affects CD 4 cells, i.e. T–cells.
- Lower ratio of T 4–T 8 cells (reversed helper to suppressor cells ratio).
- AIDS related complex ARC = 2 clinical findings and 2 hematological findings.
- HIV patients are potential candidates for conventional periodontal Rx procedures to include periodontal surgery and implant placement.
- **Clinical diagnosis and radiographic criteria**—
  - The complete R/G survey of mouth requires a minimum of 14 intra-oral films and 4 posterior bitewing films.
  - OPG provides an informative overall R/G picture of distribution and severity of bone destruction in PD disease. But for PD diagnosis, and Rx planning, a complete intra-oral series is required.
  - Halitosis—is primarily caused by volatile sulfur compounds, specifically hydrogen sulfide and methyl mercaptan, which result from the bacterial putrefaction of proteins containing sulfur aminoacids.
  - Proximal contact relations can be checked by clinical observation and by dental floss.
- **Level of attachment**—is the distance from the base of pocket to the CEJ.
- **Pocket depth**—distance from the base of the pocket to the gingival margin.

GINGIVAL DISEASES

- Gingivitis = is the inflammation of gingival with no attachment loss.

Stages	Predominant cells	Important features
Initial lesion/ subclinical	PMN cells	
Early lesion	Lymphocytes	JE and Sulcular Epith show rete peg formation.
Established lesion	Plasma cells	

- Gingival pigmentation from systemically absorbed metals results due to perivascular precipitation of metallic sulfides in the subepithelial CT. Pigmentation occurs only in areas of inflammation, where the increased permeability of irritated blood vessels permits the seepage of the metals in the surrounding tissues.
- Bismuth = bluish black discoloration of the gingival margin in the areas of pre-existent gingival inflammation.
- Lead = Burtonian's line, i.e. linear steel–grey gingival pigmentation.
- Mercury = linear gingival pigmentation.
- Increased melanin pigmentation in the oral cavity is seen in:
  - Addison's disease—caused by adrenal dysfunction.
  - Peutz–Jeghers synd.
  - Albright's syndrome, i.e. polyostotic fibrous dysplasia.
- Gingival abscess—localized collection of pus limited to the marginal gingival or interdental papilla. (AIPG—2004).
- Periodontal abscess involves the supporting periodontal tissues.

Drug induced gingival enlargement

- Seen with **phenytoin** (anti-convulsant); **cyclosporine** (immuno-suppresent); **nifedipine** (calcium channel blocker).
- It occurs in the areas where teeth are present, and **not in the edentulous areas;** the enlargement disappears in the areas from which the teeth are extracted.

- Besides phenytoin, other hydantoins known to induce gingival enlargement are ethotoin and mephenytoins.
- Other anticonvulsants that have the same side effects are succinimides, methsuxinimide and velproic acid.
- Cyclosporine may be substituted by another immuno-suppressant ***Tacrolimus*** that causes much less severe gingival overgrowth.
- Attached gingival is involved in idiopathic gingival enlargement.
- Gingival enlargement is seen in pregnancy—known as pregnancy epulis/angiogranuloma.
- Epulis–inflammatory tumor like gingival enlargement.
- Pyogenic granuloma—gingival enlargement that is considered an exaggerated response to minor trauma.
- Gingival enlargement seen in leukemia patients occurs commonly in acute leukemia, but may also be seen in subacute leukemia. It seldom occurs in chronic leukemia.

ANUG

- Is inflammatory destructive disease of gingival.
- Etiology: **fusiform bacillia** and **spirochetes**.
- Characteristic lesions-punched out crater like depressions at the crest of I/D papilla, covered by a pseudomembrane and demarcated by a pronounced linear erythema.
- Vincent's angina: fusospirochetal infection of the oropharynx and throat.

PERIODONTAL INDICES

Index—defined by Russel in 1961, as a numerical value describing the relative status of a population on a graduated scale, with a definite upper and lower limit, designed to permit and facilitate its comparison with other population, classified by the same criteria and method.

It estimates only the relative prevalence or occurrence of the clinical condition.

Properties of an index

1. Clarity, simplicity and objectivity—the index should be reasonably easy to apply so that there is no undue time lost during field examinations. The criteria for the index should be clear and unambiguous, with mutually exclusive categories.
2. Validity—it should measure what it is intended to measure, so that it correlates with the clinical stage of disease under study.
3. Reliability/Reproducible—ability of an index to measure condition in the same subject repeatedly and obtain the same score each time.
4. Quantifiability—should be amenable to statistical analysis, so that the status of a group can be expressed by a number.
5. Sensitivity—i.e. detect reasonably small shifts.
6. Acceptability—the use of the index should not be painful or unacceptable to the subject.

Types

1. Reversible—measures cumulative changes that can be reversed from diseased to healthy, e.g. Gingivitis index.
2. Irreversible—measures the cumulative conditions that cannot be reversed, e.g. Caries index.

GINGIVAL INDICES

1. PMA index—Given by Schour and Massler in 1948.

The primary impetus which led to the development of the PMA index was the need for some quantitative method of recording readily observable inflammatory conditions of the gingivae to replace the then gross assessment of gingivitis in both children and adults as mild, moderate or severe.

The index was intended to survey gingival changes in relatively large groups for epidemiological purposes and study. The basic philosophy used in the development of PMA index was very similar to the DMF index, i.e. the number of gingival units affected were counted rather than the severity of inflammation.

Facial surface of gingiva around a tooth was divided into 3 scoring units:

1. Mesial dental papilla (P).
2. Marginal gingiva (M).
3. Attached gingiva (A).

Criteria

P 0 Normal; no inflammation.

1+ Mild papillary engorgement; slight increase in size.

2+ Obvious increase in size of the papillary gingival; haemorrhage on pressure.

3+ Excessive increase in size with spontaneous haemorrhage.

4+ Necrotic papilla.

5+ Atrophy and loss of papilla.

M 0 Normal; no inflammation visible.

1+ Engorgement; slight increase in size; no bleeding.

2+ Obvious engorgement; bleeding upon pressure.

3+ Swollen collar; spontaneous haemorrhage; beginning infiltration into attached gingivae.

4+ Necrotic gingivitis.

5+ Recession of the free marginal gingivae below the CEJ due to the inflammatory changes.

A 0 Normal; pale rose; stippled.

1+ Slight engorgement with loss of stippling; change in colour may or may not be present.

2+ Obvious engorgement of attached gingivae with marked increase in redness. Pocket formation present.

3+ Advanced periodontitis. Deep pockets evident.

P, M and A values for all tooth were totaled separately and then added together to express the PMA score per person.

Advantages

(i) Main usefulness of this index was in the examination of children in whom the early stages of gingivitis were usually seen without obvious changes in the other periodontal tissues.

(ii) Broad application in epidemiological surgery and clinical trials.

(iii) Served as the basis for many other indices.

2. Gingival component of PDI—By Ramfjord in 1959.

Teeth examined $\frac{6 \quad 14}{41 \quad 6}$

Criteria

0 – Absence of inflammation.

1 – Mild to moderate inflammatory changes not extending all the tooth.

2 – Mild to moderately severe gingivitis extending all around the tooth.

3 – Severe gingivitis characterized by redness, swelling, tendency to bleed and ulceration.

$$\text{PDI Score: } \frac{\text{Sum of score of all six teeth}}{\text{No. of teeth examined}}$$

Importance—used in epidemiologic surveys, longitudinal studies on periodontal disease and clinical trials of therapeutic or preventive procedures.

3. Gingival index—By Loe and Silness in 1963.

Most frequently index of gingivitis nowadays.

Scoring surfaces are:

1. Buccal
2. Mesial
3. Distal
4. Lingual

Criteria

0 – Normal gingiva.

1 – Mild inflammation, slight change in colour, slight edema, no bleeding on palpation.

2 – Moderate inflammation, redness, edema and glazing, bleeding on probing.

3 – Severe inflammation, marked redness and edema, ulcerations; tendency to spontaneous bleeding.

Scoring

0.1–1.0 Mild gingivitis.

1.1–2.0 Moderate gingivitis.

2.1–3.0 Severe gingivitis.

Totaling the score around each tooth and dividing by 4 yields the GI score for the tooth. Totaling all the scores and dividing by the number of teeth gives the GI score per person.

Advantages

1. Distinguishes clearly between those with little or no gingivitis.
2. Used to determine prevalence and severity of gingivitis both in epidemiologic surveys and in an individual.

4. Modified gingival index—By Lobene and associates.

Modification of gingival index in which the bleeding criteria is eliminated making the index non-invasive.

Criteria

0 Absence of inflammation.

1 Mild inflammation slight change in colour, little change in texture of any portion of the marginal or papillary gingival unit.

2 Mild inflammation, criteria as above, but involving the entire marginal or papillary gingival unit.

3 Moderate inflammation, glazing, redness, edema and/or hypertrophy of the marginal or papillary gingival unit.

4 Severe inflammation, marked redness, edema and/or hypertrophy of the marginal or papillary gingival unit, spontaneous bleeding congestion or ulceration.

Advantage

The criteria for mild and moderate inflammation is well defined, which increase the index sensitivity in the lower portion of the scoring scale.

5. Periodontal screening examination—By O'Leary and co-workers (1963).

They used a combined gingival periodontal index, in which the mouth is divided into 4 posterior and 2 anterior segments. The gingival scoring for each segment is based upon the gingival unit with the greatest severity in each segment providing the score for that segment.

Criteria

0 Normal gingiva.

1 Slight to moderate inflammation not surrounding any particular tooth.

2 Similar inflammation but completely surrounding one or mor teeth.

3 Marked inflammation.

4 Presence of buccal or lingual recession.

Adv- O'Leary gingival evaluations lend themselves mainly to broad surveys.

6. End point method of assessing gingivitis—By Fischman and co-workers (1973).

The rationale of this index was that the time it took for a subject with pre-existing gingivitis to reach an arbitrary level of gingivitis would be a measure of the efficacy of a preventive agent. This arbitrary level of gingivitis could be defined in terms of the Loe index. The authors felt that this system would permit the evaluation of the potential therapeutic agents in groups with pre–existing gingivitis.

One of the criticisms of this system is that it measures deterioration in gingival health and not an improvement, although the criteria could be reversed in terms of the end-point.

Adv: It permits the evaluation of the therapeutic agents without the need to empirically search for an optimum time period to evaluate a drug's effect.

7. Suomi and Barbano (1968), suggested an index based upon a 3 point system of 0, 1 and 2, scoring both facial and lingual units for each of 12 segments of the mouth (molar, premolar and anterior for each quadrant). Although this index separates subjects well on the presence or absence of gingivitis, it is found to be too limited in its description of the severity of gingivitis.

INDICES OF GINGIVAL BLEEDING

1. Sulcus bleeding index—By Muhlemann and Mazor in 1958.

Index used bleeding on probing as an indicative of gingival inflammation.

Criteria

0 No inflammation, no bleeding on probing.

1 Bleeding from gingival sulcus on gentle probing tissue otherwise appears normal.

2 Bleeding on probing, change in colour due to inflammation.

3 Bleeding on probing, change in colour and slight edema.

4 Bleeding on probing, change in colour and obvious edema.

5 Bleeding on probing, change in colour, spontaneous bleeding, marked edema, with or without ulceration.

Sulcus bleeding index is determined by averaging all of the scores for the individual.

2. Bleeding point index—By Lenox and Kppezyk in 1973.

Developed to assess in patient's oral hygiene performance. It determines the presence or absence of bleeding interproximally and on the facial and lingual surfaces of each tooth. A periodontal probe is drawn horizontally through the gingival crevice of a quadrant and the gingiva is examined for bleeding after 30 seconds.

3. Gingival bleeding index—By Carter and Barnes in 1974.

This index also assesses the presence or absence of gingival bleeding, but only at the interproximal sites and using unwaxed dental floss. All interproximal areas having a mesial and distal sulcus are considered to be susceptible to gingival inflammation and these areas are recorded as total areas at risk. Although these involve two sulci, they are scored as one gingival unit. The mouth is divided into six segments and flossed in the following order—upper right, upper anterior, upper left, lower left, lower anterior and lower right. Gingival bleeding score is obtained by noting total units of bleeding and the total susceptible areas at risk.

4. Gingival bleeding index—By Ainamo and Bay in 1975.

Easy and suitable way for the practitioner to assess patient's progress in plaque control. Presence or absence of bleeding is determined by gentle probing of gingival crevice with a periodontal probe. Appearance of bleeding within 10 seconds indicates a positive score, which is expressed as percentage of total number of gingival margins examined.

The authors felt that this index was well suited for epidemiological studies, short term clinical tests and in the daily practice of dentistry.

5. Papillary bleeding index—(PBI) By Muhlemann in 1977.

Criteria

0 No bleeding.

1 Bleeding some seconds after probing

2 Bleeding immediately after probing.

3 Bleeding on probing spreading towards the marginal gingiva.

Barnett and Colleagues (1980), modified the Muhlemann PBI by precisely defining the placement of the probe at the mesial line angle of the tooth and gently sweeping the probe forward into the mesial papilla. They timed the appearance of bleeding and graded it as follows:

0 No bleeding within 30 sec of probing.

1 Bleeding between 3 and 30 sec of probing.

2 Bleeding within 2 sec of probing.

3 Bleeding immediately upon probe placement.

The authors showed modified PBI to be more sensitive than the visual aspects of the GI in assessing changes in gingival health.

6. **Interdental bleeding index** (Eastman IBI)—By Caton and Palson in 1985.

A triangle shaped toothpick made of soft, pliable wood is inserted interproximally from the facial surface, depressing the interproximal papilla by up to 2 mm. It is inserted and removed 4 times and the presence or absence of bleeding within 15 seconds is noted.

IBI score is determined by dividing no. of bleeding site by no. of sites evaluated.

7. **Index used by NIDR**

Assesses gingival inflammation by the presence or absence of bleeding.

This index is based on the objective that bleeding is a more objective sign than colour change and provides evidence of recent plaque exposure.

Two sites per tooth (mesial–buccal interproximal and mid buccal on all teeth excluding molars; and mesial buccal interproximal and mid-buccal of the mesial root of molars) on one half of the maxillary arch and the contralateral half of the mandibular arch are examined after excess moisture is dried with air.

Left or right arch selection is randomly decided.

NIDR probe is inserted 2 mm into the gingival sulcus at the mid-point of the buccal and than gently down into the mesial-buccal interproximal area. Total numbers of bleeding site divided by total sites examined and multiplied by 100 gives the percentage of sites with gingival bleeding.

Criteria

0 No bleeding present.

1 Bleeding after NIDR probe is placed in sulcus up to 2 mm and drawn along the inner surface of sulcus.

8. Bleeding Index—By Edwards in 1975.

In this index a dental tape is wrapped around a proximal tooth surface in a bucco-lingual manner and inserted into the base of the crevice. This procedure is repeated twice. If no bleeding occurs after 15 sec, a score of 0 is recorded and 1 if bleeding occurs.

PLAQUE INDICES

Most of these indices utilize a numerical scale to measure the extent of the surface area covered by plaque.

1. Plaque component of PDI—Given by Ramfjord in 1959.

Index teeth examined $\frac{6 \quad 14}{41 \quad 6}$

Surfaces examined—interproximal, facial and lingual surfaces.

Criteria and score:

0 Absence of Plaque.

1 Plaque at interproximal surface and not covering more than 1/3 of tooth surface.

2 Plaque covering more than 1/3rd but less than 2/3rd of the tooth surface.

3 Plaque covering more than 2/3 of the tooth surface.

Advantage

Index is suitable for longitudinal studies of periodontal disease.

Shick and Ash modified the original criteria of Ramfjord by excluding consideration of the interproximal areas of teeth and restricting the scoring of plaque to the gingival half of the facial and lingual surfaces of the index teeth.

Score

0 Absence of dental plaque.

1 Dental plaque in the interproximal area at the gingival margin covering less than one third of the gingival half of the facial or lingual surfaces of the tooth.

2 Dental plaque covering more than one-third, but less than two third of the gingival half of the facial or lingual surface of the tooth.

3 Dental plaque covering two thirds or more of the gingival half of the facial or gingival surface of the tooth.

$$\text{Plaque score} = \frac{\text{Total score}}{\text{No. of teeth examined}}$$

2. Quigley Hein Plaque Index—(1962).

It measures plaque on the gingival third of the facial surfaces of the anterior teeth using basic fuchsin as disclosing solution.

0 Absolutely no plaque.

1 Single line of plaque.

2 Clear line of plaque along large extents of the gingival margins.

3 Plaque on only the cervical third of crown.

4 Plaque extending on the middle third of the crown.

5 Plaque extending into the occlusal third of crown.

$$\text{Q.H index} = \frac{\text{Sum of scores}}{\text{No. of surfaces evaluated}}$$

3. Turesky-Gillmore-Glickman modification of the Quigley-Hein Plaque index—(1970).

Plaque is assessed on the facial and lingual surfaces of all the teeth after using a disclosing agent.

0 No plaque.

1 Separate flicks of plaque at the cervical margin of the tooth.

2 A thin continuous band of plaque (up to 1 mm) at the cervical margin.

3 A band of plaque wider than 1 mm, but covering less than one third of the crown.

4 Plaque covering at least one-third but less than two thirds of the crown.

5 Plaque covering two thirds or more of the crown.

$$\text{Plaque score} = \frac{\text{Total score}}{\text{No. of teeth examined}}$$

Advantages

1. Relatively easy to use because of the objective definition of each numerical score.
2. Can be applied to longitudinal studies and clinical trials of preventive and therapeutic agents.

This index is one of the two indices of choice when assessing plaque in clinical trials.

4. Plaque index—By Sillness and Loe in 1967.

Uniqueness of this index is that it ignores the coronal extent of plaque on the teeth surface area and assesses only the thickness of plaque at the gingival area of the tooth.

It does not exclude or substitute for teeth with gingival restoration or crowns.

Tooth scoring units = distofacial, facial, mesiofacial and lingual.

Scores and Criteria

0 No plaque in the gingival area.

1 A film of plaque adhering to the gingival margin and adjacent area of the tooth. The plaque may be recognized only by running a probe across the tooth surface.

2 Moderate accumulation of soft deposits within the gingival pocket and on the gingival margin and/or adjacent tooth surface that can be seen by the naked eye.

3 Abundance of soft matter within the gingival pocket and/or on the gingival margin and adjacent tooth surface.

$$PI = \frac{\text{Sum of individual scores}}{\text{No. of surfaces examined}}$$

Index can be used for longitudinal studies and clinical trials.

5. Simplified oral hygiene index

Given by Greene and Vermillion in 1960 and later modified by them to include only six tooth surfaces, representative of all the anterior and posterior segments of the mouth.

The imprecise term 'debris' was used because it was not practical to distinguish among plaque, debris and materia alba.

It measures the surface area of tooth covered by debris.

Index teeth are facial surfaces of 3, 18, 14 and 24 and lingual surfaces of 19 and 30.

A mouth mirror and a sickle shaped explorer is used.

The explorer is placed on the incisal third of the tooth and moved towards the gingival third.

Scores and Criteria

0 No debris or stain present.

1 Soft debris covering not more than one-third of the tooth surface or the presence of extrinsic stains without other debris, regardless of surface area covered.

2 Soft debris covering more than one-third, but not more than 2/3 of the exposed tooth surface.

3 Soft debris covering more than 2/3 of the exposed tooth surface.

$$\text{Debris index score} = \frac{\text{Total score}}{\text{No. of surfaces examined}}$$

Interpretation of scores:

0.0–0.6 Good

0.7–1.8 Fair

1.9–3.0 Poor

6. **Patient hygiene performance index** (PHP)—Given by Podshadley and Haley in 1968.

First index developed for the sole purpose of assessing an individual's performance in removing debris after toothbrushing instructions.

Same six teeth are used as in OHI-S.

Each tooth surface is divided into five areas–3 longitudinal thirds with the middle third subdivided horizontally into thirds.

Presence or absence of debris is recorded as 1 or 0 using the six surfaces.

Index is easy to use and can be quickly performed.

Index can be applied to individual patient education.

7. **Navy-plaque index**—Given by Elliott in 1972.

Index teeth are $\dfrac{6 \quad 14}{41 \quad 6}$

Each tooth surface is divided into 9 scoring units.

Criteria

0 Absence of plaque.

1 Plaque present.

$$\text{Navy plaque index} = \frac{\text{Totalling all 9 subdivision scores for 6 teeth}}{\text{No. of tooth surfaces examined}}$$

8. **DMPI system**—by Cancro (1983).

This index places more emphasis on the gingival or cervical portion of the tooth as well as the interproximal areas. These areas are frequently missed by the toothbrush and may be used to study the effects chemical agents brought to the tooth by such vehicles as toothpaste or mouthrinse without interference by the mechanical action of toothbrushing.

Each area is scored as

0 Absence of plaque

1 Plaque covering 1/3rd of the area.

2 Plaque covering 2/3rd of the area.

3 Plaque covering the entire area.

The remaining area is scored as 1 or 0 depending on the presence or absence of plaque.

Plaque score can be represented as sums per tooth, per quadrant, or per area of all teeth.

Recent studies have shown that this index is easily learned by hygienists and is reproducible in clinical trials.

9. Bonded bracket index—By Ciancio, et. al. in 1984.

This index assesses plaque in orthodontic patients.

It scores bracket associated plaque as follows.

0 No plaque on bracket or tooth surface.

1 Plaque on brackets only.

2 Plaque on brackets, tooth, no extension to gingiva.

3 Plaque on bracket, tooth, extension to papilla.

4 Plaque on bracket, tooth, partial coverage to gingiva.

5 Plaque on bracket, tooth, full coverage to gingiva.

CALCULUS INDICES

1. Calculus component of simplified oral hygiene index

Calculus is assessed by gently placing an explorer into the distal gingival crevice and drawing it subgingivally from the distal contact area to the mesial contact area.

Scores and Criteria

0 No calculus present.

1 Supragingival calculus covering not more than one-third of the exposed tooth surface.

2 Supragingival calculus covering more than one-third, but not more than 2/3rd of the exposed tooth surface or the presence of individual flicks of subgingival calculus around the cervical portion of the tooth or both.

3 Supragingival calculus covering more than two-thirds of the exposed tooth surface or a continuous heavy band of subgingival calculus around the cervical portion of the tooth or both.

$$\text{CI} = \frac{\text{Total score}}{\text{No. of surfaces examined}}$$

2. Calculus component of periodontal disease index

Teeth recorded $\frac{6 \quad 14}{41 \quad 6}$ (facial and lingual surfaces)

Score and Criteria

0 Absence of calculus.

1 Supragingival calculus extending only slightly below the free gingival margin (not more than 1 mm).

2 Moderate amount of supragingival and subgingival calculus or subgingival calculus alone.

3 An abundance of supragingival and subgingival calculus.

$$\text{Calculus score per person} = \frac{\text{Total score}}{\text{No. of teeth examined}}$$

Advantages

1. Has a higher degree of examiner reproducibility.
2. Can be quickly performed.
3. Best application in epidemiologic surveys and longitudinal studies.

3. **Probe method of calculus assessment** (Volpe and Manhold Index, 1961).

- Index was developed for longitudinal studies of the quantity of supragingival calculus formed.
- A periodontal probe graduated in mm is used to measure the vertical extent of calculus deposits on the lingual surfaces to mandibular incisors and canines.
- This index has a high degree of inter- and intra-examiner reproducibility.

4. **Calculus surface index**—By Ennever in 1961.

Index teeth—Mandibular incisors.

Surfaces examined—All four surfaces.

Criteria

0 Absence of calculus.

1 Presence of supra/sub-gingival calculus.

Maximum score can be 4 × 4 = 16.

Adv: Used in short-term (< 6 weeks) clinical trials of calculus inhibiting agents.

5. **Marginal line calculus index**—By Muhlcmann and Villa in 1967.

- This index was developed to assess the accumulation of supragingival calculus on the gingival third of the tooth or more specifically, supragingival calculus along the margin of gingival.
- Used in short-term clinical trials of anti-calculus agents.
- Calculus content is observed along the previously cleaned lingual gingival margin of the mandibular incisors.
- Scoring is given in percentage.

6. **Calculus index used by NIDR**

Unlike gingival assessment, calculus under assigns only one score per tooth, after examining both the mid-buccal and mesial-buccal inter proximal sites, on one half of the maxillary arch and contralateral mandibular arch.

Criteria

0 Calculus absent.

1 Supragingival calculus, but no sub gingival calculus is present.

2 Supra calculus, or sub gingival calculus only, is present.

Indices to measure periodontal destruction.

1. **Gingival sulcus measurement component of PDI**—By Ramfjord in 1967.

A university of Michigan probe # 0 probe is used for the purpose. The probe should be held with a light grasp such that the angle formed by the working end of the probe and the long axis of the crown of the tooth is approximately 45°.

Only buccal and mesial measurements are undertaken since it was found by Jamison and Ash in separate extensive analysis, that there is no significant loss of accuracy in the PDI index from omitting the distal and lingual scores. Also omitting lingual and distal scores enhances reproducibility in buccal and mesial scoring. The crevicular measurements are made in the following manner: The distance from the free gingival margin to the cemento-enamel junction and the distance from the free gingival margin to the bottom of the gingival crevice or pocket is measured for the buccal and mesial aspect of each tooth examined. The buccal measurements should be made at the middle of the buccal surfaces. The mesial measurement should be made at the buccal aspect of the interproximal contact area with the probe touching both teeth if there is a neighbor tooth present.

If the gingival margin is on enamel, measure from gum margin to CEJ and record the measurement. If the epithelial attachment is on the crown and the CEJ cannot be felt by the probe, record the depth of the gingival crevice on the crown. Then record the distance from the gingival margin to the bottom of the pocket if the probe can be moved apically to the CEJ without pain or resistance. The distance from the CEJ to the bottom of the pocket can then be found by subtracting the first from the second measurement.

If the gingival margin is on the cementum, record the distance from the CEJ to the bottom of the gingival crevice as a plus value. Both loss of attachment and actual crevice depth can be assessed from these scores.

2. Periodontal index—By Russel in 1956.

- This index considers periodontal diseases as a slowly progressing, continuous disease process extending from gingivitis to advanced periodontal disease.
- This index was intended to estimate the intent of deeper periodontal disease by determining the presence or absence of gingival inflammation and it's severity, pocket formation and masticatory function.
- It is an epidemiologic index with a true biologic gradient since it measures both the reversible and irreversible aspects of periodontal disease.

Score criteria		Add. radiographic criteria
0	Negative. There is neither overt inflammation in the investing tissues or loss of function owing to destruction of supporting tissues.	Normal radiographic appearance.
1	Mild gingivitis. There is an overt area of inflammation in free gingival, but this area does not circumscribe the tooth.	
2	Gingivitis. Inflammation completely circumscribes the tooth, but there is no apparent break in epithelial attachment.	
4	(Used when radiographs are available.)	Early notch like resorption of the alveolar crest.

Score Criteria	Add. radiographic criteria
5 Gingivitis with pocket formation. Epithelial attachment is broken and there is pocket formation. No interference with normal masticatory function. The tooth is firm and has not drifted.	Horizontal bone loss involving the entire alveolar crest up to the length of tooth root.
6 Advanced destruction with loss of masticatory function. The tooth may be loose, may have drifted, may sound dull on percussion with a metallic instrument or may be depressible in the socket.	Advanced bone loss involving more than half of the tooth root or a definite infra bony pocket with widening of the periodontal ligament. There may be root resorption or rarefaction at the apex.

$$\text{PI score} = \frac{\text{Sum of individual scores}}{\text{No. of teeth present}}$$

Interpretation of score:

0–0.2	Clinically normal tissues.	⎤
0.3–0.9	Simple gingivitis.	⎥
0.7–1.9	Beginning destructive periodontal disease.	⎦
1.6–5.0	Established destructive periodontal disease.	⎤
3.8–8.0	Terminal disease.	⎦

Disadvantages

It tends to underestimate the true level of periodontal disease, since only a mouth mirror is used.

Importance. 1. It was used in Ten-state Nutrition survey (1968–70), National Health Survey (1960–62), National Health and Nutrition

Examination Survey (1971–74), and Hispanic Health and Nutrition Examination Survey (1982–83).

3. **Extent and severity index:** Given by JP Carlos, MD Wolfe, and Kingman in 1986.

- ♦ This index considers periodontal disease a chronic process with intermittent periods of activity and remission that affects individual teeth and site around teeth at different rates within the same mouth.
- ♦ Unlike periodontal index which uses only a mouth mirror, this index uses periodontal probe to determine the attachment levels.
- ♦ It expresses the percentage of site that exhibits disease (E for Extent) and at the same time measures mean attachment loss in mm (S for Severity). (Disease is any site with more than 1mm of attachment loss).
- ♦ Attachment loss is measured at the mesio-buccal interproximal and mid-buccal location on all teeth excluding molars and at the mesio-buccal interproximal and mid-buccal of the mesial root of molars, in one half of the maxillary arch and the contralateral half of mandibular arch.

4. **Radiographic approaches to measure bone loss**

(a) **Gingival-Bone Count Index**—Developed by Dunning and Leach in1960.

It records the gingival condition and the level of the crest of the alveolar bone. The bone level is assessed by clinical examination, but radiographs are recommended for greater accuracy. The gingival is assessed on a scale of 0 to 3, and the bone involvement is scored on a scale of 0 to 5.

The Gingival-Bone Count Index is the average gingival score per person plus the average bone score.

(b) **Periodontitis Severity Index**—Developed by Adams and Nystrom.

It consists of two components. The presence or absence of clinical inflammation is scored 0 or 1 respectively. The presence or absence of interproximal bone loss is determined radiographically using a modified Schei ruler. Each 10% increment in bone loss corresponds to a bone loss score of 1, to a maximum score of 10. The periodontitis severity index is a product of clinical inflammation score and bone loss score.

The index has promise in longitudinal studies, but is limited in epidemiologic surveys because of the need of the periapical radiographs.

INDICES TO ASSESS TREATMENT NEEDS

1. **GPI index** by O'Leary in 1967.

   G–Gingival status.

   P–Periodontal status.

   I–Irritation index (triad of materia alba, calculus and overhanging restorations).

- Modification of Ramfjord's PDI and is used for the purpose of screening person to determine the need for periodontal treatment.
- Maxillary and mandibular arch is divided into 3 segments, anterior, left posterior and right posterior.
- Each segment is assesses for the 3 components of the index.
- The objective is to determine the tooth or surrounding tissues with the severest conditions within each of the six segments.

Criteria

0 Tissue tightly adapted to teeth; firm consistency with physiologic architecture.

1 Slight to moderate inflammation, indicated by changes in colour and consistency, involving one or more teeth in the same segment, but not completely surrounding any one tooth.

2 Above changes either singly or combined completely encircling one or more teeth in a segment.

3 Marked inflammation, as indicated by loss of surface continuity (ulcerations), spontaneous haemorrhage, loss of faciolingual continuity, as any interdental papilla, marked deviation from normal contour, recession and clefts.

- Area with highest score determines the gingival score for the entire segment.

$$\text{Gingival status of mouth} = \frac{\text{Sum of gingival score of segments}}{\text{No. of segments}}$$

1. **Periodontal treatment need system** (PTNS)—By H.T. Bellini in 1973).

- This index assesses plaque, calculus, and gingival inflammation and pockets more than 5 mm, in each quadrant of mouth, and place individuals into 4 groups.

PTNS	Unit	Plaque	Calculus and /or Overhangs	Inflammation	Pocket Depth
Class O	Mouth	No	No	No	Not considered
Class A	Mouth	Yes	No	No	d ≤ 5 mm
Class B	Quadrant	Yes	Yes	Yes	< 5 mm
Class C	Quadrant	Yes	Yes	Yes	> 5 mm

2. **CPITN**—621 method according to WHO technical series publication.

- By WHO in 1997.
- Combines GPI and PTNS.
- Periodontal status is assessed by 3 indicatiors:
  (a) Presence or absence of gingival bleeding.
  (b) Supra/sub gingival calculus.
  (c) Periodontal pocket-shallow (4–5mm) or deep (6 mm or more).

CPITN probes

Epidemiological probe—Probe has markings from 3.5–5.5 mm with a 0.5 mm diameter ball at the tip.

Clinical probe—Probe has markings from 3.5–5.5 mm and from 8.5–11.5 mm with a 0.5 mm ball at the tip.

The ball prevents the probe from being pushed through inflammatory tissues at the base of pocket. Probing force is 20 gm.

Index teeth

$$\frac{17\quad 16\quad 11\quad 26\quad 27}{47\quad 46\quad 31\quad 36\quad 37}\quad \text{For 20 years and above}$$

$$\frac{16\quad 11\quad 26}{46\quad 31\quad 36}\quad \text{For upto 19 years}$$

This avoids classifying deepened crevices associated with eruption as periodontal pockets. For same reason periodontal pockets are not covered for children under 15 years of age.

Principles

1. Mouth is divided into sextants.
2. Last molar is not included.
3. It second molar is extracted and 3rd molar has shifted in its position, it can be included.
4. Tooth indicated for extraction is not included.
5. Tooth with vertical mobility due to periodontal diseases should not be included.
6. If only one tooth is present in one segment, it should be included in the adjoining segment.
7. Two or more teeth should be present in a segment for study.

Criteria

0 Healthy periodontium.

1 Bleeding observed, directly or by using mirror.

2 Calculus felt during probing, but the entire black area of probe (3.5–5.5 mm) is visible.

3 Pocket 4 to 5 mm (gingival margin on black area of probe).

4 Pocket > 6 mm (black area not visible).

Treatment needs

0 No treatment needed.

1 Oral hygiene needs improvement.

2 1+ professional scaling.

3 1+ professional scaling.

4 1+ professional scaling + complex treatment.

Advantages

1. Permits rapid examination of a population to determine periodontal treatment needs.
2. American Academy of Periodontology has proposed that the index may be used for periodontal screening and recording tool for general practioner.

Periodontitis as a manifestation of systemic diseases

Disease	Features
Papillon-Lefevre syndrome	• Characterized by hyperkeratotic skin lesions, severe destruction of periodontium and in some cases, ***calcification of dura***. • Cutaneous and periodontal changes appear together before the 4 yrs age. • It follows an autosomal recessive pattern. Parents are not affected and both must carry the autosomal gene for the syndrom to appear in child. Males and females are equally affected.
Down synd; trisomy 21	• Prevalence of periodontal disease in it is higher, i.e. almost 100% in patients younger than 30 yrs.
Chediak-Higashi	• Decreased neutrophil chemotaxis and secretion. • Neutrophil granules fuse to form large granules know as megabodies.

Periodontitis as a manifestation of systemic diseases (*Contd.*)

Disease	Features
Hypophosphatasia	• Rare; familial; skeletal disease. • C/F: rickets; poor cranial bone formation; premature loss of primary teeth; esp the incisors. • Low levels of serum alk Pase enz. • Phosphoethanolamine is present in serum and urine. • Teeth are lost with no clinical evidence of gingival inflammation and show reduced cementum formation. • In adolescent, the disease resembles localized juvenile periodontitis.
Localized aggressive periodontitis	• Age of onset is around puberty. • Involvement of first molars and incisors • A ***striking feature*** of this form is **lack of clinical inflammation** despite the p.o. deep pockets. • Amount of plaque on affected teeth is minimal. • Plaque contains elevated levels of **Actinobacillus actinomycetamcomitans** and in some patients, Porphyromonas gingivalis. • **Other C/F: distolabial migration** of max incisors with concomitant diastema formation. Increased mobility of first molars; sensitivity of denuded root surfaces to thermal and tactile stimuli and deep, dull radiating pain during mastication. • **R/G: arc-shaped loss** of alveolar bone extending from the distal surface of 2nd premolar to mesial surface of the 2nd molars **Immunological defects**.

Periodontitis as a manifestation of systemic diseases (*Contd.*)

Disease	Features
	• Functional defects of PMNs, monocytes or both; these defects can impair either the chemotactic ability or their ability to phagocytose. • Hyperresponsive monocytes producing large quantity of PGE-2 on lipopolysaccharide stimulation. • Poorly functional form of monocyte receptor, Fc-gamma-RII, the receptor for IgG 2 antibodies.

Skeletal disturbances manifested in the jaws (Also refer to the section of oral pathology in volume I for details.)

Osteitis fibrosa cystica	• Also known as **Recklinghausen's dis of bones**. • Develops in advanced primary or sec. hyperparathyroidism and causes osteoclastic resorption of bone with fibrous replacement and haemorrhage with **hemosiderin deposition** creating a mass known as **brown tumor**. • It results in scattered cyst like radiolucent areas throughout the jaws and a **generalized disappearance of the lamina dura**.
Paget's disease	• **Lamina dura is absent**. • Normal trabecular pattern is replaced by hazy, fine trabecular markings or scattered radiolucent areas may contain irregularly shaped radiopaque zones.
Fibrous dysplasia	• May appear as a small radiolucent area at a root apex or as an extensive radiolucent area with irregularly arranged trabecular markings.

	• **Ground glass appearance.** • **Obliteration of lamina dura.**
Langerhans cell histiocytes	• Appear as single or **multiple radiolucent areas** which may be unrelated to the teeth or entail destruction of tooth supporting bone.
Osteopetrosis	• The **outlines of the roots may be obscured** by diffuse radiopacity of the jaws.
Scleroderma	• The **PDL is uniformly widened** at the expense of surrounding alveolar bone.

EPIDEMIOLOGY

Incidence = i.e. number of new cases occurring in a defined population during specific period of time.

I = no. of new cases of specific dis. During a given time period × 1000/population at risk.

Prevalence = all current cases, i.e. old and new. Existing at a given point of time (point prevalence) (AIPG–2004) or over a period of time in a given population (period prevalence).

P = no. of all current cases of specified dis existing at a given point or period time × 1000/estimated population.

Relationship = prevalence = incidence × mean duration.

Cross-sectional study = single examination of a cross section of population at one point in time.

Longitudinal study = observations are repeated in the same population over a prolonged period of time by follow up examinations.

Case control study, i.e. retrospective study

- ♦ Both exposure and outcome/disease have occurred before the start of the study.
- ♦ Study proceeds backwards from effect to cause.

- Study uses a control or comparison group to support or refute an inference.

Cohort study, i.e. prospective study

- Cohort—A group of persons exposed to the same sort of environment.
- Proceeds forward from cause to effect.
- A study began in 1970 with a group of 5000 adults who were asked about their Gutka consumption; the occurrence of cancer was studied in this b/w 1990–1995. This is an example of cross-sectional study/retrospective cohort study/concurrent cohort study/case–control study.
- **Epidemic** = the unusual occurrence in a community or region of disease clearly in excess of expected occurrence.
- **Endemic** = constant p.o. of a disease or infectious agent within a given geographic area or population group.
- **Sporadic** = sporadic means scattered; cases occur irregularly from time to time.
- **Pandemic** = an epidemic affecting a larger proportion of population and occurring over a wide geographical area such as section of a nation, a continent or the world.
- **Sensitivity** = proportion of subjects with the disease **who test positive.**

  Se = no. of subjects who test positive/no. of subjects with disease.
- **Specificity** = proportion of subjects without the disease **who test negative.**

  Sp = no. of subjects who test negative/no. of subjects without disease.

Question

The usefulness of a screening test in a community depends on (AIPG-2004).

Sensitivity/specificity/reliability/prediction values _____.

Normal development of a child

Prenatal: Embryofetus	End of 2nd week to 1 month From 1 mo till birth
Postnatal	
Neonate	2 wk to 1 mo
Infant	1 mo to 1 yr
Preschool	1 yr to 3 yrs
Primary school	4 yrs to 8 yrs
Middle school	8 yrs to 12 yrs
Pubertal	13 yrs to 15 yrs

Self notes:

GINGIVAL INFLAMMATION

Stage	**Lesion**
I	Initial
II	Early
III	Established
IV	Advanced

Main features of different stages of gingivitis

Stage I	**Stage II**	**Stage III**
Also known as initial lesion	Also known as early lesion	Also known as established lesion
Of 2–4 days duration	Of 4–10 days duration	Of 2–3 wks duration
Acute inflammation		Chronic inflammation
Main cells are PMNs	Lymphocytes antibodies	Plasma cells which produce

Main features of different stages of gingivitis (*Contd.*)

Stage I	Stage II	Stage III
Vascular changes, i..e. dilatation of capillaries is the first response	Erythema, i.e. colour change is seen; Bleeding on probing.	Colour modified due to congested blood vessels, Hb breakdown, etc.
Loss of perivascular collagen	Collagen destruction esp of circular and dento-gingival fibers	Increased collagenolysis due to enz collagenase
Most coronal portion of JE is altered	JE shows rete pegs formation	Increased rete pegs
Esp Fibrin present		Increased levels of enz alk and acid Pases.

Important points

- Gingivitis is the **most common** type of gingival disease.
- **Chronic marginal gingivitis/simple gingivitis** is the most common type of gingival disease.
- **Contained gingivitis** = the stage in which T-lymphocytes are preponderant. As the severity increases, the no. of B-cells increase.
- Initial response of gingival to plaque is = **subclinical**.
- First clinical **symptom**—bleeding.
- In stage II, the first clinical **sign** of gingivitis is = colour change.
- Cells of acute inflammation are—PMN and lymphocytes.
- PMNs = also cause phagocytosis in gingival.
- Intercellular spaces in JE widen through which the PMN cells migrate in the gingival sulcus.
- Bacterial composition in gingivitis is cocci and rods, which changes to spirochetes and motile organisms in periodontitis.
- Cells of chronic inflammation are—macrophages, lymphoid cells
- Collagen destruction occurs especially of circular and dento-gingival fibers are affected.
- Main fibers affected are circular and dento-gingival fibers.

- Extension of lesion into alveolar bone is the fourth stage known as advanced lesion or the stage of **periodontal breakdown**.
- 2 earliest s/s of gingivitis are—increased GCF formation and bleeding on probing.
- **Bleeding** on probing appears earlier than change in the colour, etc. It is an objective sign. Mostly, the sites which bleed are predominantly lymphocytic, i.e. stage II.
- Most common cause of abnormal gingival bleeding is chronic gingival inflammation.
- Bleeding is due to dilatation and engorgement of the capillaries, which come closer to the surface of the epithelium. And thinning /ulceration of SE.
- Bleeding sites are collagen poor and inflamed CT have cellular infiltrate rich in lymphocytes.
- Bleeding in ANUG = is due to ulceration of necrotic surface epithelium and the engorged blood vessels are exposed in the CT.
- Systemic causes of bleeding—purpura; hypoprothrombinemai, i.e. vitamin K deficiency; hemophilia; leukemia; Christmas disease; multiple myeloma; anticoagulants, e.g. dicumarol and heparin; salicylates, etc.

Surface texture

Condition	**Surface**
Gingivitis	Loss of stippling
Chronic inflammation; exudative	Surface is smooth and shiny
Chronic inflammation; fibrotic	Surface is firm and nodular
Senile atrophic gingivitis	Smooth
Chronic desquamative gingivitis	Peeling of the surface
Hyperkeratosis	Leathery
Non-inflammatory gingival hyperplasia	Minutely nodular surface

Colour change: Normal colour is coral pink.

- Black line = due to Bi, As, Hg.
- **Burtonian line** = i.e. bluish red/deep blue linear; due to Pb.
- Violet marginal line = due to Ag argyria.

Types of gingivitis

Type	Features
Acute	Painful; comes suddenly; short duration.
Subacute	Less severe phase of acute condition.
Recurrent	Reappears after treatment or spontaneously disappears and reappears.
Chronic	Slow; of long duration; painless.
Localized	Confined to gingival i.r.t. a single or a group of teeth.
Generalized	Involves entire mouth.
Marginal	Involves gingival margins.
Papillary	Involves I/D papillae but may involve margins also; earliest signs of gingivitis most often occur in papillae.
Diffuse	Affects gingival margins + AG + I/D papillae.
Localized marginal	Confined to one or more areas of marginal gingival MG.
Localized diffuse	Extends from the margin to mucobuccal fold but limited in areas.
Localized papillary	Confined to one or more interdental spaces in a limited areas.
Generalized marginal	i.e. GM i.r.t. all the teeth are involved.
Generalized diffuse	Involves entire gingival; the **alveolar mucosa/ AM is also affected**; so the demarcation b/w AM and AG is lost.

SULCULAR FLUID

- Also known as gingival crevicular fluid, i.e. GCF.
- Is an inflammatory exudates, not a continuous transudate.
- Very little or no fluid found in strictly normal gingival.
- Collected by microcapillary pipette or absorbing strips.
- **Brill technique** = strip is placed inside the sulcus or pocket.
- **Loe and Holm Pederson technique** = strip is placed at the entrance of the pocket.
- Measurements are done by periotron.
- JE and SE are permeable to substances of M wt upto 1 million.
- Glucose conc is 3–4 times greater than in serum.
- Total protein conc is very less as cp to serum.
- Main Ig present are = G, M, A.
- C3 and C4 also present.
- **Protective role** = as cleansing agent; antibacterial agent; due to WBCs, Abs and adhesive actions.
- **Circadian rhythm** = GCF increases from 6 AM to 10 PM; and then decreases.
- Female sex hormones increase GCF as they increase vascular permeability, e.g. in pregnancy; oral contraceptives; ovulation, etc.
- Vigorous gingival brushing increases GCF.
- GCF increases during healing after the PD surgery.
- Tetracycline/doxycycline excreted in GCF; and so it is preferred in gingival diseases.
- **Main WBCs** found in GCF are **neutrophils,** i.e. PMN cells approx 92%, these are phagocytic and protective; these are also present in saliva, where their main source is gingival sulcus.
- Ratio of T-cells to B-cells is 1:3, which is the reverse of serum, i.e. 3:1.

Saliva (Also refer to section of physiology and dental histology in vol 1 and 2.)

- Antibacterial factors: lysozymes, Lactoperoxidase–thiocynate system/i.e. LPT; antibodies.
- LPT system is bactericidal to certain strains of Lactobacillus and Strept. By preventing accumulation of lysine and glutamic acid.
- Main antibodies in saliva = secretory IgA.
- **Main antibodies in GCF** = IgG.
- IgA of parotid saliva can inhibit attachment of oral mucosal and dental surfaces.
- Major enz in saliva is **parotid amylase**.
- Certain glycoproteins bind to many plaque–forming bacteria which aids in formation of plaque.
- Certain glycoproteins having BLOOD GROUP REACTIVITY inhibit sorption of bacteria to tooth surface and mucosa.
- Most important **salivary buffer**—is bicarbonate–carbonic acid system.
- **Coagulation factors** present in saliva are 8–12 factors.
- **Principal cells** are PMN cells; WBCs reach saliva by passing through gingival sulcus lining.
- **Xerostomia** = it is seen in Sjogren's syndrome; Mikulicz disease; sarcoidosis; irradiation, etc. it causes increases dental caries; gingival diseases, etc.

Normal clinical features of gingiva

Colour	• Normal colour is coral pink; esp of AG and MG. • AG is demarcated from adjacent alveolar mucosa by mucogingival line MGL. • Alveolar mucosa is red; shiny and smooth. • H/E = epithelium of alveolar mucosa is thin/ non-keratinized; no rete pegs present. • CT of alveolar mucosa = loosely arranged; more numerous blood vessels.

Normal clinical features of gingiva (*Contd.*)

Contour	• MG—collar like fashion and follows scalloped outline on facio-lingual surfaces. • Gingival margin is knife-edged.
Consistency	• Firm and resilient, tightly bound to underlying bone except free margin. • Collagenous lamina propria/CT and gingival fibers cause firmness.
Surface texture/ stippling	• Orange peel appearance of surface due to stippling. • AG is stippled; MG is not. • Central part of I/D papilla is stippled; but its margins are smooth. • Less on lingual surface than the facial surface. • Varies with age; absent in infancy; begins to disappear in old age. • Is produced due to papillary layer projecting into elevations on the epithelial surface. • Is a form of adaptive specialization or reinforcement for function and is a feature of healthy gingiva. • Degree of keratinization and prominence of stippling are related. • It disappears in gingival disease due to oedema.
Keratinisation	• It is also a protective adaptation to function. • There is a CT based genetic determination of the type of epithelial surface.
Position	• Is the level at which gingival margin is attached to the tooth. • Varies with eruption of tooth but depth of gingival sulcus is maintained by remodeling of OE, JE, REE.

Continuous tooth eruption

- Eruption continues throughout life.
- It has active and passive phases.
- **Active eruption** is the movement of tooth towards OP; it is coordinated with attrition.
- **Passive eruption** is exposure of tooth by apical migration of gingival; is a **pathological process**.
- **Anatomic crown** = part of the tooth covered by enamel.
- **Anatomic root** = part of the tooth covered by cementum.
- **Clinical crown** = part of the tooth projecting in oral cavity.
- **Clinical root** = part of the tooth covered by PD tissues.
- When tooth reaches the OP at its functional antagonist, the clinical crown is approx 2/3rd of the anatomic crown.
- **Passive eruption** is divided in 4 stages:

Stage	JE position	Base of gingival sulcus
I	On enamel	On enamel
II	Partly of enamel partly on cementum	On enamel
III	On cementum	At CEJ
IV	On cementum	At cementum; a part of cementum is exposed.

- Proliferation/migration of JE on root is due to degeneration of gingival and PDL fibers and their detachment from the tooth.
- Distance b/w apical end of JE and alveolar crest remains same throughout continuous tooth eruption, i.e. 1.07 mm.
- Exposure of tooth by apical migration of gingival is know as gingival recession/atrophy.

DENTIFRICES

Components	% age	Functions
Detergent, e.g. sodium lauryl sulfate;	1–2	• Lowers the surface tension. • Loosens the debris/stains for easy removal. • Foaming action.
Abrasive	25–60	• Abrasive action on deposits.
Binder, e.g. alginate; cellulose, etc.	1–2	• Prevents separation of solid and liquid ingredients. during storage.
Humectant, e.g. glycol; sorbitol, etc.	20–40	• Retains moisture and prevents hardening on exposure to air.
Flavoring agent, e.g. peppermint oil; cinnamon oil, menthol, etc.	1–1.5	• Helps to mask the less pleasant flavors of other ingredients.
Water	15–50	• To create gel or paste consistency.
Preservative, sweetener and colouring agents	2–3	• Preservative to prevent the bacterial growth, e.g. alcohol, benzoates, formaldehyde, etc. • Sweeteners give pleasant taste, e.g. sorbitol, glycerine, etc. • Colours give attractiveness, e.g. vegetable dyes.
Therapeutic agents	0–2	• Fluorides = anticaries, e.g. NaF, etc. • Plaqueinhibitors, e.g. chlorhexidine, triclosan, etc.

DENTIFRICES (*Contd.*)

Components	% age	Functions
		• Desensitizing agents = occlude the open dentinal tubules, e.g. stannous fluoride; potassium nitrate; strontium chloride, etc. • Tartar controlling agents = inhibit the formation of calculus supragingivally, e.g. disodium pyrophosphate; zinc citrate, etc.
Recently incorporated therapeutic agents		• Anti-plaque = triclosan; chlorhexidine; stannous fluoride; vitamin P factor; sanguinarine. • Anti-tartar = enz pyrophosphatase. • Anti-calculus = 0.3% triclosan; 2% gentrez.
PM tooth brush, i.e. proton magnesium brush		• No tooth paste required. • Electrically operated. • It uses saliva to conduct an electric shock to remove plaque.

GINGIVAL ENLARGEMENT

Localized	Limited to the gingival adj to a single tooth or group of teeth.
Generalized	Involves the gingival throughout the mouth.
Marginal	Confined to MG only.
Papillary	Confined to I/D papillae.
Diffuse	Involves MG, AG and I/D papillae.

GINGIVAL ENLARGEMENT (*Contd.*)

Discrete	An isolated tumor like growth.
Drug induced	Esp by phenytoin; cyclosporine and nifedipine; it is generally gingival hyperplasia, i.e. increased no. of cells; lesion is mulberry shaped; firm pale; minutely lobulated; does not occur in edentulous area; fibroblast to collagen ratio is normal; elongated rete pegs and hyperplasia of CT occurs; only GM and I/D papillae are involved, (as cp to idiopathic gingival hyperplasia, in which MG, AG and I/D papillae are involved).
Leukemic enlargement	Is due to dense infiltration of immature and proliferating leukocytes; it is mainly found in acute or subacute leukemia but seldom in chronic leukemia. Gingival is bluish red and moderately firm.

- Systemic administration of phenytoin accelerates the healing of gingival wounds in non-epileptics by decreasing collagen degradation due to production of an inactive fibroblastic collagenase. But may cause megaloblastic anemia and a folic acid deficiency (AIPG—95).
- Cyclosporine is immuno-suppresent drug to prevent organ transplant. It reversibly inhibits helper T-cells;

ANUG

- Also known as trench mouth; **Vincent's infection,** etc.
- **Vincent's angina** = i.e. with involvement of the throat and larynx also.
- Punched out; crater like depressions at the crest of the I/D papillae extending to the marginal gingival; surface covered by gray pseudomembranous slough.
- Metallic taste; thick pasty saliva; constant radiating gnawing pain; foul smell.

- It **does not lead to formation of PD pockets,** because the necrotic changes involve the JE; and a viable JE is required for formation of the pockets.
- Caused by **spirochetes (borrelia vincenti) and fusiform bacilli (treponema)**. Specific cause of ANUG has not been established.
- **4 zones** of the lesion are seen as:
  - zone 1 **bacterial zone** = most superficial.
  - zone 2 **neutrophil rich** zone.
  - zone 3 **necrotic** zone.
  - zone 4 zone of **spirochetal infiltration.**
- Mostly, intermediate sized spirochetes are found.
- There is increased levels of IgG and IgM antibodies to intermediate sized spirochetes and B. melaninogenicus subsp intermedius.
- Depression of host defense mechanism—Depressed PMN chemotaxis and phagocytosis.
- **Role of cortisol** = stress causes increased secretion of cortisol, which is associated with **depression of lymphocytes and PMN functions,** which may predispose to ANUG.
- ANUG is non-contagious but transmissible.
- It is more common in children with Down syndrome than in other retarded children.
- In agranulocytosis–inflammation is very less than ANUG, which is due to decreased host resistance and decreased number of PMN cells.
- Streptococcal gingivostamatitis is caused by strept. Viridans.
- Gonococcal stomatitis is caused by Neisseria gonorrhoeae.
- Acute herpetic gingivostomatitis is caused by herpes simplex virus HSV. It most frequently occurs in children younger than 6 yrs of age. Inclusion bodies are found in nucleus of the cells, which may be colony of virus particles. It is contagious and may be present as subclinical infection.
- Vesicles of Acute herpetic gingivostomatitis; H. zoster; varicella/ chicken pox reveal eosinophilic intranuclear inclusion bodies in the peripheral cells.

Differences b/w slow progressing and rapidly progressing periodontitis

Slow progressing periodontitis	Rapidly progressing
In 50–60 yrs age	In 20–35 esp in young adults
Associated with abundant plaque	Scantier plaque
Slow pace of development	Rapid bone destruction
No defects in neutrophils functions	Defective neutrophils and monocytes chemotaxis

Types of marginal periodontitis according to severity and degree of tissue destruction:

- Mild if 2–4 mm loss of attachment.
- Moderate if 4–6 mm loss of attachment.
- Severe if more than 7 mm loss of attachment.

♦ Juvenile periodontitis occurs in children and adolescents.

♦ Post juvenile periodontitis occurs in adults, i.e. 18–30 yrs age.

♦ Refractory periodontitis = cases not responding to treatment or recurring after treatment.

♦ Generalized juvenile periodontitis = e.g. in Papillon-Lefevre syndrome; hypophosphatasia; agranulocytosis and Down's syndrome, etc.

Extension of gingival inflammation

♦ It extends along collagen fibers and follows the course of blood vessels and loose tissues. Interproximally, it spreads in the loose CT and transseptal fibers and then in the bone at the crest of interdental septum. It leads to **horizontal bone loss**. The site at which it enters the bone depends on the location of vascular channels; facially and lingually, it may spread along outer periosteal surface.

- In TFO, the inflammation spreads b/w transseptal fibers directly into the PDL. It leads to **vertical bone loss** in TFO.
- Rate of bone loss—0.2 mm/yr on facial surfaces; and 0.3 mm/yr on proximal surfaces. Loss of attachment precedes the loss of alveolar bone by 6–8 mos.
- Osteoclast remove the inorganic part of the bone, while mononuclear cells remove organic part of the bone. During bone resorption, fatty marrow is replaced by fibrous marrow. Periodontal destruction is **episodic**. During destructive activity, T-cells change to B-cells and plasma cells. During healing, bone is formed adj to sites of bone resorption to buttress weakened bony trabeculae, which is known as **Buttressing bone formation**. The shelf like thickening of alveolar margin is known as **lipping**.
- The newly formed osteoid is more resistant to resorption as it is non-calcified, than the mature bone.
- Radius of action of bone resorption factors is 1.5–2.5 mm. Beyond 2.5 mm, they do not have any effect. Interdentally, the angular defects can only occur in spaces wider than 2.5 mm. On facial surfaces of anterior teeth, the bone thickness is lesser and so only horizontal bone loss occurs.

Furcation involvement

- Mandibular first molars are most common sites and the maxillary premolars are the least common.
- Diagnosis is done by Naber's probe which is a blunt probe.

Different gradings

Grade I	Incipient bone loss
Grade II	Partial bone loss
Grade III	Total bone loss
Grade IV	Total bone loss with gingival recession. It is also known as visible furcation.

- Furcation areas are most sensitive to injury from excessive occlusal forces.

JUVENILE PERIODONTITIS

- 2 types, i.e. localized and generalized.
- Causes of generalized JP—Papillon-Lefevre syndrome; Downs syndrome; nerutopenia; leukemia; hypophosphatasia; prepubertal periodontitis.
- Papillon-Lefevre syndrome = hyperkeratotic and ichthyosis skin lesion; severe loss of periodontium; calcification of dura; the cutaneous and periodontal lesions appear before the age of 4 yrs; primary teeth are lost by 5–6 yrs of age; and permanent teeth by 15 yrs of age; there is no osteoblastic activity; autosomal recessive.
- Downs syndrome = is trisomy 21; mental and growth retardation; high incidence of PD dis and gingivitis esp in lower anterior regions; decreased resistance to infection; defective T-cell maturation and chemotaxis; increased no. of B. melaninogenicus.
- Hypophosphatasia = abnormal alk Pase activity; early loss of primary teeth esp incisors.
- **Prepubertal periodontitis** = occur during or after eruption of primary teeth; neutrophil and monocytic defects; extreme acute inflammation of gingival tissues and rapid bone loss.

LOCALISED JP; LJP = is a disease of periodontium occurring in an otherwise healthy adolescent, which is characterised by a rapid loss of alveolar bone about more than one tooth of the permanent teeth; the amount to destruction manifested is not commensurate with the amounts of local irritants.

- **Main bacteria** involved = Actinobacillus, actinomycetemcomitans and capnocytophaga.
- Site = esp the first molars and incisors area which are the first erupted teeth, with least destruction of canine-premolar area; bone loss is bilaterally symmetrical.
- Rapid bone loss; 3–4 times than in the typical periodontitis.
- Bone loss is vertical and arc shaped.
- Absence of clinical inflammation in p.o. deep PD pockets.
- Plaque does not tend to mineralize.
- Mobility and migration (esp distolabial migration of max incisors) of involved teeth.

Histopathology

- Bacteria invade the CT reaching the bone surface.
- Mainly plasma and blast cells accumulate.
- More **unattached plaque** is present; plaque is non-mineralized.
- Epithelial attached subgingival plaque is responsible for LJP.
- There is **functional chemotactic defect of PMN** as the main cause.

Destructive mechanisms are:

- **Inhibition of PMN chemotaxis**; and hence pahgocytosis is reduced.
- Due to endotoxins and leucotoxins produced by the microbes.
- Due to production of fibroblast inhibitory factors.
- Collagen destruction by proteolytic enzymes.
- By direct lytic action.

Treatment options

- LJP has better prognosis than GJP.
- Surgery and antibodies are required, because microbes remain in the tissues even after scaling and root planning.
- Scaling, root planning, curettage, bone grafts, etc.
- Antibiotics = tetracycline 250 mg qid for 14 days every 8 weeks; bone loss was stopped.
- Transportation of 3rd molar to 1st molar site
- Extraction of teeth is the last resort.

Host response: the basic concepts

- Difference b/w tissue/host collagenase and bacterial collagenase is that former destroys the collagen completely, while latter just splits the collagen, which have the tendency to reunite when bacteria are removed.
- Monocytes form macrophages, which give cell mediated immunity.

- T-cells provide cell mediated immunity.
- B-cells provide humoral immunity.
- B-cells/B-lymphocytes form plasma cells in spleen and lymph nodes.
- Plasma cells form Ig, which give **systemic humoral immunity**.
- Plasma cells form Abs, which give **local humoral immunity**.
- Ig has 2 parts, i.e. Fc and Fab. Fc is heavy chain and is complement binding site, while Fab is light chain and is Ab binding site.
- **Secretory IgA** is more resistant to digestion by proteolytic enzymes than other Igs.
- IgA is in salive.
- IgM is first formed after infection.
- IgE appears in allergies; is reaginic Ab.
- IgG is most abundant; known as blocking antibody.

Tissue responses

- Type I/anaphylaxis = (mast cells + IgE complex) reacts with Antigen/Ag—and then histamine, etc. are released which lead to tissue damage.
- Type II/cytotoxic = cell's Ag reacts with Ab, e.g. RBC, autoimmune disease and produce hemolysis of cells.
- Type III/Arthus' reaction = Ag reacts with Ab and lead to local tissue damage due to lysosomal enzymes.
- Type IV/delayed hypersensitivity—CMI = lymphocytes react with Ag and so lymphokines are released. Here, no Abs are involved.

PLAQUE: Also known as **microcosm**

- It is a thin, transparent film on the tooth surfaces which are not properly cleaned, consisting of bacteria; leucocytes; desquamated epithelial cells; etc.
- It is complex, metabolically interconnected highly organized system.

- It appears as a thin tenacious gelatinous film on the tooth surface, which accumulates within 24–48 hrs after removal to its normal thickness.
- An important component of plaque is **acquired pellicle,** which is a glycoprotein derived from saliva and adsorbed on tooth surface and it covers the whole tooth and facilitates plaque formation. It does not have any bacteria; but may serve as a nutrient for bacteria; it is formed within 30 min after removal and within 24 hrs to its normal thickness (0.1–0.8 microns). It is acellular.
- ***Materia–alba*** can be removed with water jet but plaque cannot be.
- In plaque; most numerous organisms were aciduric streptococci in caries process.
- PH of plaque in caries active person is approx 5.5.
- ***3 main organism in plaque*** are strept mutans; veillonella and actinomyces.
- *S mutans* synthesise **Glucan** from dietary sucrose. This glucan/ dextran is insoluble, sticky gel, inert and resistant to attack by bacterial hydrolytic enzymes, which causes plaque to adhere to the tooth surface and acts as a barrier against the diffusion of salivary buffers which tend to neutralize the acid produced by the bacteria.
- **Sucrose** gives rise to glucose and fructose. Glucose forms dextrans and fructose forms levans.
- Dextrans are maximum carbohydrate in plaque.
- Plaque is mainly bacteria, i.e.70–80%.
- 1 cu.mm = 1 mg plaque = contains 10^8 bacteria.
- Types of plaque—supragingival and subgingival.
- Supragingival is—coronal and marginal types.
- Subgingival is—tooth associated, i.e. attached; epithelium associated; and unattached.

Bacterial adherence

In gingival sulcus	On enamel	On tongue
Bacteroides	Str mutans	Str salivarius
Spirochetes	Str sanguis	A. naeslundii
	Lactobacilli	
	Actinomyces viscosus	

Composition of plaque according to its age—with accumulation of plaque and development of gingivitis, there is both qualitative and quantative change in plaque.

1 day	Cocci
3 days	Rods
5–7 days	Filaments
7–10 days	Spirochetes
3 wks	Corn cob appearance
2 mos	Bristle brush appearance
Early gingivitis	Actinomyces filaments
Long standing gingivitis	Fusobacterium and veillonella
On active sites	B gingivalis; B intermedius; A actinomycetamcomitans
On Treated sites	Esp str. sanguis
Adult periodontitis	B gingivalis

- Salivary IgA—prevents bacterial attachment.
- Most nutrients for the formation of supragingival plaque are provided by saliva. Strept and actinomyces are initial colonizers, they use salivary carbohydrates as nutrients.

Attached plaque/tooth associated subgingival plaque	1. Mainly G + bacteria predominate. 2. G(–) rods in apical part 3. Cocci and filaments are perpendicular to tooth surface. 4. They cause: calculus formation; **root caries** and resorption and alveolar bone loss **(slow** progressing PD diseases). 5. Apical border of plaque is **some distance from JE** and that gap is filled up with WBCs.
Epithelial associated subgingival plaque	1. **Extends upto JE** 2. Mainly consist of G (–) rods; cocci and spirochetes. 3. Causes **rapid alveolar bone destruction.** 4. **No root caries.** 5. Extremely periodontopathic. 6. Has higher virulency. 7. May penetrate epithelium and CT.
Unattached plaque	1. Has G(–) rods; cocci. 2. Extends to JE. 3. Is associated with gingivitis.
In LJP and rapidly	1. Tooth associated plaque is minimal; progressing periodontitis but epithelial associated plaque is extensive. 2. Plaque is very virulent. 3. Epithelial associated plaque is more dangerous.

- Microbes are 43 millions to 5.5 billions/ml; average is 750 millions.
- Most of the salivary bacteria are derived from dorsum of the tongue.

- Str sanguis and other G + cocci are the major bacteria which initiate supragingival plaque.
- At healthy sites, especially G + cocci, e.g. str. sanguis mainly and A. viscosus facultative bacteria are present.
- In patients with PD diseases, influence of supragingival microbes and plaque–control procedures appear to be limited to approx 4 mm into the pocket.
- Subgingivally, main source of Ig and C is GCF.
- Athymic rats show increased bone loss.
- Progressive PD dis are associated with B-cells dominated lesions.
- After scaling and root planning, increased Abs levels occur esp to Bacteroides.

Major bacteria which initiate supragingival plaque	Str sanguis and other G + cocci.
In healthy sites	G + cocci, e.g. str sanguis mainly and facultative A. viscosus
Initial gingivitis	By A viscosus and A israelii, G + rods. Bacterial succession is required to produce disease, i.e. from G + cocci to G + rods to G(–) rods.
Pregnancy gingivitis	Bacteroides intermedius and capnocytophaga; are anaerobes. It is associated with increased levels of estrogen and progesterone, because these hormones serve as nutrients for these species.
ANUG	Borrelia vincenti; Bacillus fusiforme.
Slow progressing periodontitis	By A israelii; and A naeslundii; by tooth attached plaque.
In subgingival plaque	Increased G(–) capnophilic and anaerobes.

Rapidly progressing PD	By B gingivalis; B intermedius; Wollinella recta; Eikenella corrodnes; Actinobacillus actinomycetamcomitans;
Refractory periodontitis	By B gingivalis; B intermedius; Actinobacillus actinomycetamcomitans;
LJP	Main microbes are sacchrolytic, capnophilic, anaerobic G(–) rods; e.g. **Actinobacillus actinomycetamcomitans** is the most common microbes; which can penetrate into **connective/ gingival tissues**; they produce leucotoxins; epitheliotoxins; collagenase, etc. for its spread into the CT; so antibiotics are must for the Rx. Other microbe is capnocytophaga. There is altered chemotactic effect.
Prepubertal PD	Occurs during or after eruption of primary teeth; most common microbe is Actinobacillus actinomycetamcomitans; also capnocytophaga and B intermedius. Severe defect of PMN and macrophages.
Mainly G(–) facultative anaerobes are main bacteria associated with PD disease	e.g. bacteroides species, i.e. B gingivalis; B intermedius; Wollinella recta; Eikenella corrodnes; Actinobacillus actinomycetamcomitans.

Pathogenic mechanism of bacteria in PD diseases

Invasion

Production of exotoxins

Role of cell constituents, i.e. endotoxins; surface components; capsule, etc.

Production of enzymes.

Evasion of immunologic host responses.

Host-bacteria interaction

Endotoxins	1. Penetrate gingival epithelium. 2. Alternate path of complement system is activated—occurs at C3 but C1, 4, 2 is byepassed. 3. Cause localised Schwartzman reaction. 4. Activate factor 12 causing intravascular clotting. 5. Is cytotoxic. 6. Cause bone resorptin.
Hyaluronidases	1. Influence gingival permeability by allowing apical proliferation of JE along the root surface and increases intracellular gaps. 2. Bacteroidcs and A actinomycetamcomitans produce collagenases. 3. Phopholipase A may initiate alveolar bone resorption as a precursor of prostaglandins.
Ig	Are deactivated or destroyed by proteases.

Immune findings in periodontal diseases

ANUG	1. Periodontal chemotactic defects. 2. Increased Ab titers to B intermedius.
Adult periodontitis	1. Increased Ab titers to B gingivalis, etc. 2. Immune complex present in tissues. 3. CMI to gingival bacteria. 4. Immediate hypersensitivity to gingival bacteria.
LJP	PMN chemotactic defect and depressed phagocytosis increased Ab titers to A actinomycetamcomitans
GJP	PMN chemotactic defect and depressed phagocytosis increased Ab titers to B gingivalis
Prepubertal	PMN and monocytic chemotactic defect.
Refractory periodontitis	Reduced PMN chemotaxis

Facts about immunoglobulins

Reaction	Ig	Cells, etc.
Anaphylactic/regain dependant reaction	IgE	From mast cells, basophils
Cytotoxic	IgM, IgG	
Immune complex/ Arthus reaction	IgM, IgG– lysozymes	Complexes occur in tissues and blood vessels
Cell mediated/ delayed hypersensitivity	Lymphokines, Osteoclast activating factors	T-cells

Neutrophil associated PD diseases

Neurophil disorders associated with PD disease	1. Diabetes mellitus. 2. Papillon-Lefevre syndrome. 3. Down syndrome. 4. Chediak-higashi syndrome. 5. Drug induced agranulocytosis. 6. Cyclic neutropenia.
PD diseases with neutrophil disorders	1. ANUG. 2. LJP. 3. Prepubertal periodontitis. 4. Rapidly progressing periodontitis. 5. Refractory periodontitis.

Cellular predominance

In healthy sites	G + cocci
In early gingivitis	T-cells predominate
In advanced gingivitis	Plasma cells predominate
In periodontitis	B-cells predominate
T4:T8 ratio	2:1 in gingivitis 1:1 in periodontitis < 1 in AIDS (reversed ratio due to destruction of T4-cells)

CALCULUS

- Calculus is mineralized plaque.
- It helps to keep plaque in close contact with the gingiva.
- 2 types: supragingival; subgingival.
- **Supragingival calculus** = coronal to the gingival margin; whitish yellow in colour; hard clay-like consistency; easily detached from tooth; esp present on the lingual surface of lower incisors opposite Whaton's duct; buccal surface of maxillary molars opposite Stensen's duct; also called **salivary,** because it is derived from saliva.

- **Subgingival calculus** = below the crest of the marginal gingival; is not visible in oral cavity; dense dark brown colour; hard in consistency; firmly attached to tooth; also called **serumal,** because it is derived from GCF and blood serum.
- **Supragingival calculus** has 70–90% inorganic component; mainly consisting of calcium phosphate.
- **The ratio of** Ca to P is higher subgingivally, and the Na content increases with the depth of PD pocket.
- Calculus is mineralized plaque, which starts b/w 1–14 days of plaque formation. At 2 days, it is 50% mineralized, and at 12 days, it is 60–90% mineralized. Microbes are not required for calculus formation.
- Plaque cannot mineralize in acidic atmosphere. Calcification starts in the inner surface of supragingival plaque and in the attached component of subgingival plaque; **filamentous bacteria increase** with the calcification.
- Average daily formation of calculus is 0.10–0.15% of dry wt.
- Material-alba = is an acquired bacterial coating; is clearly visible without the use of disclosing agents. It can be flushed away with a water spray. It lacks a regular internal pattern which is seen in plaque.

Dental stains

Brown	Fe; pigmented pellicle. Tobacco stains are dark brown; tenacious.
Black	Fe; Ag; chromogenic bacteria, e.g. Actinomyces (main cause); B melaninigenicus. Black stains which occur on human primary teeth is typically associated with low incidence of caries.
Green	Cu; Ni. Penicillium and Aspergillus. Usually occur on the facial surface of the maxillary anteriors.

Dental stains (*Contd.*)

Orange	Serratia marcescens and Flavobacterium lutescens.
Metallic	**Mn-black stains.** **Hg-greenish black.**
Chlorhexidine stains	Retention is due to its affinity to sulfate and acidic groups yellowish to brownish colour appears.

Old bacteria with new terminology

Bacteroides gingivalis	Porphyromonas gingivalis
Bacteroides intermedius	Prevotella intermedius
Bacteroides	Prevotella melaninogenicus
Wolinella recta	Campyobacter recta

Classification of mobility of the teeth

Grade I	0.5–1.0 mm facially or lingually.
Grade II	1–2.0 mm facially or lingually.
Grade III	> 2 mm in horizontal or vertical/apical direction.
Physiologic mobility	Shows circadian rhythm, i.e. highest in morning, lowest in evening greater in females; increases in pregnancy; decreases in lactation; most mobile are upper incisors.

Gingival grafting procedure

Condition	Procedure
Long narrow gingival defect on a single tooth.	Best is laterally positioned flap.
Pockets extending to MGJ; thick manageable pocket wall.	Apically positioned flap.
Soft friable pocket wall.	Gingival extension procedures with free gingival graft
Absence of AG with no pockets only recession is present with non pathologic dehiscence.	Free gingival graft.

Interdental embrasures

Type I	No gingival recession	Dental floss is indicated.
Type II	Moderate papillary recession	I/D brush like proxa brush, miniature bottle brush indicated.
Type III	Complete loss of papilla	Unitufted brush indicated

Differences b/w gracey and universal currets

Area of use	Area specific	Universal; anywhere.
Cutting edge	Only outer edge; used with pull stroke	Both edges are used
Curvature	2 planed; curvature is upwards and sidewards	One plane instrument
Blade angle	Offset of 60 degrees	90 degrees
Side specificity	For left and right side separate	No specificity

Suturing techniques

Technique	Indications
Direct or loop sutures	Need for coverage of I/D bone with I/D papilla. When bone graft is used.
Figure of eight	When flaps are not in close adaptation due to apical flap displacement of non-scalloped incisions.
Sling ligation	When flap involving 2 I/D spaces and opposite flap not reflected.
Horizontal mattress suture	Used in wide I/D spaces to adapt the I/D papilla against the bone.
Anchor suture	Closing of flap mesial or distal to tooth as in mesial or distal wedge procedure.
Periosteal suture	Used to hold apically displaced partial thickness flap.

Special days

2003	International year of fresh water.
11th April	National safe motherhood day.
11th July	World population day.
14th Nov	World's diabetes day.
16th Sept	International ozone day.
1st July	Doctor's day.
1st Oct	Senior citizen day.
1st Oct	International blood donation day.
21st May	Anti-terrorism day; Rajiv Gandhi's death day.
22nd March	World water day.
22nd May	World biodiversity day.

Special days (*Contd.*)

24th March	World TB day.
26th June	International day vs drug abuse.
26th Sept	World's heart day.
27th Sept	World tourism day.
2nd Sunday of May	International mother day.
31st May	World no-tobacco day.
4th May	World asthma day.
5th June	World environment day.
7th April	World health day.
7th April	WHO day.
8th March	International women's day.
Road safety	Theme of world health day 2004.

- White ribbon alliance for safe motherhood/India: WRAI.
- National nutrition week—1–7th sept 2004.

Common occlusal interferences

Position	Maxillary cusps	Mandibular cusps
RCP	Mesial inclines of lingual cusps (CR); these are to be removed first	Distal inclines of lower cusps and MR of PM and molars
Protrusive prematurities	Distofacial inclines	Mesiofacial inclines
Mediotrusive or balancing contact	Inner inclines of lingual cusps or non-working (not a pathologic interference)	Inner inclines of buccal cusps
Laterotrusive or working	Inner inclines of buccal cusps	Inner inclines of lingual cusps

VARIOUS DENTAL MEDICAMENTS

Component	**Function**
EDTA	Chemical reaming of root canals;
Disodium edetate	Chelating agent for reaming RCs
Parachlorophenol + thymol + camphor	Antiseptics for RC disinfection
Dexamethasone	Decreases inflammation of RCs
Chlorohexidine digluconate 20% and ethyl alcohol	For RC decontamination by acting on anaerobes
Iodoform paste	Acute and chronic infections of RC Esp in deciduous teeth Does not interfere with permanent teeth
Calcium hydroxide	RC decontamination; due to its high pH Helps sec dentin formatin Has a chemical neutralizing effect on acids from cements/mouth
Endomethasone	RC sealer; has ZnO + eugenol; Antiseptic; thymol iodide + para-formal-dehyde Anti-inflammatory; corticosteroids Radiopaque; barium sulfate
Tetrachloroethylene	RC filling remover
Pulp sedative for pulpitis	Lidocaine HCl as anesthetic Creosote as sedative Phenol/eugenol as antiseptic and disinfectant
Pulp vitality testing	Tetrafluororethane and ethyl alcohol
KNO_3; HEMA; sodium fluoride	For Rx of dentinal hypersensitivity
Fluoride Rx	Knutson's tech; at 3, 7, 10, 13 yrs age

VARIOUS DENTAL MEDICAMENTS (*Contd.*)

Antiseptic for hands	By chlorohexidine gluconate + methyl parahyeroxybenzoate + propyl parahyeroxy-benzoate
Disinfection of instruments	Aldehyde + quaternary ammonium compounds + corrosion inhibitors
Disinfection of impression material	By ampholytic surfactants + isopropyl alcohol (bactericidal, fungicidal, viricidal) also 2% glutraldehyde solution for 10 min.

Nutritional deficiencies

Vitamin C deficiency = known as scurvy; retardation of wound healing; increased susceptibility to infections; haemorrhagic lesions into ms of extremities and joints; defective formation and maintenance of collagen; retarded osteoid formation.

Relation of vitamin C deficiency and PD diseases.

- Low levels of vitamin C influence the metabolism of collagen in periodontium, and so affect the ability of tissues to regenerate and repair.
- It interferes with bone formation leading to loss of periodontal bone.
- It increases the permeability of oral mucosa and of crevicular epithelium.
- Vit C is required to maintain the integrity of the PD vasculature.
- Vit C deficiency interferes with the ecologic equilibrium of bacteria in plaque and so increases the pathogenicity of plaque.
- PD fibers least affected by vitamin C deficiency are those below the JE and above the alveolar crest.

Vitamin D deficiency = it may lead to rickets in infants and osteomalacia in adults.

Osteoporosis of alveolar bone; reduction in the width of PDL; defective mineralization of osteoid and cementoid; generalized partial to complete disappearance of lamina dura; increased radiolucencies of trabecular interstices, etc.

Hypervitaminosis D = increased osteoblastic activity; osteoscelerosis; dystrophic calcification in PDL; hypercementosis and ankylosis of many teeth.

Calciphylaxis = is a condition of induced systemic hypersensitivity, in which tissues respond to appropriate changing agent with local calcification.

Hormonal influences on periodontium

Hypothyroidism	Causes cretinism in infants and myxodema in adults. Delayed physical and mental development occurs. Increased weight; feeling of cold; non-pitting edema of subcutaneous tissues; low BP and BMR. Chronic PD dis with severe bone loss.
Hyperthyroidism/ thyrotoxicosis	High BP; cardiac enlargement; loss of wt; high BMR; heat intolerance; exophthalmos; increased growth and development; early eruption of teeth. Osteroporosis of alv bone; increased size of marrow spaces and increased width of PDL.
Hypopituitarism	Due to deficiency of hormone by anterior pituitary. Retardation of growth of all tissues; dwarfism; delayed eruption of teeth; skeletal Class II relation of jaws; underdeveloped sinuses esp frontal sinus.
Hyperpituitarism	Due to increased secretion of hormone by anterior pituitary. Acromegaly or gigantism occurs; disproportionate growth of facial and body

Hormonal influences on periodontium (*Contd.*)

	bones; skeletal Class III jaw relation esp increased size of mandible. Marked overgrowth of alveolar process; increased size of dental arches; spacing b/w teeth; hypercementosis.
Hypoparathyroidism	Due to accidental removal of parathyroid gland. Hypocalcemia and tetany occurs; if it occurs in infancy, it causes enamel hypoplasia.
Hyperparathyroidism	Generalized demineralization; bone cysts; giant cells tumor; serum Ca conc. increased; serum P level decreases. Tooth mobility; malocclusion; alveolar osteoporosis; widening of PDL; absence of lamina dura.
Diabetes mellitus	Hypofunction of beta cells of islets of Langerhans; glucose levels of blood and GCF high; a decreased camp levels in GCF; (camp reduces inflammation, so in diabetics, there is more inflammation). Altered response of PD tissues to local irritants; Altered flora of oral cavity; decreased salivary flow. Reduction in defense mechanism, increased susceptibility to infections; increased bone loss. Tendency of abscess formation; diabetic periodontoclasia; greater loss of attachment; increased tooth mobility.

Hormonal influences on periodontium (*Contd.*)

	H/E: thickened walls and narrowed lumen of arterioles; increased thickness of basement membrane of capillaries. Main bacteria: S epidermidis; staphylococci. Immunology—infections are due to PMN deficiencies resulting in impaired chemotaxis; defective phagocytosis, etc.
Gonads	Progesterone produces dilatation of gingival microvasculature, which increases susceptibility to injury and exudation; Estrogen-counteract tendencies of hyperkeratosis of epithelium and fibrosis of vessel walls; also stimulates bone formation and fibroplasia. Testosterone—retards downgrowth of sulcular epithelium over the cementum; restores osteoblastic activity; increases cellularity in PDL.
Pregnancy	Gingivitis increases during 2nd or 3rd month and decreases during 9th month depending on the levels of hormones; gingival is edematous; pitting; bright red to bluish red in colour; raspberry appearance. Main microbe is B intermedius, it can substitute progesterone or estradiole for vit K as growth factor. Progesterone produces dilatation of gingival microvasculature and stasis, which increases susceptibility to injury and exudation.

Hormonal influences on periodontium (*Contd.*)

	Destruction of gingival mast cells by increased sex hormones and release of histamines may lead to increased inflammatory response.
HEMATOLOGIC EFFECTS ON PERIODONTIUM	
Leukemia	Immature leukocytes infiltrate the gingival corium leading to enlargement esp of I/D papilla. Highest incidence is in cases of acute monocytic leukemia; then acute myelomonocytic leukemia. Not found in edentulous patients. Gingival colour is bluish red and cyanotic. Gingival bleeding is due to thrombocytopenia, which is due to replacement of bone marrow by leukemic cells; it also decreases the tissue resistance to infections and leads to ulceration.

VARIOUS DISCLOSING AGENTS: it is a solution which when applied to teeth makes, visible by staining roughness and foreign matter on the teeth". Eg.

- Iodine preparations
- Mercurochrome preparations
- Bismark brown (Easlick's disclosing solution)
- Basic fuchsin
- Merbromin
- Erythrosine
- Fast green
- Fluorescin
- Plak lite : uses UV light as light source
- Two tone solutions

11

MCQs in Periodontics

Part I

1. **The primary reason for splinting teeth is:**
   A. As a preventive measure
   B. For esthetics
   C. To immobilize excessively mobile teeth for patient comfort
   D. To aid a patient in home care

2. **All of the following are advantages of placing a periodontal dressing after surgical procedures except:**
   A. Protects the surgical wound
   B. Minimizes patient discomfort
   C. Enhances the healing rate to the tissues
   D. Helps maintain tissue placement
   E. Helps to prevent postoperative bleeding

3. **Which focal sign of acute inflammation listed below is caused by increased capillary permeability?**
   A. Redness (Rubor)
   B. Heat (Calor)
   C. Swelling (Tumor)
   D. Pain (Dolor)

4. **Which of the following vitamins functions in collagen formation?**
   A. B

B. C
C. D
D. A

5. Most root amputations involve the:
A. Mandibular first and second premolars
B. Maxillary first and second molars
C. Maxillary canines
D. Maxillary and mandibular third molars

6. Which of the following are important factors that must be evaluated before performing a laterally repositioned flap?
A. The presence of bone on the facial surface of the donor tooth
B. The thickness of the gingiva at the donor site
C. The width of attached gingiva at the donor site
D. All of the above

7. Cervical line contours are closely related to the attachment of the gingiva at the neck of the tooth. The greatest contour of the cervical lines and gingival attachments occurs on
A. The distal surface of anterior teeth
B. The distal surface of posterior teeth
C. The mesial surface of anterior teeth
D. The mesial surface of posterior teeth

8. The alveolar process is that part of the maxilla and mandible that houses the teeth. It consists of two main parts. Which part is a thin layer of lamellar bone that surrounds the root to the tooth and is where the periodontal ligament fibers attach?
A. Alveolar bone proper
B. Supporting alveolar bone

9. The air syringe is used during scaling to locate the epithelial attachment. When the explorer is used to detect subgingival calculus it should be grasped firmly.
A. The first statement is true, the second is false
B. The first statement is false; the second is true
C. Both statements are true
D. Both statements are false

10. Which of the following are objectives of gingival curettage?
A. To eliminate or reduce inflammation (edema)
B. To remove chronically inflamed tissues
C. To reduce pocket depth and promote better tissue architecture
D. All of the above

11. The effectiveness of tooth brushing is best measured by:
A. The amount and location of plaque
B. The caries experience
C. The tooth brushing frequency
D. The condition of the toothbrush

12. Which of the following home care aids consists of a plastic handle that will reccive round polished toothpicks and permits the patient to cleanse the teeth at gingival margins, where accessible, and in the areas of difficult access?
A. Dental floss
B. Perio Aid
C. Stim-U- Dent
D. Proxa brush

13. Which of the following is the main function of cementum?
A. Compensation for tooth wear
B. Reparative
C. To attach the principle fibers of the periodontal ligament to the tooth
D. Protection

14. When probing, the tip of the periodontal probe should always be kept in contact with the tooth. Four measurements are recorded for each tooth.
A. Both statements are true
B. Both statements are false
C. The first statement is true, the second is second is false
D. The first staten ent is false, the second is second is true

15. The characteristic cell components of chronic inflammation include all of the following except:
A. Lymphocytes
B. Plasma cell

C. Polymorphonuclear leukocytes
D. Macrophages

16. The acquired pellicle could become stained by all of the following except:
A. Chromogenic bacteria
B. Cariogenic bacteria
C. Food
D. Chemicals

17. The main goal of osseous recontouring (surgery) is:
A. To cure periodontal disease
B. To eliminate the existing microflora
C. To eliminate periodontal pockets
D. To change the existing microflora

18. Which graft listed below is one in which the transplant is connective tissue without an epithelial covering?
A. Free gingival graft
B. Free mucosal autograft
C. Neither of the above
D. Both of the above

19. The narrowest band of attached gingiva is found:
A. On the lingual surfaces of maxillary incisors and the facial surfaces of maxillary first molars
B. On the facial surfaces of mandibular second bicuspids and the lingual surface of canines
C. On the facial surfaces of the mandibular canines and first bicuspids and the lingual surfaces of the mandibular incisors
D. None of the above

20. Parts of the free gingiva include all of the following except:
A. Gingival margin
B. Free gingival groove
C. Mucogingival junction
D. Gingival sulcus
E. Interdental (interproximal) gingiva

21. What should be done if a patient experience sensitivity while being scaled with an ultrasonic scaling device?
A. Proceed to another tooth and often return to the sensitive tooth later in the appointment
B. Make necessary adjustments to the water spray
C. Use less pressure
D. All of the above

22. Which of the following instruments is best for performing root planing procedures?
A. An ultrasonic instrument
B. A hoe
C. A periodontal curette
D. Periodontal files

23. Periodontal disease in multiple sites in patients who continue to demonstrate attachment loss after apparently appropriate periodontal treatment is referred to as?
A. Gingivitis
B. Localized juvenile periodontitis
C. Refractory periodontitis
D. Rapidly progressive periodontitis

24. In a healthy sulcus, which bacteria below are most abundant?
A. Actinobacillus actinomycetemcomitans and Bacteroides forsythus
B. Streptococcus species and Actinomyces species
C. Treponema species and Capnocytophaga species
D. Prevotella intermedia and Prophyromonas gingivalis

25. Water irrigation devices have been shown to:
A. Produce a transient bacteremia in patients with gingival inflammation
B. Stimulate a new epithelial attachment
C. Remove acquired tooth pellicle
D. Cause no harm to the gingival tissues

26. Which of the following brushing techniques emphasizes placing the bristles of the toothbrush at a 45° angle on the tooth and pointing apically so that the bristles enter the gingival sulcus?
A. Charter's technique

B. Stillman technique
C. Roll technique
D. Bass technique (Sulcular)

27. All of the following will reduce the abrasive action of a polishing agent except?
A. Using an agent with nice large particles
B. Using an agent containing particles that are dull and round
C. Applying the polishing agent with firm pressure and increasing to a heavy constant pressure
D. Polishing at a low speed with light pressure

28. All of the following are indications for the use of an apically respositioned flap except:
A. Moderate or deep pockets
B. Patients at risk for root caries
C. Furcation -involved teeth
D. Crown Lengthening

29. Which cells listed below are the first ones to emigrate into gingival sulcus as a result of inflammation in the initial lesion of gingivitis?
A. Mast cells
B. Lymphocytes
C. Polymorphonuclear neutrophils PMNS's
D. Plasma cells

30. The most common clinical sign of occlusal trauma is:
A. Caries
B. Migration of teeth
C. Periodontal disease
D. Tooth mobility

31. Which of the following conditions predisposes a patient to the development of inflammatory periodontal disease or exacerbation of an existing disease?
A. Pregnancy
B. Neutropenia
C. Agranulocytosis
D. Leukemias
E. All of the above

32. A variation of the laterally repositioned flap is called
   A. A coronally repositioned flap
   B. A double papilla flap
   C. Apically repositioned flap
   E. Nine of the above

33. Which group listed below of the principal fibers of the periodontal ligament runs perpendicular from the alveolar bone to the cementum and resists lateral forces?
   A. Alveolar crest
   B. Horizontal crest
   C. Oblique
   D. Apical
   E. Interradicular

34. Of the choices listed below, which one describes the boundaries that define the attached gingiva?
   A. From the gingival margin to the interdental groove
   B. From the free gingival groove to the gingival margin
   C. From the mucogingival junction to the free gingival groove
   D. From the epithelial attachment to the cementoenamel junction

35. Which of the following are indications for the use of ultrasonic scaling devices?
   A. Supragingival calculus removal
   B. Subgingival debridement
   C. Initial debridement of a patient with ANUG
   D. Gross scaling prior to extractions
   E. Removal of orthodontic cement, bonding material, and overhanging restorations
   F. All of the above

36. Name the type of curettage that is performed when the soft tissue wall of a pocket is removed by the offset cutting edge of a curet during a root planing procedure.
   A. Non-definitive curettage
   B. Coincidental curettage
   C. Closed sub gingival curettage
   D. Open sub gingival curettage

37. The most accepted theory as to the cause of root sensitivity is the

A. Baeyer's theory
B. Chemo-isosmotic theory
C. Hydrodynamic theory
D. Quantum theory

38. Which of the following is a constituent of gram-negative microogranisms and has been suggested as an important agent in the pathogenesis of inflammatory periodontal disease?

A. Exotoxin
B. Endotoxin
C. Plaque
D. Carbohydrates

39. Pseudopocketing is a condition in which pocketing occurs without:

A. Bleeding
B. Exudate
C. Attachment loss
D. Inflammation

40. Which of the following is a condition in which there is expansion of the marginal tissue coronally rather than an apical movement of the epithelial attachment?

A. The periodontal pocket
B. The gingival pocket
C. An infrabony pocket
D. All of the above

41. Which of the following refers to an excessive occlusal force being applied to a tooth or teeth with normal supporting structures (no periodontal disease)?

A. Primary occlusal trauma
B. Secondary occlusal trauma
C. Tertiary occlusal trauma
D. None of the above

42. What should be done if the periodontal probe comes into contact with an obstacle once it has been inserted into the gingival sulcus

A. Remove the probe and then reinsert it in another area
B. Push the probe beyond the obstacle
C. Attempt the move past the obstacle and then continue to move the probe apically
D. Record the measurement where the probe stopped
E. Remove the probe and reinsert a much thinner one.

43. A modified Widman flap is:

A. A partial - thickness flap
B. A full - thickness flap
C. An epithelial graft
D. None of the above

44. All of the following statements concerning B cells are true, except:

A. They mature in the bone marrow and migrate to lymphoid organs
B. They are found in the germinal centers of the spleen and lymph nodes
C. They are progenitors of plasma cells
D. Are involved in humoral (antibody-mediated) and cell-mediated immunity
E. They function to search out, identify, and bind with specific antigens

45. There are various distal flap approaches used for retromolar reduction. The simplest is the:

A. Gingivectomy
B. Gingivoplasty
C. Distal wedge
D. None of the above

46. When measuring the pocket depth with a periodontal probe it may not stop at the bottom or base of the pocket. How far it reaches will depend on which of the following factors?

A. Size of the probe
B. The force exerted

C. The dimensions of the pocket
D. Access to the pocket
E. Degree to the pocket
F. The presence of deposits
G. The accuracy of the examiner in reading the probed measurements
H. All of the above

47. The periodontal ligament is composed primary of:
A. Elastic fibers
B. Reticulin fibers
C. Collagen fibers
D. Spindle fibers

48. Which of the following cells may be found in the periodontal ligament?
A. Fibroblasts
B. Osteoblasts
C. Cementoblasts
D. Macrophages
E. All of the above

49. Which of the following are possible uses of the periodontal file?
A. Calculus removal where access is limited
B. Incision placement
C. Final smoothing of the tooth surface
D. Curettage

50. Which of the following is most significant in regard to the prognosis of a periodontally involved tooth?
A. Pocket depth
B. Attachment loss
C. Anatomical crown length
D. Bleeding upon probing

51. Which of the following is a progressive proliferation of the gingiva, particularly the collagenous elements?
A. Inflammatory gingival enlargement
B. Hereditary gingivofibromatosis

C. Both of the above
D. Neither of the above

52. All of the following statements concerning calculus are true, except:
A. It is calcified or mineralized bacterial plaque
B. It forms on natural teeth, dentures and other dental prostheses
C. The surface is very rough and is covered by a layer of bacterial plaque
D. Inorganic material makes up about 10-15% of the composition while organic material and water make up about 70-90% of the composition
E. Its main role in periodontal disease is to serve as a collection site for more bacteria

53. Which of the following is the key etiologic agent in initiation of gingivitis and periodontal diseases?
A. Calculus
B. Plaque
C. Tooth brush abrasion
D. Saliva

54. All of the following types of oral mucosa are nonkeratinized except.
A. Buccal mucosa
B. Inferior surface of the tongue
C. The soft palate
D. The hard palate
E. Floor of the mouth

55. The free gingival graft is most commonly used for which purpose listed below
A. To halt gingival recession
B. For crown lengthening
C. To increase the width of gingiva either on the facial or lingual surfaces of the teeth
D. None of the above

56. Which of the following has been shown to be the most effective antimicrobial agent for reducing plaque and gingivitis long-term?

A. Stannous fluoride
B. Phenolic compounds
C. Chlorhexidine
D. Quaternary ammonium compounds

57. The junctional epithelium in health is:

A. A collar-like band of stratified columnar epithelium 2-5 cells thick near the sulcus and 1-2 cells thick at the apical end
B. A collar-like band of stratified squamous epithelium 10-20 cells thick near the sulcus and 2-3 cells thick at the apical end
C. A collar-like band of simple columnar epithelium 5-10 cells thick near the sulcus and 20-25 cells thick at the apical end
D. A collar-like band of pseudostratified columnar epithelium 2-5 cells thick near the sulcus and 10-15 cells thick at the apical end

58. Which of the following signs and symptoms are typical of a perioendo abscess?

A. Radiographic involvement of the periodontium and periapex
B. Significant probing depths
C. Percussion sensitivity
D. Pulpal sensitivity
E. All of the above

59. Which surgical procedure below is directed towards reshaping the gingiva and papilla of a tooth for correction of deformities and to provide the gingiva with normal and functional form?

A. Gingivoplasty
B. Gingivectomy
C. Free mucosal graft
D. None of the above

60. How should a periodontal probe be adapted in an interproximal area?

A. It should be parallel to the long axis of the tooth at the point angle

B. It should be parallel to the long axis of the tooth at the contact area
C. It should touch the contact area the tip should angle slightly beneath and beyond the contact area
D. It should be perpendicular to the long axis of the tooth, in front of the contact area

61. The periodontal ligament fibers are anchored into cementum and bone by
A. Purkinje's fibers
B. Sharpey's fibers
C. Spindle fibers
D. Gray fibers

62. Surrounding each tooth is a specialized epithelium known as
A. Connective tissue attachment
B. Periodontal ligament attachment
C. Junctional epithelium
D. Nasmyth's membrane

63. How an instrument shank is designed influences the intended use of the instrument. It is recommended that an instrument with a rigid shank be used for removal of heavy calculus deposits.
A. Both statements are true
B. Both statement are false
C. The first is true, the second is false
D. The first is false, the second is true

64. While scaling subgingivally, the tip of the curet breaks off. All of the following are appropriate actions to take to try and remove this tip, except:
A. Use a push stroke to force the tip out of the sulcus
B. Gently examine the gingival sulcus
C. Take a periapical radiograph of the area
D. Place the patient in an upright position

65. In health, the crest of the alveolar bone lies at a level approximately
A. 3-4 mm below the level of the CEJ's of adjacent teeth
B. 1-2 mm below the level of the CEJ's of adjacent teeth

C. 4-5 mm above the level of the CEJ's of adjacent teeth
D. 2-3 mm above the level of the CEJ's of adjacent teeth

66. Which of the following needs to be evident in order to make a diagnosis of periodontitis?
A. Bleeding
B. Pocket depths of 5 mm or more
C. Radiographic evidence of bone loss
D. A change in tissue color and tone

67. All of the following are considered to be the basic principles of flap management except:
A. Conserve the attached gingiva so that after healing there is adequate width of gingiva
B. Make the flap uniformly thick so that it is not very flexible and can be easily sutured to place
C. Avoid flap necrosis (by avoiding desiccation or maltreating the flap or injuring the blood supply)
D. Design the flap sufficiently long and deep to permit it to be retracted fully and with ease
E. Avoid excessive use of relieving incisions coupled with narrow two- three-or four- toot flaps

68. Which of the following etiologic factors is the most common cause of gingival recession?
A. Gingival inflammation
B. Tooth brush injury (abrasion)
C. Faulty tooth alignment
D. Anatomic abnormalities
E. Deleterious habits

69. All of the following statements concerning the periodontal ligament are true, except:
A. It is highly vascular and cellular connective tissue that surrounds the roots of the teeth and bridges the cementum with the alveolar bone
B. It is shaped like an hour glass with the narrowest portion at the middle of the root
C. The average thickness in the adult is 2.0 mm and it increases with age

D. It acts as a cushion by ameliorating the impact of the forces generated during mastication on the alveolar bone.

70. Infrabony pockets (or defects) are generally classified by:

A. The number of bony walls that were destroyed by periodontal disease
B. The number of bony walls left surrounding the tooth
C. The number of bony walls that will remain after surgery
D. Periodontal probe readings

71. Which of the following is the objective of instrument sharpening ?

A. To produce a "wire edge" on the cutting edge
B. To sharpen infrequently to extend the life of the instrument
C. To produce a sharp cutting edge without changing the original design of the instrument
D. To round the cutting edge slightly to prevent tissue trauma

72. Which of the following is true of hoes:

A. They are not designed for removal of heavy calculus
B. It is impossible to adapt them to curved tooth surfaces
C. They are only able to be adapted to facial mesial surfaces
D. Sharpening is not possible

73. The frequency of maintenance visits for a patient who has had pervious periodontal treatment should be dependent upon which factor listed below?

A. On whether or not the patient feels that frequent visits will help maintain his/her periodontium.
B. On the appearance and clinical condition of the gingival tissues.
C. On the amount of attachment loss prior to the periodontal treatment.
D. On the presence of inadequate amount of plaque.

74. Which of the following is the most common error when performing periodontal probing?

A. Using the wrong type probe
B. Incorrectly reading the periodontal probe
C. Excessively angling the probe when inserting it interproximally beyond the long axis of the tooth
D. Forgetting to also probe the lingual of every tooth

75. Gingival change evident during pregnancy probably result from the effect of which of the following?
A. Estrogen
B. Progesterone
C. Histamine
D. None of the above

76. What is guided tissue regeneration?
A. A soft tissue graft used to correct mucogingival junction involvement
B. Placement of a membrane (such as Gore-Tex) over a bony defect
C. A free gingival graft used to increase the amount of attached gingiva
D. Placement of an autograft to treat a bony defect

77. Which of the following is the main objective of root planing?
A. To remove chronically inflamed tissues
B. To change the bacterial microflora
C. To prove optimally smooth root surfaces
D. To eliminate pockets

78. When extensive scaling and root planing must be performed, the best approach would be
A. A series of appointments set up to scale and root plane a segment or quadrant of teeth at a time (thoroughly and completely)
B. Gross debridement (sub and supragingival) of the entire mouth, following by a series of appointments for fine scaling and polishing

79. Which of the following is the primary purpose of a night guard that is worn for the treatment of periodontal trauma?
A. To stabilize the dentition
B. To provide patient comfort
C. To modify the nature of the habit (bruxism) or redirect the forces into non-traumatic pattern
D. To act as a splint after periodontal surgery

80. A bone grafting procedure is least likely to be successful in a:
A. One-walled defect
B. Two-walled defect
C. Three-walled defect
D. Through - and - through furcation defect

81. All of the following are goals that a clinician strives to attain by performing flap procedures except:
A. Pocket elimination
B. Regrowth of alveolar bone and reattachment of connective tissue at more coronal levels
C. To cure periodontal disease
D. Establishment or retention of gingival of adequate width
E. Establishment of an adequate soft and hard tissue contour

82. Bruxism is a pathologic manifestation of:
A. Erosion
B. Abrasion
C. Attrition
D. Resorption

83. Which immunoglobulin listed below is most abundant in the gingival exudate common in gingivitis:?
A. IgA
B. IgG
C. IgD
D. IgE

84. The primary reason for the failure of a free gingival graft is:
A. Infection
B. Edema
C. Disruption of the vascular supply before engraftment
D. None of the above

85. Which group of gingival fibers listed below resist rotational forces that are applied to a tooth?
A. Transseptal fibers
B. Dentogingival fibers
C. Alveologingival fibers
D. Circumferential fibers
E. Dentoperiosteal fibers

86. The periodontium includes:

A. The gingiva
B. The periodontal ligament
C. The cementum
D. The alveolar and supporting bone
E. All of the above

87. Which of the following cells participates in the early phase of inflammation for example, the early lesion of gingivitis?

A. Eosinophils
B. Kupffer's cells
C. Mast cells
D. Epithelioid cells

88. All of the following are examples of an endogenous intrinsic stain except?

A. Tobacco stain
B. Tetracycline
C. Amelogenesis imperfecta
D. Systemic fluoride

89. Which of the following are specific contraindications to the selection of gingival curettage as a definitive surgical procedure?

A. Gingival tissues that are firm and fibrotic
B. When the lateral gingival wall is extremely thin
C. Wide or tortuous infrabony pockets
D. In bi- and trifurcation involvement
E. All of the above

90. All of the following bacteria have been found to be the chief periodontal pathogens except:

A. Prophyromonas gingivalis
B. Bacteroides forsythus
C. Eubacterium
D. Campylobacter rectus

91. The normal, healthy mouth consists mainly of:

A. Obligate anaerobes
B. Facultative anaerobes

C. Acidogenic bacteria
D. All of the above

92. Bone destruction in the furcation has been such that a probe can be passed through the furcation from the buccal to the lingual and vice versa . This furcation involvement would be classified as
A. Type I
B. Type II
C. Type III
D. None of the above.

93. Which of the following are contraindications to selective grinding in the natural dentition?
A. When pulp chambers are large
B. In the presence of tooth sensitivity
C. When major occlusal discrepancies may require orthodontics or reconstruction
D. In patients who are poor candidates for full month reconstruction because of psychologic factors
E. All of the above

94. Toothbrush trauma (abrasion) usually occurs on which teeth listed below?
A. Centrals and laterals
B. Canines and premolars
C. Second and third molars
D. First and second molars

95. In acute gingivitis:
A. Gram-negative anaerobic organisms predominate
B. Gram-negative aerobic organisms predominate
C. Gram-positive organisms predominate
D. Spirochetes predominate

96. Which factor below has been shown to be a prime etiologic factor in inflammatory periodontal disease?
A. Open or loose contacts
B. Food impaction
C. Calculus
D. Poorly designed fitting prosthesis

97. Young plaque is dominated by:
A. Gram-positive cocci
B. Gram-positive rods
C. Gram-negative rods
D. Filaments

98. Which of the following statements are true concerning supragingival and subgingival plaque?
A. Subgingival plaque is attached or loosely adherent; supragingival plaque is attached or tooth associated
B. Subgingival plaque is dominated by gram-negative rods; supragingival plaque is dominated by gram-positive cocci
C. Subgingival plaque has more anaerobes than supragingival plaque
D. All of the above statements are true concerning supragingival and subgingival plaque

99. What is the term used to describe a stain which originates from a source outside the tooth and remains on the exterior surface of the tooth?
A. Exogenous intrinsic
B. Endogenous extrinsic
C. Exogenous extrinsic
D. Endogenous intrinsic

100. All corners of a periodontal flap should be:
A. Sharp
B. Rounded
C. It doesn't matter whether the corners of a periodontal flap are sharp or rounded
D. None of the above

101. Gingival fibers are found within the:
A. Attached gingiva
B. Free gingiva
C. Mucogingival junction
D. Attached and free gingiva

102. Which of the following instruments are designed primarily for the removal of subgingival calculus deposits in all tooth surfaces?
A. Gracey curets
B. Universal curets
C. Chisel scalers
D. Sickle scalers

103. All of these bacteria have been found to be the principal bacteria associated with acute necrotizing ulcerative gingivitis (ANUG) except?
A. Prevotella intermedia
B. Spirochetes
C. Fusobacterium species
D. Porphyromonas gingivalis

104. Which of the following are clinical criteria used for diagnosing gingivitis?
A. Color of gingiva
B. Contour of gingiva
C. Size of gingiva
D. Bacterial plaque and calculus
E. All of the above

105. The base of the pocket (epithelial attachment) is coronal to the crest of the alveolar bone in a?
A. Infrabony pocket
B. Suprabony pocket
C. Both of the above
D. Neither of the above

106. When evaluating an osscous defect, the only way to determine the number of walls left surrounding the tooth is by:
A. Periodontal probing
B. Radiographs
C. Exploratory surgery
D. Testing for mobility

107. Which of the following is the best way to distinguish between a periodontal abscess and a periapical (pulpal) lesion?
A. Radiograph

B. Pulp testing
C. Hot and cold tests
D. Asking the patient the nature of the pain

108. The most important aspect of Phase I (initial therapy) of periodontal treatment planning is:
A. Extraction of hopeless teeth
B. Oral Hygiene Instructions
C. Occlusal adjustment
D. Splinting

109. The reshaping or recontouring of nonsupportive bone is called:
A. Ostectomy
B. Osteoplasty
C. both of the above
D. None of the above

110. The vascular phase of acute inflammation involves all of the following cells except:
A. Platelets
B. Tissue mast cells
C. Eosinophils
D. Basophils

111. Which of the following describe how an ultrasonic scaling device removes calculus deposits:
A. Blunt, shearing action of the tip
B. Vibratory action of the tip
C. Pressure of the water
D. High frequency sound

112. Which structure listed below is the inner layer of cells of the junctional epithelium and attaches the gingiva to the tooth?
A. Mucogingival junction
B. Free gingival groove
C. Epithelial attachment
D. Gingival pocket

113. All of the following statements are true concerning desquamative gingivitis, except:

A. It is a chronic gingival disease characterized by erythematous erosive, vesiculobullous and /or desquamative involvement of the free and attached gingiva
B. The majority of patients are males between the age of 20 and 30
C. While many diseases and conditions have been associated with this gingival disease, the majority are dermatologic
D. Topical corticosteroids (Triamcinolone, e.g., kenalog in Orabase) are effective in treating the oral lesions

114. An exploratory stroke is used to remove calculus. A waling stroke is utilized during periodontal probing.

A. Both statements are true
B. Both statements are false
C. The first statement is true, the second is false
D. The first statement is false, the second is true

115. Which of the following are considered to be pedicle grafts?

A. Apically repositioned flaps
B. Laterally repositioned flaps
C. Coronally repositioned flaps
D. All of the above

116. Which type of cementum is found on the apical third of the root?

A. Cellular
B. Acellular

117. Which statement below is true?

A. Periodontitis is the same as gingivitis
B. Periodontitis usually does not begin as gingivitis
C. Periodontitis always begins as gingivitis
D. All of the above.

118. All of the following bacteria have been found to be the principle bacteria associated with juvenile periodontitis, except:

A. Actinobacillus actiomycetemcomitans (AA)
B. Capnocytophaga species

C. Wolinella recta
D. Prevotella intermedia
E. Eikenella corrodens

119. All of the following bacteria have been found to be principle bacteria associated with rapidly progressive periodontitis, except:

A. Porphyromonas gingivalis
B. Actinobacillus actinomycetemcomitans (AA)
C. Capnocytophaga species
D. Prevotella intermedia
E. Fusobacterium nucleatum
F. Eikenella corrodens
G. Campylobacter rectus

120. All of the following statement concerning bacterial plaque are true, except:

A. It is the key etiologic agent in the initiation of gingivitis and periodontal disease
B. It is an accumulation of a mixed bacterial community in a dextran matrix
C. It forms on a cleaned tooth within minutes
D. It is composed of solids (80%; 95% of which are bacteria) and water (20%)
E. There are two categories: supragingival and subgingival plaque
F. Different bacteria may be found in plaque (cocci, rods and filaments) and their proportions change with time, diet and location.

Answer Key to MCQs in Periodontics Part I

1	C	2	C	3	C	4	B
5	B	6	D	7	C	8	A
9	D	10	D	11	A	12	B
13	C	14	C	15	C	16	B
17	C	18	B	19	C	20	C
21	D	22	C	23	C	24	B
25	A	26	D	27	A	28	B
29	C	30	D	31	E	32	B
33	B	34	C	35	F	36	B
37	C	38	B	39	C	40	B
41	A	42	C	43	B	44	D
45	C	46	H	47	C	48	E
49	A	50	B	51	B	52	D
53	B	54	D	55	C	56	C
57	B	58	E	59	A	60	C
61	B	62	C	63	A	64	A
65	B	66	C	67	B	68	B
69	C	70	B	71	C	72	B
73	B	74	C	75	B	76	B
77	C	78	A	79	C	80	D
81	C	82	C	83	B	84	C
85	D	86	E	87	C	88	A
89	E	90	B	91	D	92	C
93	E	94	B	95	C	96	C
97	A	98	D	99	C	100	B
101	B	102	B	103	D	104	E
105	B	106	C	107	B	108	B
109	B	110	C	111	B	112	C
113	B	114	D	115	D	116	A
117	C	118	C	119	C	120	D

Part II

1. **Which of the following features about free gingival groove is incorrect?**
   A. It demarcates free and attached gingiva
   B. It is present in only 40–50% of the population
   C. It remains stationary throughout life.
   D. All the above are correct

2. **The cementum over palatal root of maxillary first molar is supplied by**
   A. Posterior superior alveolar nerve
   B. Middle superior alveolar
   C. Greater palatine nerve
   D. None of the above

3. **In what percentage of furcations is the furcation entrance narrower than a standard size curette?**
   A. 52%
   B. 58%
   C. 67%
   D. 85%

4. **Which areas of the gingiva are stippled?**
   A. Attached gingiva only
   B. Attached gingiva + centre of interdental papilla
   C. Attached gingiva + col
   D. Attached gingiva + entire interdental papilla

5. **In a supra-erupted tooth,**
   A. Anatomic crown > Clinical crown
   B. Anatomic crown < Clinical crown
   C. Anatomic crown = Clinical crown
   D. Either of the above

6. **Sharpey's fibers are terminal portions of principal fibers that are embedded in**
   A. Cementum only
   B. Alveolar bone only

C. Both in cementum and alveolar bone
D. None of the above

7. Collagen molecule is characterized by
A. Triple helical structure
B. 64 nm striation pattern
C. Amino acids hydroxyproline and hydroxylysine
D. All of the above

8. The first group of periodontal ligament fibers to develop
A. Transseptal
B. Apical
C. Alveolar crest
D. Oblique

9. The intrinsic fibers of cementum are
A. Same as sharpey's fibers
B. Formed by fibroblasts
C. Formed by cementoblasts
D. All of the above

10. Woven bone is
A. Bone adjacent to periodontal ligament that contains sharpey's fibers.
B. Made of dense cortical bone
C. Made of Cancellous bone
D. Formed by calcification of immature bone

11. Periosteum is
A. Composed of single layer of osteoblasts
B. Tissue lining internal bony cavities
C. Double layered, with outer layer being composed of osteoblasts
D. Double layered, with inner layer being composed of osteoblasts

12. The characteristic feature of Sulcular Epithelium is
A. Stratified squamous keratinized epithelium with rete pegs
B. Stratified squamous non-keratinized epithelium with rete pegs
C. Stratified squamous non-keratinized epithelium without rete pegs
D. Stratified squamous keratinized epithelium without rete pegs

13. The collagen type present in basal lamina is

A. Type I
B. Type III
C. Type IV
D. Type VI

14. The oblique fibers of periodontal ligament run from

A. Cementum to bone in a coronal direction
B. Bone to cementum in a coronal direction
C. Bone to cementum perpendicular to the long axis of the tooth
D. None of the above

15. The calcified masses present in periodontal ligament are

A. Epithelial rests of Malassez
B. Cementicles
C. Denticles
D. Both (a) and (b)

16. Which of the following statements are true?

A. Periodontal ligament is thin mesially while cementum is thin distally.
B. Periodontal ligament is thin diatally while cementum is thin mesially.
C. Both are thin mesially.
D. Both are thin distally.

17. Alveolar bone proper is

A. Made of Cancellous bone.
B. Seen as lamina dura istologically.
C. Also called as cribriform plate.
D. All are true

18. The receptors for Parathormone are located on

A. Osteoblasts
B. Osteoclasts
C. Osteocytes
D. In bone matrix

19. The lymphatic drainage of cementum of manbdibular incisors is

A. Submental

B. Submandibular
C. Submaxillary
D. None of the above

20. Actinobacillus actinomycetemcomitans is a
A. Gram – ve rod
B. Gram + ve rod
C. Gram + ve cocci
D. Gram – ve cocci

21. The most common serotype of Actinobacillus actinomycetemcomitans implicated in Aggressive periodontitis is
A. Serotype A
B. Serotype B
C. Serotype C
D. Serotype E

22. Interproximal attachment loss is generally a consequence of
A. Tooth brush trauma
B. Bacteria-induced periodontitis
C. Self inflicted injury
D. Tobacco use

23. The "raspberry- like appearance" of gingiva is seen in
A. Gingival disease in Vit. C deficiency
B. Gingival disease in diabetes
C. Gingival disease in pregnancy
D. Gingival disease in puberty

24. Regarding osseointegration, which of the following statements are true?
A. It is the direct contact of implant with the bone at EM level
B. It is the direct contact of implant with the bone at light microscopic level
C. All clinically successful implants show 100% osseointegration
D. All of the above

25. The success of free gingival graft depends on
A. Survival of epithelium
B. Survival of connective tissue

C. Sloughing of epithelium
D. Sloughing of connective tissue

26. Miller class III recession denotes
A. Recession that does not extend to the mucogingival junction
B. Recession extends to or beyond mucogingival junction with bone/soft tissue loss in interdental area
C. Recession extends to or beyond mucogingival junction without bone/soft tissue loss in interdental area
D. Recession extends to or beyond mucogingival junction with severe bone/soft tissue loss in interdental area

27. Free gingival graft is used to
A. Increase the width of attached gingiva
B. Achieve root coverage
C. Deepen the vestibule
D. Both (a) and (b).

28. Coronally displaced flap
A. Increases the width of attached gingiva
B. Requires the presence of sufficient width of attached gingiva
C. Can be used to deepen vestibule
D. Has no relation with attached gingiva

29. The minimum width of attached gingiva necessary for gingival health is
A. 0.5 – 1mm
B. 1–2 mm
C. 2–3 mm
D. No established particular width

30. The presence of cul-de-sac indicates what degree of furcation involvement?
A. Grade I
B. Grade II
C. Grade III
D. Grade IV

31. The best way to evaluate the success of regenerative osseous surgery is
A. Probing

B. Radiographic assessment
C. Surgical re-entry
D. Sounding

32. Osteoinduction is
A. Development of new bone by cells contained in the graft
B. A physical process in which graft as a scaffold
C. A chemical process by which BMP's in the graft convert neighbouring cells into osteoblasts
D. None of the above

33. The freeze drying process in the manufacture of bone allografts
A. Decreases graft antigenicity
B. Exposes the BMP's in the graft
C. Increases the graft survival time
D. Reduces the chances of infection

34. Alloplasts are
A. Grafts obtained from different species
B. Grafts between same species
C. Grafts between twins
D. Grafts of inert synthetic materials

35. Osteoplasty is
A. Removal of tooth supporting bone
B. Bone reshaping with removal of tooth supporting bone
C. Bone reshaping without removal of tooth supporting bone
D. Same as ostectomy

36. The resorption time for chromic gut sutures is
A. 8–10 days
B. 12–15 days
C. 18–25 days
D. 45–60 days

37. The procedure of choice for moderate to severe periodontitis in maxillary anterior region is
A. Papilla Preservation Flap
B. Modified Widman Flap
C. Undisplaced Flap
D. Scaling and Root Planing

38. The flap of choice for osseous regenerative procedures is

A. Sulcular Incision Flap
B. Papilla Preservation Flap
C. Modified Widman Flap
D. Apically Displaced Flap

39. The ideal result of pocket therapy is obtained by

A. Surgical removal of pocket wall
B. Extraction of tooth side of pocket
C. Retraction/shrinkage of pocket
D. New attachment techniques

40. Listerine is

A. 0.12% chlorhexidine
B. 0.2% chlorhexidine
C. An essential oil mouthwash
D. Sanguinarine containing mouthwash

41. Actisite is

A. Tetracycline containing fiber
B. 10% doxycycline
C. 2% minocycline
D. 25% metronidazole

42. Periostat has

A. 20 mg tab of Doxycycline hyclate
C. No anti-bacterial action
C. An anti collagenase action
D. All of the above are true

43. Interproximal spaces with no papillae are best cleaned by

A. Dental floss
B. Interproximal brushes
C. Single-tufted brushes
D. Any of the above can be used

44. The recommended brushing technique for any patient is

A. Fones
B. Modified stillman
C. Charters
D. Bass

45. Increasing the power setting of an ultrasonic scaler incrases
A. Frequency of oscillation
B. Amplitude of oscillation
C. Water spray
D. All of the above

46. The instrument of choice for subgingival scaling and root planing is
A. Gracey curettes
B. Universal curettes
C. Sickle scalers
D. Hoe

47. Gracey curette no 11–12 is used on
A. Buccal surface of premolars
B. Facial and lingual surface of posterior teeth
C. Mesial surface of posterior teeth
D. Distal surface of posterior teeth

48. Kirkland knife is used for
A. Facial/lingual incision
B. Interdental incision
C. Electrosurgical purpose
D. Any incision

49. For 2 patients with comparable levels of remaining connective tissue attachment and alveolar bone, prognosis is
A. Better for the older patient
B. Better for the younger patient
C. Same foe both
D. Prognosis is not affected by age

50. The restorative margins that accumulate maximum amount of plaque are
A. Supragingival
B. Subgingival
C. Equigingival
D. All margins accumulate same amount of plaque

51. Prognosis is established
A. After diagnosis but before treatment plan
B. Before diagnosis and treatment plan
C. After diagnosis and treatment plan
D. Before diagnosis but after treatment plan

52. The mobility of a tooth is checked by holding the tooth between
A. Index finger and the handle of mouth mirror
B. Index finger and thumb
C. The handles of two metallic instruments
D. Both (a) and (c)

53. The stroke with which a probe is used is called
A. Push stroke
B. Pull stroke
C. Walking stroke
D. Exploratory stroke

54. In cases of inflamed periodontium,
A. Biologic depth > Probing depth
B. Biologic depth < Probing depth
C. Biologic depth = Probing depth
D. Probing depth is always more irrespective of the inflammation

55. The parameter that is of utmost importance in determining the periodontal status is
A. Bleeding on probing
B. Pocket depth
C. Presence of pus
D. Clinical attachment level

56. The width of keratinized gingiva is
A. Same as that of attached gingiva
B. Combined width of attached and marginal gingiva
C. Half the width of attached gingiva
D. Same as width of marginal gingiva

57. The most common oral lesion in HIV is
A. Oral hairy leukoplakia
B. Kaposi sarcoma

C. Linear gingival erythema
D. Candidiasis

58. Linear gingival erythema seen in HIV patients is characterized by
A. Microflora resembling that of periodontitis.
b. Involvement of attached gingiva
C. Involvement of alveolar mucosa
D. All the above

59. The first bacteria to colonize dental pellicle is
A. Actinomyces
B. Fusobacteria
C. Staphylococcus aureus
D. Streptococcus sanguis

60. Enlargement of attached gingiva is seen in
A. Drug-induced gingival enlargement
B. Pubertal gingival enlargement
C. Idiopathic gingival enlargement
D. Pregnancy-associated enlargement

61. Gingival enlargement attributed to allergy is
A. Plasma cell gingivitis
B. Idiopathic gingival enlargement
C. Pyogenic granuloma
D. Drug-induced enlargement

62. In patients with gingival enlargement caused by cyclosporine, the drug substitute that can be given is
A. Tegretol
B. Baclofen
C. Tacrolimus
D.

63. The microorganism indicated in pubertal gingivitis is
A. Capnocytophaga + Prevotella intermedia
B. Campylobacter
C. Fusobacteria
D. Actinomyces

64. The etiological factors for ANUG are

A. Microorganisms
B. Smoking
C. Stress
D. All of the above

65. Which of the following about primary herpetic gingivo-stomatitis is not true?

A. It is primarily an infection of the oral cavity
B. Mostly, it is asymptomatic.
C. After infection the virus ascends via nerves and persists in the neuronal ganglia as latent HSV.
D. Usually seen in older age group patients.

66. The base of the pocket is located apical to the level of the adjacent alveolar bone. The pocket is

A. Suprabony
B. Supraalveolar
C. Subcrestal
D. None of the above

67. The classic "strawberry gums" appearance of gums is seen in

A. Wegener's granulomatosis
B. Plasma cell gingivitis
C. Pemphigus
D. Erythema multiforme

68. Angular bony defects are classified on the basis of

A. Number of osseous walls remaining
B. Number of osseous walls destroyed
C. Number of tooth involved
D. Number of tooth surfaces involved

69. The presence and configuration of osseous defects can be best determined by

A. Sounding
B. Radiographs
C. Surgical exposure
D. All of the above

70. The direction of migration of maxillary incisors in Localized aggressive periodontitis is
A. Mesio-labial
B. Disto-labial
C. Mesio-lingual
D. Disto-lingual

71. The BANA hydrolysis for bacterial identification is based on enzyme detection. The enzyme detected is
A. Collagenase
B. Hyaluronidase
C. Trypsin
D. Lysozyme

72. The predominant Ig found in saliva is
A. Ig G
B. IgA
C. Ig M
D. Ig D

73. The main Ig in GCF is
A. Ig G
B. IgA
C. Ig M
D. Ig D

74. Periogard is a chairside detection test for
A. Aspartate aminotransferase
B. Neutral serine protease
C. Trypsin-like enzyme
D. collagenase

75. Phase IV of periodontal treatment begins
A. Immediately after phase I
B. Immediately after phase II
C. After phase III is completed
D. After completion of the entire periodontal therapy only.

76. Attachment of gingival/periodontal fibers to the tooth surface from which they were separated during preparation for a full veneer crown is called
A. New attachment

B. Re-attachment
C. Regeneration
D. Epithelial adaptation

77. The tissue cells which are critical for new attachment are
A. Oral epithelial cells
B. Gingival connective tissue cells
C. Bone cells
D. Periodontal ligament cells

78. An absolute contra-indication for periodontal treatment is
A. Diabetes
B. HIV infection
C. Pregnancy
D. None of the above

79. For hypertensive patients, appointments should be preferentially scheduled at
A. Morning
B. Afternoon
C. Late evenings
D. Either of the above

80. Side-effects of Chlorhexidine include
A. Increased calculus formation
B. Tooth staining
C. Dysgeusia
D. All the above

81. Chlorhexidine is a potent anti-plaque agent. It has no action on established plaque.
A. Both statements are true.
B. Both statements are false.
C. First is true, second is false.
D. First is false, second is true.

82. The most effective and stable grasp for periodontal instrumentation is
A. Pen grasp
B. Modified pen grasp

C. Palm and thumb grasp
D. Modified palm and thumb

83. The most commonly used finger for finger rest is
A. Thumb
B. Index finger
C. Middle finger
D. Ring finger

84. The effective angulation of an instrument for gingival curettage is
A. > 45°
B. 45°–90°
C. < 90°
D. 0°

85. Gracey curettes use a single cutting edge. The edge used is
A. Outer
B. Inner
C. It depends on the area on instrumentation
D. Gracey curettes use both the cutting edges.

86. Intraoral finger-on-finger rest is used for
A. Maxillary posterior region
B. Mandibular posterios region
C. Maxillary anterior region
D. Mandibular region

87. In the treatment of ANUG, antibiotics are
A. Routinely prescribed
B. Restricted to patients with systemic complications
C. Never prescribed
D. Given by i.v. Route only.

88. Phase I periodontal therapy includes all of the following except
A. Treatment of occlusal trauma
B. Odontoplasty
C. Restoration of carious tooth
D. Restoration of tooth by FPD.

Answer Key to MCQs in Periodontics Part II

1. (C) It is the mucogingival junction that remains stationary throughout life.
2. (D) Cementum is avascular, lacks nerve supply and lymphatic drainage.
3. (B)
4. (B)
5. (B) Anatomic crown is the actual crown of the tooth which is demarcated from the root by cemento-enamel junction. Clinical crown is the portion of the tooth visible in the oral cavity. In supra-erupted tooth Anatomic crown < Clinical crown. The reverse is true of incompletely erupted tooth.
6. (C)
7. (D)
8. (A)
9. (C) The cemental matrix contains two types of fibers- extrinsic and intrinsic fibers.

   Extrinsic fibers are sharpey's fibers. The intrinsic fibers are the fibers of cemental matrix and formed by cementoblasts.
10. (C) Woven bone is immature bone. It is made of Cancellous bone. Choice a refers to bundle bone
11. (D) Periosteum is double layered, with the inner layer being composed of osteoblasts surrounded by osteoprogenitor cells and an outer layer fich in blood vessels and nerves, and composed of collagen fibers and fibroblasts.
12. (C)
13. (C)
14. (A)
15. (B) Although epithelial rests are present in the periodontal ligament, they are not calcified. Cementicles are calcified masses but they are formed by the calcification of the epithelial rests.
16. (C)

17. (C) Alveolar bone proper is dense cortical bone that lines the tooth sockets. It is seen as a thin radio-opaque line in radiographs called as lamina dura. In histological sections, it appears perforated so called as cribriform plate.
18. (A) Since parathormone promotes bone resorption, it is very common mistake to assume that the receptors for the hormone must be located on osteoclasts. But actually, they are present on the osteoblasts.
19. (D) Cementumis an avascular tissue that also lacks nerve supply and lymphatic drainage.
20. (A)
21. (B)
22. (B) Attachment loss facially/lingually is generally a consequence of toothbrush abrasion while interprtoximal attachment loss is generally a consequence of bacteria-induced periodontitis.
23. (C)
24. (B) Osseointegration denotes direct contact of bone with the implant at the light microscope level. Seen at the EM level, a cell free amorphous layer 20–1000nm thick composed of glycosaminoglycans and proteoglycans is present at implant-bone interface. Moreover, clinically successful implants show 30 to 95% osseointegration.
25. (B) During the healing phase, there is sloughing of epithelium but it is by no means necessary for graft survival.
26. (B) (a) is Class I, (c) is Class II and (d) is Class IV.
27. (D) Mainly, free gingival graft is used to augment the width of attached gingiva. It can be used for root coverage but the graft does not perfectly blend with the recipient site creating an esthetic mismatch. Finally, it cannot be predictably used to deepen the vestibule.
28. (B) Coronally displaced flap is used for root coverage when sufficient width of attached gingiva is present apical to the defect.
29. (D) There is no established particular width of attached gingiva that can be considered best for gingival width. In patients with

very good oral hygiene, gingival health can be maintained even in the absence of attached gingiva.

30. (B) This is the Glickman's classification of furcation involvement based on the horizontal component of furcation destruction.
31. (C) All the four techniques can be used to evaluate the bone topography but the best method is surgical re-entry.
32. (C) (a) is Osteogenesis and (b) is Osteoconduction
33 (A) There are two processes involved-graft decalcification which exposee the BMP's in the graft to enhance its osteogenic potential and freeze drying of the graft which basically reduces the graft antigenicity and the chances of infection.
34. (D) (a) is Xenograft, (b) is allograft and (c) is Isograft
35. (C) If the tooth supporting bone is removed, the procedure becomes an ostectomy.
36. (D)
37. (D) In maxillary anterior region, a non-surgical procedure is the procedure of choice and therefore first choice would be Scaling and Root Planning. When a surgical procedure is unavoidable, then the first choice flap is papilla preservation Flap.
38. (B) Papilla Preservation Flap affords complete coverage of the surgical site thereby promoting graft stabilization.
39. (D) Although any of these could be used for pocket elimination, the ideal result would be obtained by new attachment, i.e. regeneration of lost periodontium.
40. (C)
41. (A) (b) is Atridox, (c) is Dentamycin or Periocline, (d) is Elyzol. Also available is a chlorhexidine chip (Periochip). All these are local drug delivery systems.
42. (D)
43. (C) Embrasures spaces with no gingival recession are cleaned using dental floss. Larger spaces with exposed root surfaces require the use of an interproximal brush.
44. (D) Fones method is recommended for children. Modified stillman is used for cleaning in areas with progressive gingival

recession and root exposure to minimize abrasive tissue destruction. Charters method is used in areas of healing wounds after periodontal surgery.

45. (B) The frequency of oscillation of a particular scaler is fixed. Also, there is a different control to regulate the amount of water spray.
46. Generally, curettes are the instruments of choice for subgingival scaling and root planning and even among the curettes, gracey curettes are preferred over universal curettes.
47. (C) 1–2 and 3–4: anterior teeth; 5–6: anterior teeth and premolars; 7–8 and 9–10: posterior teeth: facial and lingual; 11–12: posterior teeth: mesial; 13–14: posterior teeth: distal.
48. (A) Orbans knife is used for interdental incision
49. (A) This is because despite the better healing capacity of the younger patient, same amount of destruction occurred over a relatively shorter period of time compared to the older patient.
50. (C) Both supra and sub-gingival margins are better than equigingival margins in terms of plaque accumulation.
51. (A)
52. (D) Using both the fingers gives a false sense of mobility due to the softness of the finger pads.
53. (C) Generally, all instruments are used with a pull motion except for chisels. Exploratory stroke is used by the explorer.
54. (B) Biologic depth is same as histologic depth.
55. (D)
56. (B)
57. (D)
58. (D)
59. (D)
60. (C)
61. (A)
62. (C)
63. (A)

64. (D)
65. (C)
66. (C)
67. (A)
68. (A)
69. (C) Although any of the method can be used for determination of osseous defects, the best method is surgical exposure.
70. (D)
71. (C)
72. (B)
73. (A)
74. (A)
75 (A)
76. (B)
77. (D)
78. (D)
79. (B)
80. (B)
81. (C)
82. (B)
83. (D)
84. (B)
85. (A)
86. (A)
87. (B)
88. (D)

12

Prosthodontics

Fixed Partial Dentures

Crown = is an artificial replacement, which restores the morphology, function and contour of coronal part of the tooth.

Full veneer crown

Partial veneer crown

Intracoronal cast restoration—fits within the crown largely.

Inlay = intracoronal restoration with mild/moderate extensions.

Onlay = intracoronal restoration with an occlusal veneer is known as onlay.

Bridge = FPD—Permanently attached to remaining teeth.

Abutment = tooth serving as an attachment for a bridge.

Pontic = artificial tooth suspended between abutments.

Retainer = i.e. restorations which are cemented to the prepared abutment teeth.

Connecter = i.e. between pontic and retainer.

HISTORY OF THE PATIENT

1. Reactions to drugs especially LA and antibiotics.
2. Uncontrolled HT = No Rx till controlled.
   - Patients with HT/coronary heart disease = No adranline should be given, because adrenaline leads to = BP/increased HR.

3. Rheumatic fever = then pre-medicate the patient.
4. Epilepsy = provide Protection.
5. Diabetes = leads to Periodontal breakdown/Abscess formation.
6. Hyperthyroidism = should be controlled to avoid stresses.
7. TMJ S/S.

Diagnostic casts

1. Should be mounted on semiadjustable articulator.
2. Mandibular cast should be set in most retruded position.

Abutment

It bears additional forces (which were normally absorbed by missing tooth).

Ideally = it should be VITAL tooth.

Ante's law = PDL surface area of supporting teeth should be more than the teeth being replaced.

C:R ratio = ideal is 1:2; but 1:1 is acceptable.

Dislodging forces on a bridge retainer act in MD direction.

Dislodging forces on a single restoration act in BL direction.

Secondary abutment

- To bolster the primary abutment.
- To solve C:R ratio problem.
- Must have at least as much RSA root surface area and as favorable C:R ratio as the primary abutment.
- The retainers on secondary abutments will be placed in tension when pontic flexes and primary abutment acts as fulcrum.
- To avoid torquing, the secondary retention should extend a distance from primary inter-abutment axis equal to the distance that the pontic lever Arm extends in opposite direction.

Pier abutments = i.e. tooth having edentulous area on both sides.

- **Rigid connectors** = i.e. solder joints is preferred method of FPD.
- Bucco-lingual movements range from = 56–108 microns.

- Intrusion movement ranges to = 28 microns.
- **Non-rigid connnector** = is a broken stress mechanical union of retainer and pontic, most commonly used is T-shaped key (on pontic) with dovetail key–way on retainer.

The location of stress-breaker on pier abutment—5 unit FPD = should be placed on the middle-abutment = it prevents it to act as a fulcrum.

- Keyway of the connector should be placed within the NORMAL DISTAL CONTOURS OF MIDDLE abutment.
- And the key should be placed on the mesial side of first molar pontic = it helps to seat the key into key way in mesial movement of teeth under occlusal leads.
- Rx of choice for a mesially tilted tooth = orthodontic uprighting.
- Long axes of the prospective abutments should converge by no more than 25–30°.

Canine replacement bridge = V. difficult.

- Maxillary lateral incisor and first premolar are weakest teeth.
- Maxillary canine bridge is subjected to more stresses than mandibular canine bridge, because forces are transmitted labially (outward) in the maxillary arch against the inside of the curve (i.e. its weakest point).
- On mandibular canine, forces are directed inward/lingually against the outside of curve (i.e. strongest point).

Cantilever bridge—which has an abutment's at one end only.

- Used only when there is minimum/no occlusal contact on the pontic.
- e.g. maxillary lateral incisor FPD with maxillary canine as abutment.
- But it is destructive.

Simple bridge = is one which replaces a single tooth.

Absolute maximum number of posterior teeth, which can be safely replaced with a bridge = 3 (except upper and lower incisors).

A C:R (crown to root ratio) of 3:1.0 is desirable.

OCCLUSION

Mandibular movements = are 3 dimensional.

1. Horizontal = i.e. in sagittal plane, when retruded mandible produces PURE ROTATONAL opening/closing movement around the hinge axis, extending through both condyles.
2. Vertical = occurs in horizontal plane, when mandible moves in lateral excursion. C rot. is a vertical axis extending through the **working side condyle.**
3. Sagittal = on lateral excursion, the non-working side condyle travels downward and forward, a downward arc rotating about an AP/sagittal axis passing through the **non-working condyle**.
   - **Pure rotational movement** = occur in lower compartment of TMJ.
   - Also some **gliding/translation** = occurs in the upper compartment of TMJ.
   - **Lateral movement** = non-working condyle moves medially and forward and downward.

Working condyle moves laterally/slightly posteriorly = it is known as **Bennett movement.**

Determinants of mandibular movement

- ♦ Anteriorly = U/L teeth
- ♦ Posteriorly = TMJ
- ♦ Overall = neuro-muscular system
- ♦ Posterior teeth = provide vertical stops for mandibular closure; guide mandible into position of maximum inter cuspation.
- ♦ Anterior teeth = guide the mandible in Right and Left lateral excursions and in straight protrusive movements.
- ♦ Dentist has no control over posterior determinants.
- ♦ Dentist has direct control over the teeth determinants by orthodontic tooth movements selective grinding; so ICP and (AG) anterior guidance can be altered.

- The closer to a determinant a tooth is located, the more it will be influenced by that determinant. A tooth placed near the anterior region will be influenced greatly by AG and less by TMJ.

OCCLUSAL INTERFERENCES = 4 types:

- Centric
- Working
- Non-working
- Protrusive

1. **Centric interferences** = is a Premature Contact which occurs when mandible closes with condyles in a retruded, superior position in the glenoid fossa.
2. **Working interferences** = i.e. when there is a contact between maxillary and mandibular posterior teeth on the same side of arches as the direction, in which mandible is moved.
3. **Non-working interferences** = occlusal contact between maxillary and mandibular teeth on the side of arches opposite the direction, in which mouth has moved in lateral excursion.
4. **Protrusive interference** = a Premature Contact between the mesial aspect of mandibular posterior teeth and distal aspect of maxillary posterior teeth.

Normal maximum ICP is approx 1.25 ± 1 mm forward of the RCP (Retmdeol cuspal position).

- **Optimal occlusion** = i.e. which requires a minimum of adaptation by the patient.
- In normal occlusion = reflex function of neuro-muscular system guides the mandible in CO.
- **Articulator** = the principle employed is the mechanical replication of the path of movement of posterior determinants, i.e. the TMJ.
- **Border movement** = the outer limits of all excursive movements made by mandible. They are controlled by ligaments.
- **Non-adjustable articulator** = is capable of only a HINGE opening; it is of smaller size.

- **Semi-adjustable articulator** = larger size; it reproduces the direction and end point, but not the intermediate track of some condylar movements (Anatomical distance of axis of rotation with the teeth is closely natural as compared with the smaller in non-adjustable articulators). Intercondylar distance does not have total adjustability. Used for bridge work.

Fully adjustable articulator—reproduces:

- ♦ Entire border movements.
- ♦ Curvature and direction of condylar movements.
- ♦ Immediate side shift.
- ♦ Completely adjustable intercondylar distance.
- ♦ Used for extensive Rx only.

Arcon articulator

- ♦ Condylar element is on lower member of articulator.
- ♦ Mechanical fossa on the upper member.
- ♦ Good for FPD but not for CD.
- ♦ Centric position is less easily maintained on arcon.

Non-arcon

- ♦ Condyle element on Upper part.
- ♦ Condylar path on Lower part.
- ♦ Best for CD.

Transfer of hinge axis

- ♦ Done by face bow.
- ♦ Most accurate method = trial and error method.

Hinge axis = at a point 13 mm anterior to the middle of the superior edge of tragus on a line from tragus to outer canthus of eye.

Pantograph tracings = for recording the condyle movement and border movements of mandible.

- Best done with fully adjustable articulators.

Definitions

1. **Bilateral Balanced Occlusion**
   - Maximum number of teeth should contact in all excusive positions of mandible.
   - Esp. used in CD where contact on non-working side is important to prevent tipping of denture.
   - But not in natural teeth, because it leads to excessive wear and stresses on teeth.
   - Based on work of Spee and Monsoon.
2. **Unilateral BO** = widely accepted and used.
   - Based on work of Schuyler.
   - Cross arch balance is not necessary in natural teeth.
   - Here, all teeth on working side should be in contact during lateral excursion, and no contact on non-working side.

♦ So the group functions of teeth distributes LOAD on working sides.

♦ It also saves CENTRIC HOLDING CUSPS (which are mandibular buccal/maxillary lingual cusps) from excessive wear.

3. **Mutually protected occlusion**—also known as canine—protected occlusion or organic occlusion.
   - Based on the work of Stuart, Stallard, Lucia, etc.
   - Here, the anterior teeth bear all the load and posterior teeth get discluded in many excursion movements of mandible and vice versa.
   - Position of maximum inter-cuspation coincides with retruded position of mandible.
   - MOST-WIDELY ACCEPTED occlusion because of greatest ease of fabrication and patient tolerance.
   - But if Periodontal bone loss of anterior teeth is there, the mouth should be protected to group functions (i.e. unilateral balance).

PRINCIPLES OF CROWN PREPARATION

(a) Preservation of tooth structure = minimal cutting; maintain marginal topography of tooth.

(b) Retention and resistance.
(c) Structural durability.
(d) Marginal integrity.

Retention

- Prevents removal of restoration along the path of insertion or long axis of tooth preparation.
- Axial walls of preparation must be parallel or slightly tapered to permit the restoration to seat.
- A taper of 6° is optimal between opposing walls (2.5–6.5°).
- There is an INVERSE relation between taper and retention.
- Greater the surface area of preparation greater is the retention.
- Larger teeth have better retention than smaller teeth.
- Increase Surface Area by making grooves/boxes, etc.
- Retention increases by geometrically limiting the no. of paths of insertion. Maximum retention is with one path only.
- Basic unit of retention = 2 opposing axial walls with a 6° taper.

Resistance

- Prevents dislodgement of restoration by the forces directed in apical/oblique direction and prevents any movement of restoration under occlusal forces.
- The walls of preparation should be at right angle to the direction of forces for better resistance.
- Buccal and Lingual walls of the proximal box must meet the wall at 90°.
- A flare/bevel is added at cavosurface margins if gold is used. It helps in burnishing and adaptation of the restoration.

Path of insertion—An imaginary line along which the restoration will be drawn off or inserted on preparation.

- In maxillary posterior area = it should be parallel to long axis of tooth.
- In anterior teeth = should be parallel to incisal half of labial surface.

- Mesio-distal path should = parallel to the contact areas of tooth.

Structural durability—For adequate bulk of metal in restoration:

- There should be 1.5 mm occlusal clearance on functional cusps (i.e. lingual upper and buccal lower cusps).
- On non functional cusps = 1.0 mm.
- **Functional cusp bevel** = a wide bevel on LINGUAL inclines of maxillary lingual cusps and buccal inclines of mandibular buccal cusps to provide space for an adequate bulk of metal in the area of heavy occlusal contact.
- If bevel is not used = an over cut axial surface will occur.
- Offset; occlusal shoulders; isthmus; proximal grooves, boxes provide rigidity and durability.

Isthmus—Connects the boxes.

Offset—Ties the grooves together.

MARGINAL INTEGRITY

- For cast gold restoration—The finish line should be acute-angle = good for burnishing and adaptation.
- BUTT joint/shoulder finish line is poorest for Au (gold).
- For veneer gold restorations = best is **CHAMFER;** it exhibit LEAST stresses.
- **SHOULDER** = for porcelain—jacket crowns; wide ledge provides resistance to occlusal forces and minimizes stresses. Not good for gold.
- **BEVEL** = (modified) SLOPING shoulder; does not meet the axial walls and cavosurace at 90°, but makes an obtuse angle with axial wall; Good for porcelain fused to metal crowns. Good for labial finish lines for PFM in esthetic areas. Less stress conc. on PFM.
- As gingival finish line on proximal box of inlays/onlays and MD 3/4 crowns; labial finish line in PFM.
- But more cutting of axial wall is required for this type of finish line as compared to shoulder, to give bulk for both metal and porcelain.

KNIFE EDGE = or feather-edge.

- Permits acute margin of Gold and seems to be the IDEAL FINISH line, but can create problem—because WAX–UP is difficult for V. Thin margins;
- Can result in over-contoured restorations.
- Used on LINGUAL of mandibular posterior and on teeth with very convex axial surfaces.

FINISH LINE for Bucco-occlusal margin of maxillary partial veneer crown **and MOD onlays:**

- Narrow finishing bevel perpendicular to path of insertion.
- A contra-bevel = if heavy functions.

LOCATION OF FINISH LINE

- In areas approachable for cleaning and finishing
- Mesial extensions = should be conservative for good cosmetic effect.
- Should be placed in enamel if possible.
- Subgingival lead to periodontitis.

Cutting should be done with HIGH SPEED AIR TURBINE; low speed cause injury to tissues and overextends the preparation.

PARTIAL VENEER CROWN (PVC)

Electric pulp testing can be done on PVC, but not on fully coverage.

Most commonly used additional retentive feature in PVC is PROXIMAL GROOVE.

The occlusal finish line in maxillary teeth terminates near the bucco-occlusal angle; in mandibular teeth the finish line is approx 1 mm gingival to the lowest occlusal contact.

FOR Maxillary PVC

- First step is occlusal reduction alone.
- Reduction at functional cusp = 1.5 mm.

- ♦ Reduction at non-functional cusp = 1.0 mm.
  - Functional cusp bevel is given.
  - Proximal grooves placed in the more inaccessible proximal surface of molar (Distal) or more esthetically critical surface of PMs (mesial).
- ♦ 2 grooves are joined by occlusal **offset** on the lingual inclines of buccal cusps. It reinforces the margins.
  - Bucco-occlusal finish line bevel = 0.5 mm.

Features and their functions

Chamfer	For marginal integrity
Axial reduction	Retention and resistance structural durability
Axial cusp bevel	Structural durability
Occlusal reduction	Structural durability
Occlusal offset	Structural durability
Buccal bevel	Marginal integrity
Flare at buccal proximal line angle	Marginal integrity
Proximal groove	Retention, resistance, structural durability.

Mandibular posterior PVC–(1) Occlusal reduction.

Clearance = 1.5·mm on buccal cusp/1.0 mm on lingual cusp.

Functional cusp bevel = terminates at bucco-occlusal finish line.

Occlusal shoulder = on buccal incline of buccal cusp; 1.0 mm wide; 1.0 mm gingival to the lowest occlusal contact on buccal surface.

No offset placed on lingual inclines of buccal cusps. 0.5 mm bevel on occlusal shoulder = for BO finish line.

Functional cusp bevel	Structural durability
Occ. shoulder	Structural durability
Buccal bevel	Marginal integrity
FLARE in prox. grooves	Marginal integrity
DCP reduction	Structural durability
Axial	Structural resistance pretension
Prox. grooves	Structural resistance pretension
Chamfer	Marginal integrity

7/8th PVC—Where distal/DB cusp is to be covered; mostly used in maxillary molars.

Reverse 3/4th crown

- Mostly done on mandibular molars.
- On teeth with severe lingual inclination.
- Non-functional cusps left uncovered.

Proximal half crown

- A PVC which has been rotated 90° so that **the distal surface**, rather than buccal, left intact.

Anterior 3/4th crown

- Path of insertion = parallel to incisal 1/3–2/3rd of labial surface (rather than long axis of tooth).
- Proximal grooves = should be lingually inclined. If inclined labially, then over-cutting of labio-incisal occurs.
- Cingulum reduced for clearance of more than 0.7 mm.
- Proximal grooves = connected by incisal OFFSET placed near the opposing occlusal contact.

FULL VENEER CROWN

It is the most retentive preparation.

It should not be used in mouths with uncontrolled caries.

First step = occlusal reduction

- 1.5 mm clearance on functional cusps.
- 1.0 mm clearance on non-functional cusps.
- A wide bevel is placed on functional cusps (Buccal inclines of mandibular buccal cusps and lingual inclines of maxillary lingual cusps).
- **Chamfer line =** ***best for bulk*** required for strength and for good adaptation also.
- **Final step** = placement of seating grooves, which prevent any MD rotation of casting also. It is placed in axial surface with greatest bulk (i.e. buccal surface of mandibular and lingual surface of maxillary teeth).

For Porcelain–Fused to Metal preparations

- **Coping** = metal casting which fits over the tooth.
- Has more strength than porcelain alone.
- Deep/more reduction done on facial surface of tooth to provide space for both Porcelain and Metal (1.2 mm).
- Reduce labial surface in 2 planes to avoid pulp exposure or over contouring; parallel to gingival half and parallel to incisal half.
- Ist step = orientation grooves followed by incisal reduction.
- Labial reduction is done extending to 1 mm lingual to the proximal contacts
- **Wings** = formed on proximal surface, where labial reduction (1.2 mm) ends and lingual reduction (0.7 mm) begins, its sole aim is **to conserve tooth structure**.
- Lingual reduction = 0.7 mm; do not over reduce junction between cingulum and lingual wall.
- Shoulder with bevel (0.2–0.3 mm bevel) is finish line on labial.
- Chamfer finish line on proximal and lingual surfaces.

- Mesial and Distal incisal notches placed for edges of coping to be rounded over for structural durability.
- **Shoulder alone** = to minimize gold collar at labio–gingival margin.

Functions of different features

Gingival bevel	Marginal integrity
Shoulder	Structural durability
Wing	Preservation of tooth structure
Chamfer	Marginal integrity
Axial reduction	Retain, resistance, structural durability
Incisal notch	Structural durability
Functional cusp bevel	Structural durability
Occlusal reduction	Structural durability

For procelain jacket crowns:

- Give best cosmetic effects; done only on INCISORS.
- But susceptible to fracture as it is brittle.
- Preparation should be long for better retention.
- If short preparation—the **half moon fracture occurs** due to stress concentration in labio-gingival areas.
- **Finish line**—shoulder of approx 1 mm; it provides bulk to the porcelain and thus helps to resist forces.
- Do not use if there is edge-to-edge bite. Porcelain being harder, tends to abrade the natural teeth in its contact.
- Do not use if opposing tooth occludes in cervical 5th of lingual surface.
- 1.5–2.0 mm reduction on incisal edge.
- Shoulder finish line = 0.8–1.0 mm; for marginal integrity (i.e. 90° angle with cavosurface margin).
- Lingual axial reduction = wall should form a **6° taper** with gingival portion of labial wall.

INTRA-CORONAL RESTORATIONS

- Intra-coronal inlay = is the **simplest cast restoration**.
- Intra-coronal restoration = uses WEDGE type of retention; which exert outward pressure on the tooth.
- Inlay = can only be used if there is a large bulk and tooth structure is intact.
- It rarely replaces the lost tooth structure without protecting the remaining tooth.
- Inlay should be modified (with occlusal coverage) to distribute the stresses to a wider area.

Class II inlays—MO/DO

Occlusal outline should avoid occlusal wear faces and occlusal contacts. Otherwise inappropriate masticatory stresses get accumulated on the restorations.

Walls of isthmus = should have 6° taper.

Isthmus = no reverse curve is required, where the buccal part of isthmus blends with proximal box.

Bevel on occlusal isthmus = begins at the junction of occlusal 1/3 and gingival 2/3rd of isthmus wall and extends outward at 15–20°.

Class V inlay

- Retention = augmented by pins in M and D sides.
- Occlusal wall = at the HOC/height of contour of crown.
- Proximal walls = till the bucco proximal line angle.
- Walls should diverge slightly to conform with the directions of enamel rods and for easy removal of wax pattern.
- Axial wall is gently curved to follow buccal surface—otherwise it may lead to over-cutting and pulp exposure.
- Pin holes = placed near the junction of occlusal 1/3rd and gingival 2/3rd of axial surface; made 2 mm deep; help in retention.
- 45° narrow bevel at walls of preparation all around; 0.5 mm wide, (for marginal integrity).

MOD ONLAYS

MOD onlay is an inlay + occlusal surface cover to prevent stress concentration.

- Should not be used as bridge retainers.
- Maxillary tooth: 1.5 mm clearance on lingual cusps and 1.0 mm clearance on buccal cusps.
- Wide bevel on lingual inclines of lingual cusps on the functional cusp.
- Occlusal shoulder = 1.0 mm wide; 1.0 mm gingival to lowest occlusal contact on lingual cusp at the level lingual-occlusal finish line.
- **In Md. teeth** = functional cusp bevel and occlusal shoulder are on buccal cusp.

MANAGEMENT OF ROOT CANAL TREATED TOOTH

Post/Dowel core preparation

- Initial step is axial reduction.
- Canal preparation = by Peeso reamer (for removing GP and enlarging the canal).
- Post/Dowel should be = 2/3–3/4th the length of the root or at least as long as the clinical crown.
- A min. of 3 mm of RC filling should remain at the apex.

Peeso reamer size	Used for
1.2 mm diameter	• Mandibular incisors • Maxillary premolars • Molars
1.4 mm diameter	• Maxillary lateral incisor • Mandibular canine
1.6 mm diameter	• Maxillary central incisor • Maxillary canine • Mandibular premolars

- Key way prepared in RC at occlusal margins. It helps in preventing the rotation of the restoration.
- **Keyway placed** at the greatest bulk; 1 mm deep; 4 mm long.
- **Contra bevel** = around occlusal external periphery of preparation; prevents fracture of tooth structures.

In maxillary premolar = there are 2 roots, Main dowel placed in BUCCAL RC and stabilizing keyway in LINGUAL RC.

In maxillary molar = Dowel is placed in PALATAL RC.

In mandibular molar = Dowel is place in DISTAL RC.

IMPRESSIONS

Gingival cord = acts by chemica l + pressure.

Contains 8% Adrenaline = local vasoconstriction; gingival shrinkage. or-Alum (aluminum potassium sulfate).

Adrenaline is contra-indicated in—CVS diseases; in patients on ganglionic blockers, etc; Hyperthyroidism; Hypersensitivity to Adrenaline. In such cases, use Alum.

Force of packing instrument should be directed towards the cord previously packed.

Impression materials

Material	Features
Agar	• Agar is a ***polymer of galactose***; obtained from sea-weed; **sodium tetraborate** increases strength of gel; and viscosity of sol. • It is approx 85% water. • Least expensive; but requires special expensive instruments. • Can loose water by **SYNERESIS** (water seeping from surface). • Can absorb water by **imbibition.** • Impression can be stored in 2% K_2SO_4, water bath, etc. but impression starts distorting when it is removed from mouth.

Impression materials (*Contd.*)

Material	Features
	• **SO Pour immediately.** • Setting of **gypsum is RETARDED** in contact with gel; and BORAX can enhance it, a SOFT CAST formed. • So K_2SO_4 added = accelerates and hardens the stone.
Polysulfide	• also known as mercaptan/Thiokol. • Accelerator = **lead peroxide** with sulfur and oil. • Polymerization is **exothermic**. • Polymerization affected by moisture and temperature. • Has much greater dimensional stability. • Polymer contracts as curing occurs, so impression should be **poured with in 1 hr**. • **Hydrophobic** = so no moisture should be there on the prepared tooth when impression is taken.
Silicone rubber base	• Most commonly used rubber base impression material. • **Reactor** = ethyl silicate and tin octoate. • **Bye-products** = Methyl and ethyl alcohol, whose evaporation causes shrinkage. • It has **less dimensional stability** than polysulfide. • Impression should be **poured as soon as possible**. • Limited shelf life due to instability of alkyl silicates in presence of organo-tin compounds.
Polyether rubber base	• A copolymer of 12-epoxy ethane and tetra-hydro-furan. • Esterification reaction = by unsaturated acid. **Sulfinate** = as **cross-linkage agent**.

Impression materials (*Contd.*)

Material	Features
	• Much larger volume of base is used than the accelerator (slightly less than 8:1). Has ***excellent D-stability*** = can be poured after a long time also. • Material has affinity for water; impression should not be stored in humidor/moist atmosphere.

Type	Advantages	Disadvantages
Reversible hydrocolloid	• No custom tray required • Some **moisture tolerated** in sulcus • Clean and pleasant • Easy to pour • **Inexpensive**	• **Must be poured immediately** • Finish lines difficult to read
Polysulfide rubber base	• No special equipment required • Finish lines easily read • **Cast pour can be delayed to 1 hr** • Can be **silver plated** • **Can be poured more than once**	• Custom tray required • **Hydrophobic** • **Objectionable odor** • Messy–clothes can be ruined by contact • Requires special care in pouring
Silicone rubber base	• No special equipment required • **Superior strength** in deep suclus • Finish lines easy read • Pleasant odor and appearance	• **Must be poured immediately** • **Hydrophobic** • Easily distorted • **Expensive**

(*Contd.*)

Type	Advantages	Disadvantages
Polyether	• No special equipment required • Fast setting • Finish lines easy read • **Pouring cast can be delayed** • **Can be poured more than once**	• Custom tray required • **Expensive** • Severe undercuts must be blocked • Requires special care in pouring

Working cast = is the cast, which is mounted on the articulator.

Die = is a model of the individual prepared tooth, on which the margin of wax pattern are finished.

Articulation of casts

- U/L arches relationship should be developed with the condyle in most postero-superior position in glenoid fossa (CR).
- Mounting for diagnosis is done with the mandible in retruded position.
- Mounting for limited Rx is done in inter–cuspal position (to avoid interferences).
- **INDEXING** = soft wax placed against upper arch and patient is asked to bite lightly to get the impression of cusp tips.

CONDYLAR GUIDANCE/CG

- TMJ influences the movements of mandible.
- CG = not under the control of operator.
- Occlusal morphology of restoration should be in harmony with movements of mandible to prevent trauma form occlusion and premature contacts (TFO and PC).

Wax patterns (Also refer to the section of dental materials in Vol. II.)

- Indirect technique is better than direct = as chair side time is avoided; margins are directly visible for finishing.
- Type I wax = for making intra-oral wax patterns.

- Type II wax = for extra-oral wax patterns.
- The wax patterns should be SLIGHTLY OVERSIZED mesio-distally = s.t. the finished casting will have adequate proximal contacts.
- Proximal contacts are located slightly to the facial of middle of the posterior teeth, except between max 6, 7, which is centreed facio-lingually.
- So the lingual embrasures are slightly larger than the facial.
- HOC on facial surfaces of all posterior teeth = in cervical 3rd.
- HOC on lingual surface of max PMs and Ms = cervical 3rd.
- HOC on mandibular teeth = in middle 3rd.
- Over contouring of surfaces promotes gingival inflamers (by collection of plaque); the under contouring does not.

Occlusal morphology

- Waxing of occlusal surface is done in the last after axial surface waxing is complete.
- Lingual cusp of upper and buccal cusps of lower posterior teeth occlude in occlusal fossa or the marginal ridges of opposing teeth. These are also known as **FUNCTIONAL cusps.**
- Buccal cusps of upper and lingual cusps of lower are also known as **non-functional cusps**; protect soft tissues; prevent food from overflowing.
- **2 types of occlusal schemes** = cusp-fossa and cusp-marginal ridge.

Cusp-fossa	**Cusp-MR**
Tooth contact is occlusal fossa only	In occlusal fossa and MR.
Tooth-to-tooth contact.	Tooth-to-2 teeth contact
Occlusal forces parallel to long axis of tooth; near the centre of tooth.	
Used for full mouth/several teeth.	Most cast restorations done in restoration daily practice.
Rarely present in natural teeth.	MOST NATURAL TYPE occlusion, in 95% of adults.

MANDIBULAR CUSP PLACEMENT

Mandibular buccal cusp	**Maxillary occlusal surface**	
	Cusp MR	**Cusp fossa**
First premolar	MMR of first premolar	Mesial fossa of first premolar
Second premolar	DMR of first premolar, MMR second premolar	Mesial fossa of second premolar
MB cusp of first molar	DMR second premolar, MMR first molar	Mesial fossa of first molar
DB cusp of first molar	Central fossa of first molar	Central fossa of first molar
Distal cusp of first molar	Non functional	Distal fossa of first molar
MB cusp of second molar	DMR of first molar, MMR second molar	Mesial fossa of second molar
DB cusp of second molar	Central fossa of second molar	Central fossa of second molar
D cusp of second molar	Not present	Non functional

MAXILLARY CUSP PLACEMENT

Maxillary lingual cusps	**Mandibular occlusal surface**	
	Cusp MR	**Cusp Fossa**
First premolar	Distal fossa of first premolar	Distal fossa of first premolar
Second premolar	Distal fossa of second premolar	Distal fossa of second premolar

MAXILLARY CUSP PLACEMENT (*Contd.*)

Maxillary lingual cusps	Mandibular occlusal surface	
	Cusp-MR	Cusp-Fossa
ML cusp of first molar	Central fossa of first molar	Central fossa of first molar
DL cusp of first molar	DMR of first molar + MMR of second molar	Distal fossa of first molar
ML cusp of second molar	Central fossa of second molar	Central fossa of second molar
DL cusp of second molar	DMR of second molar	Distal fossa of second molar

- Lingual cusp of maxillary premolars fall in Distal fossa of mandibular PM.
- ML cusps of maxillary molars fall in central fossa of mandibular teeth.
- DL cusps of maxillary molars fall at DMR of mandibular molars and distal fossa of mandibular molars.

Triangular ridges

- Extend from central groove to cusp tip. Are known as triangular, because they are much wider at their base than at the cusp tips.
- Buccolingual dimension of each occlusal table formed by the ridges should be approx 55% of the overall BL dim. of the respective tooth.
- In working movement = the buccal cusp of each maxillary PM passes distal to the buccal cusp of its counterpart in the mandibular arch. So a concavity is placed in the distal inclines of buccal cusps of mandibular premolars. This depression is the **THOMAS NOTCH**.
- During working, the MB cusp of maxillary molar passes through the buccal groove, distal to the MB cusp of mandibular molars

and DB cusp of maxillary molar pass the DB groove mandibular molars.

- Also, the lingual cusps of mandibular molars should be short enough such that they do not collide with cusps of maxillary molars.
- **Fish's mouth** = is so named because of the appearance of cusp and MR at this point.
- TRIPOD contact should be formed about the cusp tips and in the fossa. The contacts should be the point contacts.
- In non-working movement, the ML cusp of maxillary molar passes distal to DB cusp of mandibular molar (i.e. through DB groove). So a notch is formed on distal incline of DB cusp.
- Also, **DB cusp** of mandibular molar moves in a ML direction across of the buccal incline of ML cusp of maxillary molar. So a groove is placed in ML cusp of maxillary molar, directed mesiolingually from central fossa. It is the **STUART'S GROOVE.**

Rules

1. Cusp height depends on inclination of protrusive path (condyle). If inclination is steep-longer cusps required. If inclination is less steep-shorter cusps required.
2. Deep bite (I G)-longer cusps required (CH). If less bite (I G)-shorter cusps required (CH).
3. Overjet if more-shorter cusps required. If overjet less-longer cusps required.
4. If protrusive condylar path is shallow and cusps must be made short, the longer cusps can be used if anterior guidance is increased.
5. A pronounced immediate side shift-shorter cusps required. A gradual side shift-longer cusps required.
6. A pronounced immediate side shift requires shorter cusps if little IG is there. But CH can be increased if IG is increased.
7. Angle between working and non-working path is greater on the teeth located farther from condyle.

INVESTING and CASTING

(Also refer to the section of dental materials in vol. 2.)

- Gold alloy shrink = 1.5% during solidification = known as solidification shrinkage.
- Gypsum bonded investment.

  Type I = uses thermal expansion.

  Type II = hygroscopic.
- Matrix = gypsum (a-$CaSO_4$ 1/2 H_2O = 30–35) acts as binder.
- Refractory filler = Silica (quartz/cristoballite) 60–65%.
- Chemical modifiers.

Dimensional compensations = uses setting expansion SE + thermal expansion TE.

SE = is due to normal crystal growth; it can be augmented by allowing the setting to occur in presence of H_2O producing HSE; this replaces the water used during HYDRATION process and so the space between crystals is maintained and they can continue to expand outwards; maximum HSE is by immersing the ring in 100°F water bath.

TE = is achieved through normal expansion which occurs upon heating the silica and phase changes, which occur in the material.

3 purposes of investment:

1. Precisely detailed reproduction of anatomical form.
2. Strong enough to withstand the heat of burnout.
3. Compensation expansion equal to the solidification shrinkage of molten alloy.

SPRUE: 10–12 gauge.

- It provides inlet for the molten metal into the casting.
- Attached at a point of greatest bulk.
- At an angle to allow free flow of incoming molten metal.
- If used at thin areas or very small size = may lead to SHRINK SPOT POROSITY.

- For uniform expansion = the pattern should be placed in the centre of the ring and should be surrounded by a uniform thickness of the investment.
- Sprue should be long enough— s.t. highest point of wax pattern is 6 mm from the end of the ring.
- For adequate solidification = the sprue itself should not be longer than 6 mm.

Investing

- 1mm thick ASBESTOS—to act as buffer zone. It allows expansion outwards to enlarge the mold. If it is not there the expansion forces will occur towards the mold leading to contraction/distortions.
- Liner should be 3 mm shorter on both ends of the ring so as to restrict expansion near the open end of the ring.
- Wet asbestos gives extra expansion of HSE type.
- Double layer provides more expansion.
- Invest under vacuum to avoid BUBBLES.
- W/P ratio should be controlled; more water means less expansion.
- Over spatulation increases the TE.

Burn out

- To remove the wax.
- Prepares the mold for molten metal.
- Allows TE to occur.
- Higher heat technique = at 1200°F for TE.
- For HSE = 1000° F used
- First burn out at 600° F × 30 min.
- Put in inverted position, s.t. wax comes out.
- Then place at 900° or 1200° F for 1 hour.
- Allow oxygen to contact the ring for 10 min before casting is made = to ensure complete wax elimination.
- The casting should be done within 30 sec; any delay may lead to heat loss and mold contraction.
- Give 3 winds to the right hand of casting machine.

USE blue/reducing/hottest zone of flame to heat the alloy.

On proper heating—the alloy is straw yellow colour; wiggles easily; appears shiny and mirror—like; and moves with the flame.

Put some flux in molten metal—to increase fluidity and to prevent oxide formation.

Quench the ring—helps to anneal the metal for better working qualities and also disintegrates the investment for easy removal.

Pickling—done to cleanse the casting.

Phosphate bonded investment

- Used for non precious alloys and for gold-platinum alloy for PFM restorations.
- Temperature = 2100° F used (If gypsum bonded is used at higher temperature, the $CaSO_4$ is disintegrated and sulfur is released which contaminates the mold).
- Mg PO_4 + Ammonium PO_4 form Mg–Ammonium PO_4 = provide STRENGTH at room temperature.
- At high temperature = silico-phosphates produced give more strength.
- Liquid = of ***colloidal silica suspension*** is used.
- Graphite and silica are present in powder.
- More silica sol + less water = more expansion.
- Less silica sol + more water = less expansion.
- Usual ratio = 3:1 = silica sol to water ratio.
- Overall liquid powder ratio = 9.5 C.C/60 gm powder.
- It possesses poor surface—wetting characteristics.
- Setting allowed for 1 hour on bench.
- HSE (0.7%) if required = place in 100° F H_2O
- Then at 600°F × 30 mm
- Then at 1300°F × 1 hr.
- A silica crucible should be used, without asbestos, instead of clay crucible.
- Heat the alloy till white/shiny and then cast it.

FINISHING AND CEMENTATION

Beilby layer—During polishing, minute amounts of abraded surface materials are filled in the surface irregularities, forming a microcrystalline surface layer.

Abrasives—Should be much harder than the material on which it is used.

Substance	KHN
Dentin	68
Amalgam	110
Type III gold	145
Enamel	343
Cr-Co-alloy	350
Porcelain	460
Sand (flint)	800
Al_2O_3	2000
Emery	2000
Si-carbide	2500
Diamond	8200

Material	Features
Diamond	Hardest; Should be used on hard, brittle substances, e.g. Enamel/porcelain. The soft/ductile substance, e.g. Au tend to choke the abrasive particles.
Silicon carbide	Very commonly used e.g. carbornudum discs; separating discs/joe-dandy discs; wheels/points/green stones.
Emery	Is a mixture of Al_2O_3 and Fe_2O_3. Bound to paper disc. Used on gold/porcelain.

Material	**Features**
Aluminum oxide	Al_2O_3 is produced from bauxite 400 grit. Used in white polishing stones know as POLY-STONES.
Garnet	Red in colour. Silicates of Al and Fe with Mg. Co. Mn, etc. Used for metal/porcelain.
Sand	Quartz known as flint is used. Sharp cutting edges. Various grits of sand paper available.
Tripoli	Fine siliceous powder with wax. Used for initial polishing steps.
Rouge	Iron oxide Fe_2O_3. Is finest of polishing agents used on gold casting. Used on crocus discs also.

Occlusal adjustment

- U/L anterior teeth should not touch in CR; the gap should be = 0.0005″.
- Non-working side adjustments are done by removing contacts on buccal incline of maxillary lingual cusp and lingual inclines of mandibular buccal cusps.
- Working side adjustments are done by removing contacts on lingual inclines of maxillary lingual cusps and buccal inclines of mandibular lingual cusps.
- Contacts between lingual inclines of maxillary buccal cusps and buccal inclines of mandibular buccal cusps should be removed if mutually protected occlusion is required and should not be removed if group function occlusion is required.

- ♦ Protrusive interferences are removed by adjusting mesial inclines of mandibular teeth and distal inclines of max teeth.
- ♦ Surface roughness on the margin is found approx 40 micron, which can be decreased to 8 micron by petrolatum and cuttle disc polishing on a white stone. Green stone should not be used.

PONTICS

- ♦ Area of contact between ridge and pontic should be small.
- ♦ Part of pontic which is near the ridge should be CONVEX and smooth.
- ♦ Pontic should exert no pressure on ridge.
- ♦ Mesial, distal, and lingual embrasures should be WIDE open for easy cleaning.
- ♦ Pontic is narrower (esp. from lingual surfaces) than the natural tooth so as to align it on the inter-abutment axis. It helps in preventing the torquing of abutments/retainers and also plaque accumulation.

Designs of pontics

Design	Features
Saddle	• Replaces all contours of missing tooth. • Fills embrasures and overlaps the ridge with a large concave contact. • Impossible to clean. • Should never be used.
Ridge lap	• Has all CONVEX surfaces for easy cleaning. • Used in appearance zone, i.e. U/L anteriors for esthetics.
Hygienic	• No contact with the tissues; 2–3 mm gap. • Also known as SANITARY pontic. • Esp used in non-appearance zone (mandibular posteriors). • Restores occlusal function; stability of teeth;

Designs of pontics (*Contd.*)

Design	Features
	• Occluso-gingival thickness should not be less than 3 mm.
Conical/bullet/ spheroidal modified ridge lap	• Cleanable, but triangular space around the tissues may collect debris.

PIN FACINGS

Reverse pin facing = has good retention where a deep bite would force the use of very short pins in the conventional facing.

PFM facing = used when maximum esthetics is required esp in anterior teeth.

Harmony facing = is most frequently used for fabricating the maxillary posterior pontics. Is not useful if occluso-gingival dim. is short.

Pin facing = is used where occluso-gingival space is limited.

Modified pin facing = made by adding porcelain to the lingual gingival area of a pin facing.

Junction between gold and porcelain should not cross the facet of wear, otherwise heavy forces may cause dislodgement of facing.

At least 1 mm clearance should be there between porcelain and the opposing facial cusp.

SOLDERING

- **Soldering** = is joining of metal parts by a filler metal/solder.
- Bonding occurs due to wetting of joined surfaces by the solder and not by the melting of metal components.
- **Welding** = the metal parts are joined by melting and fusing together, without solder.
- **Flux** = displaces gases, removes corrosion products by either combining with them or reducing them.

- **Flux** = 55% Sodium pyroborate + 35% Boric acid + 10% Silica.
- Paste of flux should be made with petrolatum, as it burns off without leaving any residue.
- Paste made with water tend to effloresce when they are heated; it produces pits in the joints and weaken them.
- **Antiflux** = used to outline the area to be soldered to limit the flow of solder, e.g. graphite pencil; rouge suspended in chloroform.
- **Karat** = i.e. parts per 24 of a metal which is gold.
- **Fineness** = i.e. parts per 100 of solder which is gold.
- However, with solder, 18 karat means that it's to be used with 18 K gold casting alloy.
- Actual precious metal content of a solder is given by = its fineness rather than karat.
- **580 fine is the minimum fineness,** which should be used for corrosion resistance.
- Solder should have fusion range about 100–150°C below that of the metal being soldered.
- If base metal % age is increased in solder, it leads to PITTING of the joint.
- Solder should be free flowing. Ag makes it free-flow and Cu makes it sluggish.
- Soldering investment = is made of quartz with low setting expansion, should be one inch thick.
- Used to solder pontic with retainers in a bridge.
- Gap between retainer pontic should be approx 0.005″, and their surface should be parallel to each other; the solder flows in the gap by capillary action. If no gap, it leads to distortion. If wide gap, then no proper flow of solder occurs.
- Solder is fed from lingual side; buccal side is used for heating the casting during soldering.
- Preheat the invested casting to 1500°F.
- Blue zone of flame is used.
- **Do not quench** or thermal stresses/distortion may occur.

- If kept for bench cooling to room temperature—crystallization and grain growth is excessive and so weaker joint occurs.
- **Best procedure is to** bench cool for 5 min. and then quench. Minimum distortion occurs; ordering heat Rx occurs, strength and hardness increase.
- Polishing rouge, i.e. (Fe_2O_3) is also an anti-flux for soldering—so do not use it before soldering.
- In non-rigid connectors, the path of the insertion of key way is aligned with the distal abutment.

PORCELAIN

- Most esthetic material.
- Non-crystalline glasses having Si and O_2.
- It should be low fusing. The fusing temperature is decreased by reducing cross linking between Si and O_2 with the help of glass-modifiers (e.g. Potassium oxide, Na_2O and Ca-oxide but they decrease viscosity).
- So Al_2O_3 is used to maintain viscosity.

Types	Temperature in F	Temperature in C
High fusing	2350–2500 F	1290–1370
Medium fusing	2000–2300 F	1000–1260
Low fusing	1600–1950 F	860–1070

High fusing

- Used for making porcelain teeth.
- It has feldspar (70–90%) + quartz (11–18%) + Kaolin (1–10%).
- **Feldspar**—glassy, translucency, matrix.
- Quartz—refractory.
- Kaolin—Binder.

Low and medium fusing porcelains—are produced by:

- **FRITTING**
- Addition of metallic oxides (Zr, Tr, Sn) make the porcelain OPAQUE—used to mask metal coping in PFM restorations.
- Yellow colour to porcelain is given = By In
- Pink colour to porcelain = Cr/Sn
- Black colour to porcelain = Fe
- Blue colour to porcelain = Co

Porcelain jacket Crown

- 0.001″ Pt foil is adapted on the die.
- Porcelain **firing** = started at 1500° F and reach at 1900°F in six minutes—under vacuum.

PFM restorations = stronger than porcelain.

- Combine strength and accuracy of metal + esthetics of porcelain.
- Coping = is the metal casting which fits over the prepared tooth. Porcelain is fused to the coping.
- Coping is covered with 3 layers of porcelain.

1. **Opaque**—Covers metal underneath.
2. **Body**—Makes the bulk of restoration.
   —Provides most of the colour/shade.
3. **Incisal area**—Translucent layer in incisal part.

- Bonding of porcelain to metal is through OXIDE LAYER, and is adhesive.
- Bond strength increases when firing is done in oxidizing atmosphere.
- Failure occurs in porcelain rather than at Porcelain—metal interface.
- Coeff of thermal expansion of Au alloy = 14×10^{-6}/°C.
- Coeff of thermal porcelain = 2–4 × 10^{-6}/°C.
- The ideal difference should be 1×10^{-6}/°C, as a difference of 1.7×10^{-6}/°C can produce shear stresses.
- So coeff of porcelain is increased by ALKALI (e.g. lithium carbonate) to 7–8 × 10^{-6}/°C.

- Coeff of metal is decreased by adding Pd or Pt to 7–8 × 10^{-6}/°C.
- Min. different between MP of metal and porcelain should be 300–500° F to avoid flow/creep of metal. So MP of porcelain should be lower than metal.
- Most satisfactory metals with porcelain have high gold (83–87%) + Pt (6–16%).
- Also ***Sn is there to form OXIDE layer***, which gives bonding strength.
- Absolute min. thickness of porcelain is 0.7 mm and optimum thickness is 1.0 mm.
- Outer junction of metal with porcelain should be a butt joint to provide bulk to the porcelain and hence strength.
- For proper strength and rigidity—the coping should be 0.3–0.5 mm thick.
- **Occlusal contacts** = should be placed on the metal on all posterior restorations and should be **away from P-M junction**, otherwise porcelain may get fractured.
- On maxillary anteriors on lingual side, the junction should not be placed in the vicinity of those contacts with mandibular teeth. But approx 2.0 mm from the contact.
- P–M junction should not be too far incisally or porcelain may fracture and also **translucency decreases**.
- Porcelain is stronger in compression.
- Proximal contact for anterior teeth should be on porcelain for better esthetics.
- On maxillary posterior teeth, the buccal porcelain covers cusp tips and 1/3rd the lingual inclines of buccal cusp.
- On mandibular teeth = the entire occlusal surface should be in **METAL.**
- On first premolar, the mesial half of occlusal surface can be covered with porcelain, because contact is only in DISTAL FOSSA.
- Proximal contact on posterior teeth should be in **metal** except mesial surface of maxillary first premolar.

- In PFM bridges—porcelain is extended on the tissue surface of pontics to avoid plaque accumulation. The thickness should be 0.5 mm.
- Surface contaminants are removed by pickling the casting in 52% HF acid for 20 min. in a sealed polyethylene container in an ultrasonic cleaner.
- **Degassing**—removes H_2 gas from coping surface so as to avoid bubbles in porcelain. Place the coping in furnace at 1200°F in vacuum till 15 min.
- Opaque porcelain is applied first to mask the metal and to give proper shade. A 0.5 mm thickness is fired from 1200°–1750°F.

Body porcelain

- Incisal 1/3rd of restoration is built up with incisal porcelain, which has less colour and more translucency.
- The restoration should be over-contoured by 1/5th to compensate for 20% shrinkage during firing.
- Glazing = from 1200° to 1800° F firing.

SHADE MATCHING

- ♦ Should be done under more than one type of light.
- ♦ **Metamerism** = is a phenomenon of an object appearing to be of different colour when viewed in different light sources.
- ♦ **Hue** = quality which distinguishes one colour from another.
- ♦ **Chroma** = is saturation or strength of a hue.
- ♦ **Value/brightness** = is relative amount of lightness or darkness in a hue. It is the single most important factor in shade matching. Higher value means lighter shade and vice-versa.
- ♦ Observation of shade should be quick (10–15 sec.) to avoid **fatiguing** the cones in retina.
- ♦ Observer should glance at **BLUE** object while resting his eyes.
- ♦ Shade should be matched by value, saturation and hue (VSH) in that order.
- ♦ Shade should be matched before the tooth preparation is started. The tooth gets dehydrated during preparation.

Complete Dentures

General features and important points

- **Bennett movement** = condyle of working side moves laterally.
- **Bennett angle** = condyle on non-working side moves forwards and mesially.
- **Working side** = the side towards which the mandible deviates in lateral excursive movements.
- **Non-working side** = the side away from which the mandible deviates in lateral excursive movements.
- Restorations are usually built in RCP as this is the most reproducible position.
- In 80–90% of the population, RCP = is < 2 mm posterior to ICP.
- **Terminal hinge axis** = an axis passing through the lower part of the condyles, about which the condyles rotate when they are in their uppermost centred position in the glenoid fossa.
- **Retention** = is the resistance to displacement of a denture **away from the ridge**.
- **Support** = is the resistance of **vertical movement** of a denture towards the ridge.
- **Stability** = is the ability of a denture to resist displacement by functional stresses. It gives physiological comfort.
- **Saddle** = that part of the alveolus from which teeth are missing.

Overdenture—is a prosthesis that gains support form one or more abutment teeth by enclosing them beneath its fitting surfaces.

Immediate denture = is a prosthesis used to replace one or more teeth and inserted on the day of extraction of the tooth or teeth.

Complete denture

- The principal functions of periodontium are support and positional adjustment of the tooth, together with the secondary and dependent function of sensory perception.
- The most prominent feature of physiological occlusal forces is their intermittent, rhythmic and dynamic nature.
- The greatest forces acting on the teeth are normally produced during mastication and deglutition.
- Deglutition occurs about 500 times a day and tooth contacts during swallowing are of longer duration than those occurring during chewing.

Total time calculated during 24 hrs during chewing

1. Actual chewing time per meal = 450 sec.
2. Total chewing time for 4 meals = 1800 sec.
3. Each second 1 chewing stroke = 1800 strokes.
4. Duration of each chewing stroke = 0.3 sec.
5. So total chewing time = 1800 × 0.3 = 540 sec. = 9 min.

Total duration of swallowing in 24 hrs

1. Duration of 1 deglutitional movement during meals = 1 sec.
2. During chewing 3 × per minute 1/3 of movements with occlusal forces only = 30 sec.
3. Between meals, in day time is 25 per hr for 16 hrs = 400 sec.
4. During sleep, 10 per hr for 8 hrs = 80 sec.
5. So total = 540 + 30 + 400 + 80 = 1050 sec = 17.5 min.

- So the total time during which the teeth are subjected to functional forces of mastication and deglutition during an entire day amounts to ***approx 17.5 min***.
- **Masticatory forces**—44 lbs; it is very much less than can be produced by concious efforts.

- Maximum masticatory **forces by complete dentures** = 13–16 lbs.
- The mean **denture bearing area in maxillary** edentulous arch = 22.96 cm^2.
- The mean **denture bearing area in mandibular** edentulous arch = 12.25 cm^2.
- The **areas of PDL of natural teeth** = 45 cm^2 in each arch, which is more than 3.5 times the average area of the basal seat of a mandibular complete denture.
- Alveolar bone supporting natural teeth receives tensile loads through a larger area of PDL; but the edentulous residual ridge receives vertical, diagonal, and horizontal loads applied by a denture having less surface area.
- Denture wearing is almost invariably accompanied by an undesirable bone loss.
- Oro-facial and tongue ms play an important role in retaining and stabilizing the CD. It occurs by setting the teeth in the **neutral zone** in the area of the ms functional balance.
- **Centric relation**—is the most posterior relation of the mandible to the maxilla at the established vertical relation. It coincides with a reproducible **posterior hinge position** of the mandible. It depends on both structural and functional harmony of osseous structures, the intra-articular tissues, and capsular ligament of TMJ.
- Unconscious swallowing is carried out with the mandible at or near the CR position. Unconscious or reflex swallow is important during the developing dentition.
- The contact of the inclined planes of the teeth aid in the alignment of the erupting teeth.
- **Centric occlusion**—the most functional natural tooth contacts occur in a mandibular position anterior to that of CR, which is know as CO.

Morphological changes associated with edentulous state

1. Deepening of the nasolabial groove.
2. Loss of labio-dental angle.

3. Decrease in horizontal labial angle.
4. Narrowing of the lips.
5. Increase in columella-philtral angle.
6. Prognathic appearance.
7. Lip pursing.

TISSUE RESPONSE TO CD

- Soft tissue hyperplasia occurring around the borders of the CD = is fibrous; know as **epulis fissuratum**; it occurs in free mucosa ***lining the sulcus or the junction of attached and free mucosa***, due to chronic irritation from ill-fitting or overextended denture;
- **Denture stomatitis** = is chronic inflammation on basal seat; it occurs due to trauma from ill-fitting denture or a parafunctional habit. Candidal infection or irritation from residual monomer is

Changes in the size of the basal seat

Maxillary arch	Mandibular arch
Bone reduction is **upward and inwards**. Resorption from outer cortex is greater and more rapid as it is more thinner.	**Anterior area** = bone resorption occurs on labial and alveolar area; so the ridge migrates lingually and inferiorly. **Posterior area** = bone resorbed on lingual side so the ridge moves buccally.
Denture bearing surface/ basal seat becomes smaller in all dimensions.	**The mandibular arch becomes wider posteriorly**; so the failure to place the artificial teeth in the natural teeth site may hamper denture support and stability.
Maxillary arch becomes narrower with time both anteriorly and posteriorly.	Outer cortex is thicker than the lingual cortex except in the molar area.

also a cause; it is ***more common in maxillary arch***; it may be granular know as ***papillary hyperplasia*** or papillomatosis.

- To take an impression of hyperplastic tissues, ***the muco-static impression materials*** should be used.
- ***Denture sore mouth*** = is mainly due to the result of an underlying abnormal metabolic or hormonal function or nutritional deficiency.

HOUSE'S CLASSIFICATION OF PATIENTS

Types	Features
Philosophical	• *Accept the judgement of their dentist without questions.* • *Have* **ideal situation for successful Rx**. • *They know that dentist will do best.*
Indifferent	• Have ***little concern for their oral health***. • Seek Rx on the insistence of family members. • Give up the Rx easily if problems arise.
Critical	• ***Find fault in everything*** done for them. • ***Never happy*** with previous dentist as he did not follow their instructions. • Must not be allowed to direct the Rx according to them.
Skeptical	• Had bad results with previous dentist. • Doubtful that any other can help them. • Are often in poor health, e.g. severely resorbed ridges. • Dentist should take more time than usual for examining such patients.

Hard and soft tissue areas in maxillary basal seat

Ideal layer should be **firm and resilient**.

1. **Torus palatinus**—should be relieved or removed.
2. **Incisive papillae**—relieve denture here to avoid pressure on blood vessels and nerves.
3. Flabby maxillary tuberosity—should be surgically removed.
4. Zygomatic process of maxillary bone as it crosses the buccal vestibule on both sides.
5. Pterygomaxillary notch—is very important for the maximum breadth to the PPS area of the CD.

Hard and soft tissue areas in mandibular basal seat

1. **Torus mandibularis**—mostly in premolar areas on lingual side = relieve or remove.
2. Hard areas of the attachment of **mentalis ms,** which come to lie close to the alveolar crest in badly resorbed ridges—**no surgery** is indicated to remove them; relieve them by modifying the denture bases.
3. **Buccal shelf**—is made of ***cortical bone***; lies on the body of mandible b/w the buccal frenum and retromolar pad and b/w the residual ridge crest and external oblique line. It has a covering of the suctorial pad and attachment of **buccinator ms**.
4. **Retromolar pad area**—***cannot supply support***; but covered to provide border seal; should not be displaced from relaxed position as some movable structures, e.g. **buccinator, superior constrictor m, and pterygomandibular raphe** pass through it. Also fibers from temporalis ms and some mucous glands are present.
5. **Fibrous cord like ridges**—should not be displaced; do not provide any support to the CD; its surgical removal can be problematic as it detaches mucosa from the mandible, and so the mucous membrane over the ridge can get pulled forward by lip and backward by tongue.

- Teeth replacement in case of Class II and Class III m.o. requires that ***the artificial teeth should be in the position of natural teeth***.

RIDGE FORM

- Ideal ridge has a broad top and parallel sides.
- When the mandibular ridge is sharp and has sharp bone spicules then = **selective pressure impression technique** is used so that more force is placed on buccal shelf area.
- When the sharp ridge has disappeared = use **minimum pressure technique** so that occlusal forces are distributed more evenly.

RIDGE RELATIONS

- Bones of maxilla resorb primarily from the occlusal surface and the buccal and labial surfaces, so that upper residual ridge **becomes shorter Antero-Posteriorly and narrower from side-to-side**.
- Mandibular ridge resorbs primarily from occlusal surface, so mandibular **ridge in posterior part becomes wider**, because the inferior border of mandible is broader than the occlusal part. The cross section shrinkage in mandible is downward and outward;
- The cross shrinkage in anterior part is D and B first; later on the basal seat moves forward.

SHAPE OF PALATAL VAULT

- ***Most ideal form*** = which has a medium depth with a well-defined incline of the rugae area in the anterior part of the palate.
- A **flat palatal vault** = gives insufficient resistance to a forward movement of upper denture.
- A **high narrow V-shaped vault** = unfavorable for the retention of the CD.

TONGUE

- Tongue becomes larger if a loose denture is there in the mouth as the patient uses it to hold the denture in place.
- A small tongue causes a problem for mandibular CD = the small tongue drops back away from the lower anteriors and thus break the border seal.

SALIVA

- ***Ideal saliva*** = moderate flow of serous saliva.
- Excessive saliva = complicates the impression making.
- Absence of saliva/***Xerostomia*** = ***affects retention***; so reduced retention. Also the lips and cheeks stick to the denture.
- Thick and ropy saliva = gets build up below the denture bases and can force the CD out of its correct position. Also complicates impression by making voids in the cast; may cause gagging.

Pre-prosthetic considerations

- **Upper labial frenum** may have a strong band of ***fibrous connective tissues*** that attaches on lingual side of the crest of residual ridge = should be removed surgically.
- **Hyperplastic maxillary tuberosity** should be removed for better base; to reduce undercuts; avoid opening in maxillary sinus.
- **Mandibular tori** should be surgically removed to prevent undercuts; and to improve border seal.
- High mandible and low maxillary attachments reduce the denture bearing area and affect the border seal; so the **vestibuloplasty** is advised. It is restricted to interpremolar area as in the posterior area, buccinator m does not give any problem. **Most frequent site is the anterior part of the body of mandible and the mentalis m** attachment migrates to the crest of the residual ridge obliterating the labial sulcus.
- Obliterated pterygomaxillary fossa/**hamular notch** = undermines the retention and PPS; so it should be deepened surgically.
- **Mental foramen** = due to extreme resorption, it comes to lie on the crest having sharp edges 2–3 mm higher than adjacent bone; **best way** is to provide relief in the denture so that no pressure fall on the nerves.

Basal seat—foundation of the denture is know as basal seat.

Fibrous connective tissues are present in those areas, where the external forces are applied; but glandular tissues are not found in those areas.

Support for the maxillary denture

- Use that impression technique which equalizes the pressure distribution.
- Midline palatal suture and raphe = should be relieved.

Stress bearing areas

- **Primary SBA** = residual ridge; is covered with fibrous connective tissues.
- **Secondary SBA** = rugae; it can resist the forward movement of the denture; it shouldn't be distorted during impression.
- Glandular area in posterior part of palate on either side of the midline = aids in retention; should not be subjected to significant occlusal forces.

Stress bearing areas	Maxillary	Mandibular
Primary SBA	Crest of the residual alveolar ridge	Buccal shelves
Secondary SBA	Rugae	Slopes of the alveolar ridges
Non- SBA	Incisive papillae mid-palatal raphe	*Crest of alveolar ridge*

Incisive papillae (Refer selection of teeth also.)

- Lies behind and b/w the central incisors.
- Foramen carries the nasopalatine nerves and vessels; it ***should be relieved in denture*** to avoid disruption in blood and nerve supply.
- With resorption, it comes near to the crest of the alveolar ridge.
- Its location indicates the amount of the resorption.
  - **Zygomatic/malar process** = located **opposite the first molar region**. ***Relief*** is required to aid in retention and prevent the soreness.

- **Maxillary tuberosity**—if excess fibrous tissue is there, it prevents the proper location of occlusal plane.
- **Torus palatinus**—hampers in retention; ***should be relieved*** in denture; if large then it is removed surgically.
- **Maxillary labial frenum**—is a **fold of mucous membrane** in the median line; ***has no muscles***; no action of its own; should be ***relieved*** in denture.
- **Orbicularis oris m**—its tone depends on the support provided by the labial flange; its fibers pass horizontally through the lip and anastomose with fibers of buccinator m.
- **Buccal frenum**—caninus m (***levator anguli oris***) is attached below it; requires more clearance for its function. It is affected by 3 ms, i.e. orbicularis oris, buccinator, caninus.

Buccal vestibule

- Extends from buccal frenum to hamular notch; used for the buccal flange of denture.
- Its size varies with the contraction of **buccinator**.
- Thickness of distal end of buccal flange is adjusted to accommodate the ramus and coronoid process and masseter m during functions.
- ***Masseter m on contraction under heavy pressure*** reduces the size of the space available for distal end of buccal flange.
- This space is usually higher than any other part of the border.
- It is altered by lateral movement of the mandible.
- Zygomatic process is unyielding and **requires relief**.

Pterygomaxillary/hamular notch

- Is b/w tuberosity of maxilla and hamulus of medial pterygoid plate.
- Is used as boundary of posterior border of maxillary denture back to the tuberosity.
- ***No ms or ligament is present***.
- PPS is placed through the centre of this notch.

Palatine fovea

- Are formed by the collection of several ***mucous gland*** ducts.
- Are close to the vibrating line; are always in soft tissues.
- Acts as ***ideal guide for location of posterior border*** of denture.

Vibrating line of the palate

- Marks the beginning of the motion in the soft palate when patient says AH.
- PPS passes 2 mm in front of fovea palatine.
- It is not the junction of hard and soft palate; ***is always in the soft palate***.
- Vibrating line on soft palate contains glandular tissues.
- Higher the vault, the more abrupt and forward the vibrating line.
- In Flat vault—it is placed posteriorly.
- Denture should extend 1–2 mm posterior of this line.
- Denture must cover the tuberosities and extend in the hamular notch.
- Overextension of denture in hamular notch = interferes with pterygomandibular raphe, which extends from hamulus to the top inside back corner of the retromolar pad, RMP.
- On wide opening of mouth = pterygomandibular raphe is pulled forward, which dislodges the denture.
    - **Submucosa**—is devoid of fat or glandular cells; in edentulous mouth is thicker than in the attached gingiva of the dentulous mouth.
    - **Compact bone**—is best able to provide primary support for the upper denture.
    - **Mucous membrane**—on the slope of the upper residual ridge; less stress is placed on the moveable tissue of the slope of the ridge.
    - **Soft tissue of hard palate**—anterolaterally is the fatty/adipose zone; postero-laterally is glandular zone; these tissues are recorded in **resting condition**.

- **Submucosa of median palatal suture**—non resilient; little or no stress can be placed; highly sensitive; **proper relief** is provided.
- **Incisive papillae**—nasopalatine nerve and vessels; **relief** to avoid pressure on them.
- **Vestibular space**—lining mucosa is non-keratinized; elastic fibers in submucosa.
- Natural ms activity in the lips and cheeks is important for the development of the borders.
- Hamular notch contains loose areolar tissues; additional pressure can be placed on this tissue to complete PPS.
- Increased amounts of keratinized material are present in edentulous ridges, when clinical quality of the denture is good.
- Removing the dentures from the mouth for 6–8 hrs a day esp during sleep allows keratinization to increase and the signs of inflammation are reduced.

RELATED ANATOMIC STRUCTURES

Muscles of soft palate

- Levator veli palatini; tensor veli palatini; musculus uvulae; glossopalatiuns; pharyngopalatinus;
- Wall of soft palate is formed principally by the pharyngopalatinus ms.
- Posterior border of maxillary denture, which forms the PPS, rests on the soft palate upto the place where the soft palate becomes moveable.

Muscles of pharynx

- Main ms are superior, middle, inferior constrictors; stylopharyngeus; salpingopharyngeus; palatopharyngeus.
- **Superior constrictor** is the muscle of kinetic chain during **swallowing**.
- **Superior constrictor** is separated from buccinator by pterygomandibular raphe just above the buccinator m.

Nerve and blood supply

- Maxillary denture foundation gets blood from—descending palatine and posterior superior alveolar A.
- Mandibular denture—from inferior alveolar A and its branches.
- Tongue—lingual A.
- Nerves of maxillary area—nasopalatine; anterior palatine; middle palatine; inferior nasal nerve on palatal side; by anterior-middle-posterior superior alveolar nerves on buccal side.
- Mandibular area—inferior alveolar and its branches, i.e. mylohyoid; dental, incisive and mental.
- Buccinator/long buccal n supplies—buccinator, vestibule, cheeks.
- Anterior 2/3 rd of tongue by lingual n; posterior 1/3rd by 9th n.

MAXILLARY IMPRESSION

- Definition—**impression** is a record of negative form of tissues of the oral cavity.
- **5 objectives of the impression**—retention; stability; support; esthetics; preservation/health of the tissues. (PRESS)
- **Retention**—is its resistance to removal in a direction opposite of its insertion; it resists the forces of gravity and is ***in vertical direction***.
- **Stability**—is the resistance ***against the horizontal movement*** and forces.
- **Denture support**—is the resistance to vertical components of mastication and to occlusal or other forces applied in a direction towards the basal seat.
- **Factors of retention**—adhesion; cohesion; interfacial surface tension; capillarity; atmospheric pressure; oral and facial ms. (CATCAM)
- **Adhesion**—is the physical attraction ***of unlike molecules*** to each other.
- A watery saliva is quite effective; thick ropy saliva gets built up and literally pushes the denture out of position (as hydraulic pressure of saliva is more than force of adhesion).

- Amount of retention supplied by adhesion is directly proportional to the area covered by the denture.
- **Cohesion**—is the physical attraction ***of like molecules*** to each other. It occurs in the layer of saliva b/w mucosa and denture. It is directly proportional to the area covered by the denture.
- **Interfacial ST**—is the resistance to separation possessed by the film of liquid b/w 2 well-adapted surfaces; directly proportional to the size of basal surface of the denture. For best results, the impression should be minimal distortion and displacement.
- **Capillarity**—is force developed because of surface tension, it causes retention of denture, because a thin film of saliva acts as a capillary tube. It is directly proportional to the area of basal seat of the denture.
- **Atmospheric pressure**—is **14.7 psi**; the retentive force by atmospheric pressure is directly proportional to the area covered by the denture.
- **Musculature**—teeth are placed ***in neutral zone***; shape of buccal and lingual flanges should be in harmony with the movement of the ms; buccal corridor.
- **Contraction of the buccinator ms** will tend to **seat both dentures** on their basal seats.
- **Occlusal plane/OP** must be at the correct level.
- Insufficient space may be present b/w the ridges esp in the tuberosity regions. It is due to excessive fibrous tissue covering the tuberosity; it should be **removed surgically**.

Impression

- Softer materials displace the soft tissues less and require less force in their molding.
- During making the special tray, ***1 mm thick spacer*** is placed, which provides space for the final impression material. The PPS area is not covered with the spacer.
- **Border molding**—is the process by which the shape of the borders of the tray is made to conform accurately to the contours of the buccal and labial vestibules.

- ***Holes*** are placed in median palatal raphe and anterolateral and posterolateral regions of palate to provide relief.
- Distobuccal angle of the buccal flange = is molded by asking the patient to move mandible side by side.

Posterior palatal seal (PPS)

- When properly formed it will be about **1 mm thick** and about **4 mm wide**.

Making space in the tray

- Is provided for final impression material.
- Entire surface is scraped for—1 mm except PPS.
- 1.5–2.0 mm relief is given at—median palatal raphe.
- Buccal and labial borders—shortened by 1.5 mm.

MANDIBULAR IMPRESSION

- Total basal area of mandible is less than maxilla.
- With teeth loss, bony base of mandible becomes shorter vertically and narrower bucco-lingually.
- Total width of bony foundation and mandibular basal seat—becomes **greater in molar area,** because the width of the inferior border of mandible from side to side is greater than the width of mandible at the alveolar process.

Buccal flange area or buccal shelf

- Is the area b/w mandibular buccal frenum and the anterior edge of the masseter muscle.
- Is ***bounded by*** external oblique ridge laterally and by RMP distally.
- Formed by smooth ***compact bone***.
- It is the principal bearing surface of the mandibular denture (***primary stress bearing area***).
- BFA is at right angle to the direction of vertical occlusal forces.

- Some buccinator ms fibers are located under it. The fibers run antero-posteriorly parallel to bone and the denture does not resist the contracting forces of this muscle. Its contraction does not lift the denture.
- Requirements of mandibular impression—best by a **selective pressure technique**.
- Short flanges in labial anterior area—because of the attachment of various ms to the rest of ridge. These ms act nearly at right angles to the flange.
- In posterior region—crest of greatly resorbed ridges is at the level of the mental foramen, which should be relieved.

Mylohyoid ridge

- Mylohyoid ms—attaches close to the inferior border of mandible ANTERIORLY and near the superior surface of the residual ridge POSTERIORLY.
- Angle of the **posterior part of lingual flange of denture** in molar region is affected by angle of mylohyoid m. while **anteriorly, only the length of the flange** is affected by it.
- MH m moves **outward and upwards** during contraction, so the denture should not be extended into the undercut below MH ridge.
- In mandible with flat residual ridge, mylohyoid ridge is very sharp; so ***relief is provided*** in denture to avoid soreness.
- **Mental foramen**—hould be ***relieved*** to avoid impingement on mental N and vessels in case of severe resorption.
- Insufficient space b/w mandible and tuberosity—angle of mandible is frequently made more obtuse with early loss of the posterior teeth and retention of anterior teeth.
- Removal of posterior support destroys the necessary counter-balance against the muscle pull at the angle of mandible. This reduces the space b/w upper and lower posterior areas.
- **Direction of ridge resorption**—maxilla resorbs upward and inward to become smaller/**narrower progressively** due to the direction and inclination of roots of upper teeth.
- In mandible, becomes **wider progressively** with age; it inclines outward.

Buccal and labial border anatomy

- Mandibular denture should be wide posterior to buccal frenum; and narrow in anterior labial region.
- Mandibular labial frenum contains a ***band of fibrous CT,*** which helps to attach the orbicularis oris m, so the frenum is active and sensitive.
- **Mandibular labial flange**—is the part b/w labial frenum/notch and the buccal frenum/notch; it is limited, because the fibers of orbicularis oris and incivus labii inferioris ms run closely to the crest of the ridge.
- **Buccal frenum**—the denture should be trimmed functionally and less extended in this area because, buccal frenum connects as a continuous band through the modiolus to the buccal frenum in maxilla.
- Tone of the skin of the lip and orbicularis oris m depends on the thickness of the flange and position of the teeth.
- **Labial flange**—no muscle extends from the residual ridge to the lip b/w the 2 triangularis ms; so the labial flange can be extended in length and thickness to supply the necessary support for the lip.

Buccal vestibule

- **Ante's law** = the PD surface area of the abutment teeth should be at least equal to the teeth replaced. Ideal ratio is 2:1.
- **Ideal C:R ratio** = should be 1 : 2. but recommended is 2:3 ideal; the ratio should be at least 1:1.
- Maxillary first molar has the maximum root surface area/RSA, i.e. 433 sq. mm; the RSA of mandibular first molar is 431 sq. mm.
- Maxillary canines have maximum RSA among the anterior teeth, i.e. 273 sq. mm.
- Mandibular first premolar has the least RSA among the posterior teeth ie 180 sq. mm.
- Mandibular central incisors have least RSA among all the teeth, i.e. 154 sq. mm.

- **Canine replacement** = occlusal scheme should be designed to provide group function in lateral excursions to avoid stresses and never the canine guidance scheme.
- **Resin bonded bridges** = panavia–21 cement is used; it has dual affinity, i.e. it chemically bonds to both enamel and non- precious alloys.

ARTICULATORS

- An articulator is a mechanical device which represent TMJ and Jaw members, to which maxillary and mandibular casts may be attached.
- Movements of articulator should simulate mandibular positions or movements of the patient within the range of normal functional contacts.
- Condylar path is governed partly in its shape and function by the MENISCUS and it moves forward during mandibular movements under lateral pterygoid muscle.
- Path is also controlled by the shape of glenoid fossa.
- Edentulous patients give only one controlling factor (CG) to the movement of mandible.
- IG provided by anteriors is an important part of control.
- IG is always UNDER CONTROL of the DENTIST.
- IG is controlled by overjet and overbite.
- IG is more influential to control mandible movements than the CG because the condylar paths are further away from the cusp incline.

ECCENTRIC RELATION RECORDS

- Ideal amount of protrusion required for making this record is to bring anterior teeth in END-TO-END relation.
- The shape of mandible fossa is an OGEE curve, rather than a straight line.
- Mechanical limitations of most of the articulators required a protrusive movement of at least **6 mm** for adjusting CG.

- For complete registration, the lateral records are necessary to indicate the limit of range of movement as shown by GOTHIC ARCH (needle point) tracing.
- Required lateral movement is to place upper buccal cusps over the lower buccal cusps.
- When needle point of the tracing device is 6 mm from the apex-the mandible in first molar region will be approx 3 mm lateral to its CR.
- During lateral movement—the gap between occlusal surfaces of posterior teeth is more on balancing side than on working side.
- A protrusive record of 6 mm is made, because with a shorter distance, the condyle does not move down its path sufficiently to be recorded properly.

POSTERIOR PALATAL SEAL _____ / details

- Extends between pterygomaxillary/hamular notches.
- Vibrating line of soft palate is a guide for ideal posterior border of denture and is located slightly anterior to the fovea palatinae.
- CD can extend posterior to vibrating line because of the gradual slope of palate.
- A narrow PPS is attained if soft palate is more sloppy and forward in the mouth.
- A wide PPS is attained if soft palate is backwards and gradually sloping.
- Width of PPS seen as a BEAD on CD = 1.0–1.5 mm high; 1.5 mm wide; and 2 mm anterior to the posterior border of CD.
- A wide PPS can displace soft tissues more and so CD is unstable during function.

POSTERIOR TEETH ARRANGEMENT

- BO is the bilateral contact of teeth during function, regardless of mandibular position; used for stability of CD. It is essential during mandibular movements when no food is in the mouth.
- Unbalanced occlusion of CD can lead to breakdown of supporting structures.

- Dr can establish all the factors of occlusion, except the CG, which is the presentation of condylar anatomy.
- Concept of flat OP allows maximum horizontal mandibular movements with the use of NEUTRAL or ZERO DEGREE IG.
- When proper appearance of patient requires an overbite, then cusped posterior teeth should be used, e.g. C_2D_2 type of occlusion.

Factors of centric occlusion details

- CO = position of U/L arches when teeth are in maximum contact.
- CO is the normal termination of masticatory closure.
- CO and CR are same in a child; but with age, the mandible takes a different position for CR there is a difference of approx 1 mm.
- During LIGHT chewing—mandible is in habitual eccentric occlusion, which may be protrusive or lateral or combination.
- But during resistant food chewing—the mandible is completely RETRUDED.
- CR = most posterior relation of mandible to maxilla at the established VR and from which lateral movement can be made at a given degree of jaw separation.
- Eccentric occlusion–is the protrusive and lateral contacts of inclined planes of teeth when jaw is not moving.
- Articulation–is relation of teeth during movements into and away from eccentric position while the teeth are in contact. It is occlusion **IN MOTION.**

Arrangement of posterior teeth

- Vertical overlap and IG. are already established in natural teeth but in CD—it is partly in the **HANDS OF DENTIST.**
- Inclination of condylar path on balancing side is in harmony with the inclines of posterior teeth on working side.
- 2 controlling factors considered in CD occlusion are—CG and IG.
- Other controlling factors are in dentist's control within the limit of esthetics.

- ♦ The more closely the IG angle approaches zero degree, the more stable the CD due to reduction of lateral inclines.

Laws of protrusive occlusion—also know as Hanau's quints

1. Inclination of CG (CG).
2. Inclination of IG (IG).
3. Orientation of OP (PO).
4. Inclination of cusps (CI).
5. Prominence of compensating curves. (CC).
   - CG and IG control the movements of the articulator and are determined before other 3 factors, i.e. OP/CC/IC.
   - OP, cusps inclination, CC can be changed by the DENTIST to attain harmony.
   - CG is the ONLY FACTOR FIXED BY PATIENT. It is obtained by protrusive registration.
   - IG is set BY DENTIST and is influenced by amount of horizontal and vertical overlap.
   - The greater the horizontal overlap—the more it reduces the angle of inclination.
   - Less the vertical overlap—the less will be the angle of inclination.
   - Posterior teeth are closer to the action of incisal inclination than they are to the condylar inclination, so greater influence is exercised on the teeth by IG than by CG.
   - With shallow vertical, the cuspal inclinations are lowered and the rotational centre of mandible is above the level of OP The denture is more stable.
   - With steep vertical overlap and so steep cusp inclination, the rotational centre of mandible is below OP and posterior to mandible and this tends to push denture forward.
   - Rotational centre is determined by drawing the lines at right angle to the IG and CG surfaces.
   - OP orientation is also the **third fixed factors** of occlusion; because lowering/raising its level can lead to esthetic and mechanical troubles.

- Cuspal inclination of tooth is the angle between the total occlusal surface of the tooth and the inclination of the cusp i.r.t. that surface.

$$BO = \frac{CG \times IG}{CI \times CC \times PO}$$

- If CG increases, the CC increases.
- Basic inclination of cusp is steeper when distal end of lower tooth is set higher than mesial end.
- CI can be decreased when the distal end of lower tooth is set lower than mesial end.
- The factor of CC is variable as it allows the dentist to alter CH without changing form of the teeth.

LAWS OF LATERAL OCCLUSION

- 2 end factors are:
  (a) CG incline on balancing side.
  (b) Lingual inclines of maxillary buccal cusps and buccal inclines of lower lingual cusp on the working side.
- These inclines must be harmonious with the path of lower canine to meet upper canine end to end.
- Rational centre in latero-trusion is established by the lines drawn perpendicular to working side inclines, balancing side inclines and balancing side condyle.
- Lateral shift of mandible may occur due to movement of condyles along the lateral inclines of mandibular fossa. This translatory movement is know as **Bennett movement**.
- 15° is the average Bennett movement.
- Angle of inclination on working side is less in posterior area and greater towards the incisal area.
- Also inclination on working side is less compared to balancing side.
- CG is not so great a factor as the amount of IG (as it is selected by Dentist).

- Reduction of cusp inclination is a great stabilizer for CD.
- Since condyles do not move horizontally, there should be some inclination of occluding surface to harmonize with the downward movement of mandible. This cuspal clination should be as flat as possible for stability of CD.
- Cusped teeth give vertical closing forces for mastication. Zero degree cusps cannot shear food. Patients do most of the chewing in CO. A cuspless occlusal scheme eliminates the possibility of deflective occlusal contacts.
- To avoid excess forces falling on the ridge, the lateral and protrusive inclines of CD teeth should be smaller than the natural teeth.
- Teeth with steeper CI should be used with steeper IG.
- An area of freedom should be provided anterior and lateral to CR for any occlusal scheme.
- Primary consideration is to set the first PM to follow the form of residual ridge and should be set slightly buccal to canine.
- Each mandibular tooth is set s.t. the perpendicular at buccal side of crest of residual ridge would bisect the buccal cusp.

When upper teeth setting is done first

- Then the lingual cusps should fall on line indicating the crest of mandibular ridge.
- Mandibular Ist PM is last tooth to be placed, as it may require grinding.
- Also, it has only buccal cusp in occlusion and does not affect the esthetics on grinding.
- The mild spaces are left between maxillary posterior teeth s.t. mandibular teeth may be fitted properly.

Cuspless teeth setting

- Should contact maximally on a CC.
- IG should be zero.
- Protrusive lateral balance is achieved by using second molar ramp.

- No vertical overlap of anteriors.
- 3 point balance effect is achieved.
- If overbite is necessary for esthetics then overjet should also be incorporated.
- CG—zero for cuspless teeth.
- IG–should be zero.
- Posterior limit of mandibular teeth is the point at which the mandibular ridge begins to curve upward. If teeth are to be placed on this slope, they should not contact their antagonist.

Appearance and functional harmony of denture bases

3 factors concerned with functional harmony are:

1. Basal surface
2. Leverage position and occlusal surfaces of teeth.
3. Shape/form of polished surface of dentures.

Most important factor is—the occlusal surface.

Inclination of polished surfaces is determined by 2 end factors, viz.

(a) Width of the border.

(b) Buccolingual position of teeth.

- Buccal surface of mandibular dentures in the first PM region should be shaped carefully so as not to interfere with the action of modiolus.
- Fullness of buccal/labial surfaces of U/L dentures is desirable and the palatal surface should be thin to allow all the space for tongue.
- Lingual flange of mandibular CD should be least bulky except at borders. It should be concave s.t. tongue has a seating action. The buccolingual width should be smaller than the natural teeth for providing space for tongue and also for less occlusal forces to be transmitted to the basal bone.
- Roots of maxillary canine > centrals > laterals.
- But roots of mandibular canine > laterals > centrals.
- Palatal surface of upper CD should be waxed approximately 2.5 mm thick.

- Lingual contours of U/L teeth should be carved in wax to provide a natural feel to the tongue.

Complete rehabilitation of the patient: i.e. occlusal settling

- The occlusion should be checked on the very first touch, when teeth are closed together.
- Old dentures should be kept outside for 24 hours s.t. new CDs are seated on healthy, undistorted tissues.
- Errors in occlusion appear in CDs due to polymerization shrinkage and warpage of acrylic resins.
- Maxilla mandibular relations are bone-to-bone relations.
- Bone is more plastic than mucosa and so any occlusal errors.
- Also inclined plane relation of cusped teeth may change if resins absorb the water.
- The errors should always be located on remounted CDs in articulator. Soft tissues being resilient, the CDs may shift/move during closure in the mouth and may increase the occlusal errors.
- In CR = the jaw should close slowly till the first contact of a back tooth. No pressure should be applied on mandible to retrude it.
- Position of left hand should be: Thumb and fingers are partly between occlusal surfaces of U/L CDs and provide slight resistance to the closure; keep CDs seated; provide tactile sensation to know any shifting of CDs.
- Palm covers the eyes of patient s.t. he is not able to see and react to the expression of dentists.

Inter-occlusal records for remounting CDs

- Errors of occlusion should be removed in articulator after remounting and not in the mouth.
- Protrusive inter occlusal records—mandible brought forward and to bite easily on front teeth. Closure is stopped before any anterior teeth make contact.
- CR record is made by pulling of the mandible backwards and the closure must be stopped before any teeth touch.

Articulator adjustment

- The lateral CG is set after setting horizontal CG (H) by the formula—

$$L = \frac{H}{8} + 12$$

To eliminate occlusal errors

- Articulating paper should be of minimum thickness.
- During centric grinding process—the incisal guide pin should be slightly away from the table to allow for slight reduction of VD.
- Lateral errors are checked, if the IG pin rises during lateral movement—then
  - ⇒ Buccal cups of upper teeth (working).
  - ⇒ Lingual cusp of lower teeth (working side) **(Bull rule)** are reduced.
  - ⇒ On balancing side—lingual side of buccal cusps of lower teeth.
  - ⇒ Grinding to treat occlusal errors in lateral occlusions are limited to—lingual inclines of upper buccal cusps and buccal inclines of lower lingual cusps on working side and lingual inclines of lower buccal cusps on balancing side.
  - ⇒ Lingual upper and buccal lower cusps should not be ground to maintain VDO. These are the **centric cusps**. Other names of the cusps.
  - ⇒ Also, grinding is to be done only in fossae and not on the cusps.
  - ⇒ After completion—there should be uniform contacts on U/L teeth shown by articulating papers.
  - ⇒ Carborundum (abrasive) paste should not be used for it, as VDO will be reduced; area of contact of tooth surfaces is increased; decreased number and size of sluice ways occurs.

Types of errors in occlusaion

- Occlusal errors in CO = 3 types.
- Working side occlusal errors = 6 types.
- Balancing side errors = 2 types.

Occlusal errors in non-anatomic teeth

- Grinding is done on occlusal surfaces of teeth which appear tipped/displaced during processing.
- In eccentric occlusion—DB portion of mandibular 2nd molar is not ground.
- All balancing side grinding is done on lingual portion of occlusal surface of upper 2nd molar.
- Abrasive past can be used here.
- BO helps in maintaining even pressure in all parts of the arch, which maintain the CD stability in functional and para-functional activities.
- Mastication with new CDs is learnt properly in 6–8 weeks.
- Tongue helps in stability of lower denture.
- **Food is pushed inward and upward** to break it with CDs (as cp. to ***Downwards and outward in natural teeth***).

Rest to oral tissues

- Is very necessary for health.
- CDs should be left out of mouth at night to relieve stresses.
- Soft tissues should be cleaned with brushes and finger massage for stimulation and circulation.
- Adhesives and home reliners should not be used—as they change the position of CDs and lead to inadvertent stresses on residual ridges.

Follow up of CD Patients

- First appointment—24 hours after insertion.
- Check shift of CDs—if the teeth touch and slide, there is an error in CO.
- Pressure on **mental Foramen**—numbness in the lower lip at the corner of mouth.
- Pressure on **incisive papilla**—numbness in anterior part of upper jaw.

- **Gagging**—mainly due to making/breaking on PPS during function. Posterior border of upper denture should not be extended more than 2 mm past the vibrating line.
- Retromylohyoid fossa lesion = may be due to pressure due to extended borders.
- **Falling upper CD** on wide opening of mouth—it is **due to DB flange** is very thick and interferes with coronoid process of mandible during opening and lateral movement function.
- If **upper CD loosens** during smiling, it is due to excess thickness or height of flange in the region of buccal notch or posterior to it.
- Acrylic resin base material of CD absorbs water and can change size and occlusion.
- **Soreness** due to occlusal shift—is mostly on the lingual side of mandibular ridge i.r.t., canine and first premolar. Its cause is mostly the deflective occlusal contact on the balancing inclines of lower 2nd molar.

TOOTH SUPPORTED CD

(a) Overdenture

- PO healthy PDL helps maintain alveolar ridge form and bone.
- Roots are maintained in bone by RCT, etc.
- Apply fluoride solution (1% NaF neutral pH on prepared abutment teeth).
- For abutment teeth, the anterior teeth are preferred over posteriors, because the anterior alveolar ridge is more vulnerable to bone resorption/reduction.
- Also **mandibular overdenture is preferred** over maxillary teeth.

(b) Immediate denture are the dentures made before removing all the remaining teeth and is inserted immediately after the removal of the teeth.

- It acts as splint after surgery; prevents humiliating period of healing and esthetic concern, remaining teeth can act as guide for tooth selection.

- Major changes in denture supporting tissues takes 8–12 months. Bony reduction is related to denture-wearing habits and the loading of denture bearing tissues.
- It acts as a splint over the surgical area and prevents breakdown of blood clot.

(c) **Delayed dentures**—prepared dentures are inserted 1–2 weeks or more after extractions. Its objective is to prevent bacteremia during early post-operative period.

(d) **Transitional dentures**—are the interim intermediate dentures, which are given until the stability of denture supporting tissues is achieved and then a new denture is made.

- All posterior teeth are removed except bilateral opposing premolars, which serve as centric stops and prevent decrease of inter-arch distance.
- ***Dual impression technique*** is used for the impression making.
- PO posterior teeth helps determine the level of OP.
- After making a cast, the alternate teeth are cut away and replaced, starting from the central incisors.
- ***Distance between the labial surfaces of the canines*** on the cast is measured to replicate on the teeth setting for proper lip support.
- A deep overbite requires steep IG and hence sharp inclines in all anterior and posterior teeth.
- After delivery, the final occlusal corrections are not made till the healing of tissues, esp 48 hrs to 2 weeks.
- Early pressure should not be placed in the area of immediate extractions especially in anterior area which is more vulnerable to resorption.
- Patient FU is done every 3 months to determine the amount of change.
- Socket calcification takes 8–12 months after extraction, approx 20–30% of bone volume of ridge decreased during 8–12 months. Only then final refitting of denture is done.
- Extensive alveolectomy is done in Angle's C_2 D_1 type of teeth set.

Single CD opposing natural teeth

- In such cases, the objective of BO cannot always be met without altering natural teeth inclines or OP.
- Maxillary CD opposing mandibular natural teeth is more common and safer; but mandibular CD is harmful to upper natural teeth.
- Most common cause of difficulty with occlusion of maxillary denture and mandibular natural teeth is due to inclination of some parts of OP (which occur due to supra-eruption of remaining teeth) of natural teeth, which may cause the maxillary CD to rotate.
- Cross–arch balancing contacts should be developed by teeth preparation for stability.
- If IG is more horizontal, the cuspal inclines are to be decreased more and so more stable will be the CD.
- If RPD/FPD is present in lower arch and maxillary CD—then all the prosthesis should be placed at the same appointment for optimal control and OP development.
- One of the major problems with CD opposing natural teeth is ABRASION. e.g. porcelain in CD can abrade gold/Ag/acrylic and natural teeth.
- Single mandibular CD opposing a natural maxillary arch poses more problems, as leverage leads to undue resorption of mandibular bone.
- Area available in maxillary denture = 45 cm^2.
- Area available in mandibular denture = 12 cm^2.
- **Relining** = denture base material, i.e. acrylic resin is added to the existing denture base, thereby refitting the denture. Done if there is mild to moderate changes in based seat.
- **Rebasing** = the CDs require refitting and reorientation; also to compensate for vertical and horizontal changes in both dentures orientations.
- Shrinkage of bone of maxilla permits upper CD to **move U and B** i.r.t. the original position. But the occlusion may force maxillary CD forward.
- Lower denture moves **D and B** i.r.t. the mandible with shrinkage. Mandible moves forward and upward, causing abnormal stresses due to occlusal prematurities.

IMPLANTS

Types of the casts

1. Working cast.
2. Study/Diagnostic cast = poured by dental stone.
3. Refractory cast.
4. Master cast = by die stone.

Advantages of casts

1. Occlusion from LINGUAL SIDE can be seen.
2. Reference of work progress comparison.
3. Discussion with patient about the Rx plan.
4. Topographic survey of dental arch.
5. Diagnostic wax up.
6. Less chair time—Lab work without patient.
7. Records.
8. For patient awareness/presentation/lectures.
9. Discussion with other Doctors.
10. Permanent patient record.

Tissues	**Important properties/features**
Mandibular labial frenum	• Has a band of **fibrous CT** which helps to attach orbicularis oris muscle, it must be trimmed. • Mandibular denture should be wide posterior to buccal frenum and narrow in anterior labial region.
Mandibular labial flange	• Part of denture between labial frenum/notch and buccal frenum/notch is know as **mandibular.** **LABIAL FLANGE** • It is ***limited by fibers of orbicularis oris*** and incisivus labii inferiors run close to crest of ridge.

Tissues	Important properties/features
Buccal frenum	• Mandibular Buccal frenum passes through the modulus to maxillary BF; these pull actively across the denture borders and surfaces and teeth. So denture ***should be extended less*** in this region and functionally trimming done. • **Thickness of labial flange and position of lower teeth.** • Affect the lower lip; tone of skin of lip and orbicularis oris m.
Labial flange	• Can be extended in length and thickness for supporting the lip. • Because **no muscle extends** from residual ridge to lip between 2 TRIANGULARIS Ms.
Buccal vestibule	• From buccal frenum to outside back corner of RMP area and from crest of ridge to cheek. • Buccinators from modiolus to pterygopalatine raphe; lower side attached in molar region in buccal shelf area, i.e. between ridge and external oblique line. • ***Action of buccinator is in horizontal direction*** and so cannot lift the denture.
Buccal flange	• Extends from buccal frenum to ant. part of masseter; is wide in cheeks; approx ***at right angles to biting forces***. • Provides GREATEST RESISTANCE to vertical occlusal forces. • ***External oblique ridge does not govern*** the extension of buccal flange.
Masseter muscle area	• Distobuccal corner of lower buccal vestibule of mandibular denture is trimmed by action of masseter m., otherwise denture gets displaced.

	mportant properties/features
	• Anterior fibers of masseter m. pass outside the buccinator here. • Pushes inward against buccinator and suctorial pad of cheek.
Distal extension of mandibular impression	• Is defined by ramus, buccinator and retromandibular fossa/RMF. • Buccinator passes from buccal to lingual. • Buccinator attaches to pterygomandibular raphe with superior constrictor. • RMF is formed by continuation of internal and external oblique ridge.
Retromolar region and pad	• RMP must be covered by mandibular denture for perfect seal. • RMP contains glandular tissues + temporal tendon fibers + buccinator + superior constrictor + RM raphe.
Lingual border	• Should be extended below mylohyoid ridge. • Should be made parallel to mylohyoid m. during contraction.
Floor of mouth	• MH m arises from whole length of MH line. • Extends from 1 cm back of distal end of MH ridge to lingual anterior part of mandible at symphysis. • Posteriorly, its fibers continue to the hyoid bone. • MH m lies deep to sublingual gland and other structures in premolar region. • Posterior part of MH m in molar region affects lingual impression during swallowing and tongue movements. • MH m is attached more superiorly on mandible in posterior region and so it **affects the slope of lingual flange** in molar area and so flange slopes towards the tongue.

Tissues	Important properties/features
	• Lingual flange is ***extended below the palpable part*** of MH ridge to avoid direct pressure on this sharp edge of bone to reduce soreness. • Also, lingual flange completes seal in retromylohyoid fossa and guides the tongue on the top of flange. • MH is also known as ORAL DIAPHRAGM. • Sublingual glands lies above the MH m.
Lingual frenum	• Should be registered in function by functional trimming, as it comes close to the crest of the ridge.
Lingual flange	• Its lower border runs parallel to the lower edge of mandible from lingual frenum to posterior end of denture. • It is shorter in anterior part and longer in posterior part. • Posteriorly, extension is bounded partially by glossopalatine m, which lies at distal extension of RMP. • Occupies alveolo-lingual sulus (ALS). • Distal ends of ALS ends at RM curtain. • RMC is pulled forward when tongue is thrust out. • Distal end of lingual flange is partly limited by glossopalatine arch. • GP arch is formed by GP m and lingual extension of sup. constrictor m. • Lingual flange is influenced by MH m in molar region. • Ant. part of lingual flange over the sublingual gland is shallow because mobility of tissues are controlled by MH m.

Tissues	Important properties/features
	• Lingual flange is of **S shape curve** as: 1. From midline, it curves outwards following curve of residual ridge. 2. At pre-mylohyoid eminence, the flange curves away from mandible to accommodate MH m. on contraction. 3. At distal end of MH ridge, the flange turns laterally towards ramus to fill retro-mylohyoid fossa. • Distal end of lingual flange is known as retromylohyoid eminence.
Alveolo-Lingual sulcus and its 3 areas	• Is space between residual ridge and tongue; occupied by lingual flange. • Extends from lingual frenum to retro-mylohyoid curtain. • **Anterior region** = from lingual frenum to pre-mylohyoid fossa/eminence. • **Middle region** = from mylohyoid fossa to the distal end of mylohyoid ridge. 1. Sulcus curves mesially from the body of mandible. 2. Curvature is caused by prominence of MH ridge. 3. The part slopes towards the tongue which rests on the flange and helps stabilizing the lower denture. • **Posterior region** = is retro-mylohyoid space/fossa. 1. Extends from end of MH ridge to retro-MH curtain. 2. Bound by anterior tonsillar pillar on lingual side; by RMH curtain and sup. constrictor muscle on distal end; and by MH m, ramus and RMP on buccal side.

Tissues	Important properties/features
	• Denture border should contact RMH curtain. • In the border of lingual flange is a **S-shape curve**.
Buccal shelf	• Located posterior to buccal frenum and extends from crest of ridge to external oblique ridge. • Fibres of buccinator run horizontally in submucosa immediately overlying the bone. • ***Bone of buccal shelf is COMPACT bone.*** • It is ***most suitable PRIMARY STRESS BEARING AREA.*** • Impression tray is in direct contact with mucosa here and so soft tissue is slightly displaced and so additional load can be placed on the supporting tissues.
RMP area	• Non-keratinized epithelium. • Submucosa contains = glandular tissue + buccinator fibers + sup. constrictor m. fibers + pteryomandibular raphe + terminal part of tendon of temporalis m. • It should be **registered in a resting position**.

Classification of mandibular impressions

1. **Pressure impression**
   - No space for the final impression material.
   - Denture may cause ***rapid resorption of residual ridge***.
2. **Selective pressure impression**
   - Space for final impression material in some places than other.
   - Spaces with less relief will transmit more pressure in favorable part of bone, i.e. buccal shelf and vice-versa.
3. **Pressureless impression**
   - i.e. with ***least possible displacement*** of soft tissues.
   - Taken with ***very fluid type of impression materials***.

Impression making

- Metal tray selected—which provides approx 6 mm (1/4 inch) bulk of impression material over the entire basal seat area.
- A wax spacer approx 1 mm thick is placed over crest and slope of ridge.
- Buccal shelf on each side and retro—MH spaces are left uncovered –s.t. More pressure can be placed in primary stress bearing area.
- Special tray of 2–3 mm thick is made of acrylic.
- 2 additional handles, one each in molar region are placed, to be used as finger rests.
- Lingual flange is shorter anteriorly than posteriorly.
- Flange becomes longer and extend below the level of mh line in canine-premolar region at pre-mh fossa.
- Lingual flange must slope towards the tongue parallel to the fibers of MH ms in molar region.
- Distal end of lingual flange is 1cm distal to the end of MH ridge. It turns laterally towards ramus below the level of rmp and MH ridge.
- The distal end of lingual flange is activated by mouth opening and tongue protrusion to activate superior constrictor m. in retromolar/RM curtain.
- On closing the mouth against resistance, the medial pterygoid m. Gets activated against rm curtain and limits the space for border in RM fossa.
- Holes about 1/2 inch about are placed in the tray in the centre of alveolar groove.
    - In retromolar fossa.
    - Help to relieve pressure on crest of residual ridge and RMP.
- Border of tray should be 0.5–1.0 mm short for final impression material.
- Minimum tissue displacement and pressure.
- Existing dentures are left out of mouth for 24 hrs to allow the tissues of buccal seat to return to health and undistorted form.

- **Boxing**—wax should extend about 9–15 mm to provide appropriate thickness to the base of cast.
- Tongue is protruded out = to determine distal extent of lingual flange.
- Wide opening of mouth = pulls pterygomandibular raphe forward against the lingual side of part of retromolar pad—i.e. distal extension of occlusal part is defined.
- Closing month against resistance—activates medial pterygoid.

ANATOMICAL CONSIDERATIONS

- Mandibular fossa is 1″ long antero-posteriors and 3/4 inch in width medio-laterally.
- Condyles project out beyond the distal part of the fossa and can be felt in the soft tissues.
- Fossa is divided into 2 parts by the petrotympanic fissure, in which anterior tympanic branch of internal maxillary A passes.
- Chorda tympani nerve passes through the canal of Huguier (iter chordae anterius).
- Anterior part of mandibular fossa is the principal bearing surface on which the condyle presses through the disk.

Condyles (Also refer to the section of anatomy in Vol. I).

- 3/4″ wide × 1/2″ AP diameter.
- Does not fill the fossa to its AP limits.
- Condyles extend 1/2″ beyond the bony limits of the meatus laterally.
- Capsular ligament completely envelops the TMJ; attached to the rim of mandibular fossa and articular eminence to the neck of condyle; the fibers run Downward and Backward.
- **TM ligament**—fibers run Downward and Backward (D/B); extends from articular eminence and inferior border of zygomatic arch to the outer/posterior border of upper part of ramus. It limits the posterior movement of condyle.
- **Sphenomandibular ligament**—runs from the angle of sphenoid to lingula of inferior mandibular foramen; runs down on inner surface of ramus.

- **Stylomandibular ligament**—from styloid process to the medial side of angle of mandible and at its posterior border.

Articular disk: (Also refer to the section of anatomy in Vol. I).

- Made of collagen fibers.
- Concavo-convex shape.
- Extends forward over the articular eminence.
- Position and movement are controlled by capsular ligament and lateral pterygoid m.
- It has extensive movements when mandible makes wider opening lateral protrusive movements.
- Disk can't move from side to side.
- TMJ is applied by auriculo-temporal N (mostly, 90%) + deep temporal + masseteric N.

Muscles of mastication–4 (Also refer to the section of anatomy in Vol. I).

- Masseter, medial pterygoid, Temporalis ms are closing ms.
- Lateral pterygoid is a guiding m/opening m.

Temporalis m

- ***Anterior fibers*** = run along coronoid process, anterior border of ramus and some fibers in RMP area.
- ***Posterior part*** = helps to retrude the mandible and braces the condyle during lateral movement.
- **Middle parts** = elevate the mandible in centric position.
- Temporalis m does not participate in biting force.

Masseter m

- 2 parts = superficial and deep.
- Elevates the mandible mainly.
- Deep fibers aid in retrusion also.
- Trim DB/disto-buccal corner of buccal flange of CD and border converges rapidly toward RMP.

Medial pterygoid m

- First part arises from medial surface of lateral pterygoid plate and the palatine bone.
- 2nd part arises from pyramidal process of palatine bone and posterior end of maxilla.
- Inserts on lower and posterior surfaces of ramus and into medial side of angle of mandible.
- Action = mostly ELEVATION; assists in lateral and protrusive movements of mandible.

Lateral pterygoid m—2 heads

- Superior belly = from greater wing of sphenoid bone.
- Inferior belly = from lateral pterygoid plate.
- Fibers run horizontally back-wards and laterally.
- Superior belly = attaches mostly to disk and neck of condyle.
- Inferior belly = inserts at the neck of condyle.
- Principal action = protrusion of condyles.
- When one lateral pterygoid m. contracts, the mandible moves to opposite side.
- Helps in food to be engaged by the teeth.
- **Superior belly** = stabilizes/floxes the condyle/disk in specific position during elevation of mandible. But it does not elevate the mandible.

Ms of depression—3 groups of ms

1. Suprahyoid ms = digastrics, geniohyoid, mylohyoid, stylohyoid and platysma.

   –are the primary movers in opening of the mandible.
2. Infrahyoid group = stabilizes the hyoid bone s.t. suprahyoid group can be effective.
3. Lateral pterygoid ms = pull the condyles forward or medially.

Mylohyoid m—is the ***only muscle of these groups which affects the denture borders***.

- Originates from MH ridge.
- Extends from symphysis to distal aspect of 3rd molars.
- Closer to the crest of alveolar process in 3rd molar/posterior region on lingual side of mandible and travels forward.
- Runs medially and D and F.
- Inserts in midline and to the anterior cornu of hyoid bone.
- MH with geniohyoid muscles forms the floor of mouth.
- **Principal action** = assists in swallowing by raising the tongue.
- Also helps in opening of mandible.

JAW RELATIONS

- All jaw relations are BONE-TO-BONE relations.
- **Orientation relations**—establish the references in the cranium.
- **Vertical relations**—establish the amount of jaw separation.
- **Horizontal relations**—establish the front-to-back and side-to-side relation of one jaw to the other.
- **Orientation relations**—orient the mandible to cranium s.t. when mandible is in most posterior position, the mandible can rotate in sagittal plane around an axis passing through or near the condyles.
- **Face bow**—is used to record the relation of jaws to TMJ or opening axis of the jaws; the record is not a maxillo-mandibular record.

Arbitrary face bow—used in CD patients; locates approximate location of condyles axis.

- The rods are placed **13 mm in front** of external auditory meatus on a line from outer canthus of eye to top of tragus.
- It locates the axis within 5 mm of true centre of opening axis of the jaws.
- Fork of this face bow is attached to the maxillary occlusal rim.

Kinematic face bow

- The fork is attached to mandibular occlusal rim.
- Locates condylar axis MORE ACCURATELY.
- Mandible is then in CR position.
- Posterior terminal hinge axis (THA) can be located only when mandible is in its most posterior position.
- Since in edentulous mandible, the occlusal rim is not as stable when face bow is attached, so its more extensive use in edentulous patients is not possible.
- If the vertical separation/VD of casts or CD is to be reduced on the articulator, the face bow record is essential.
- Face bow transfer allows a more accurate arc of closure on articulation
- Kinematic face bow helps in finding the kinematic centre of jaw opening.
- **Hanau model face bow** and other arbitrary bows are located at a point 13 mm forward from external auditory meatus.
- **Whip mix face bow**—its ends are placed in auditory meatus instead of on condyles. THA is 15 mm anterior to the position of ends of the face bow.

VERTICAL RELATIONS

Are of 2 types – VR in occlusion VDO
– VR in rest position VDR

VDR is **physiological rest position**.

- Established by ms and gravity.
- Is the postural relation of the 2 jaws.
- Teeth do not determine its vertical level.
- All the closing and opening ms are in minimum tonic contraction only to maintain the posture.
- ***Position of Head*** is important—must be upright and not supported by head rest.
- Helps as a guide to the lost VDO.

- ***Free way space***/inter-occlusal gap IOG is = VDR–VDO difference; is 2–4 mm in first premolar region.
- IOG is essential for health of PDL.
- If IOG is not there clicking of CDs occurs; rapid destruction of residual alveolar bone due to heavy forces; tissue soreness occurs, etc.

HORIZONTAL RELATIONS

- Basic horizontal relation is CR (centric relation).
- **Centric relation**/CR is the most posterior relation of mandible to maxilla at established vertical relation.
- **Eccentric relations**—i.e. deviations from CR, e.g. lateral; protrusive, etc. in horizontal plane; but changes also occur in vertical relations. It is also occur in vertical relations. It is know as ***CHRISTIANSEN phenomenon***. It develops spaces between U/L occlusal surfaces at posterior end of occlusion rim/CD.

Factors regulating jaw motion

- Rim system.
- Guiding influence of teeth.
- Mandibular ms.
- Occlusal surfaces of the teeth in c.d. should meet evenly on both sides during centric and eccentric jaw positions (***balanced occlusion***).
- It provides stability to dentures and mandible is not deflected.
- Inclined places of teeth should pass smoothly over each other and should be harmonious with other factors regulating jaw position.
- CG and IG should not be disrupted.

TMJ

- Upper compartment = primarily TRANSLATION movements occur.

- Lower compartment = primarily ROTATION movements occur.
- TRANSLATION means all points within the body move at the same velocity and in the same direction.
- Condyles can translate anteroposteriorly by approx 3/4″ (18 mm).
- During opening/closing movements—the mandible moves in SAGITTAL PLANE around a TRANSVERSE AXIS passing through both condyles.
- In lateral excursion—mandible rotates around a vertical axis which, passing through **working condyle** and the balancing/non-working condyle moves downwards, forwards and medially. It is a form of translation occurring in superior compartment of TMJ.
- Downward movement of balancing condyle causes working condyle to rotate around a sagittal axis.

Direct lateral side shift of mandible

- Occurs simultaneously with lateral movement of mandible (Bennett 1908), known as **Bennett movement**. It is due to mesial/inward movement of balancing condyle and lateral/outward movement of working condyle.
- Is an important component of lateral jaw movement.

MUSCLE ACTIVITY

Temporalis m

- Middle/Posterior part = activity increased during hinge openings and retrusion of mandible.
- Activity decreased during uncontrolled mandibular opening.
- Posterior part braces mandible during lateral excursions to the same side.
- **Temporal m** = posterior part is more horizontal than anterior and middle.
- **ISOTONIC** contraction of posterior fibers moves the mandible in CR or to hold it in most posterior position during terminal hinge movement.

Lateral pterygoid m

- Plays MAJOR ROLE in uncontrolled mandibular opening.
- It has very little role in hinge openings movements 3.
- It moves mandible forward or side ways.
- It remains inactive during mandibular terminal hinge opening movements.
- Responsible for forward movements of condyle and mandible during uncontrolled opening movements.
- Sup. belly of lat. pterygoid = fixes and stabilizes the condyle and disk during elevation of the mandible.
- It also helps in adjusting the horizontal CG and lateral CG/Bennett movement of the articulator.

Digastric ms are = very active in uncontrolled opening, retrusion and hinge opening movements of mandible.

Suprahyoid ms = produce rotary jaw movements around a transverse mandibular hinge axis.

Important points

- For CD patients, the occlusion of artificial teeth can be perfected better on articulator than in mouth, because CDs move on basal tissues, but not on articulator.
- There is only one true CR and it coincides with the most retruded position in skull.
- **Isotonic contraction** (ms fibers shorten in length during contraction and cause movement of a part) of posterior temporalis and in combination with suprahyoid ms—position the mandible in CR.
- **Isometric contraction** (ms maintain same length during contraction and fix a part in a particular location) = maintain mandible in CR during making an inter-occlusal CR records.

Neuro-muscular regulation of mandibular movements

- Impulses from subconscious level including RAS also regulate muscle tone = plays a primary role in physiologic ***rest position*** of the mandible.

- Proprioceptors are located in PDL, mandibular ms and ligaments = provide information about ***location of mandible*** in space.
- Impulses from oral receptors travel to sensory nucleus of 5th N.
- Impulses from proprioceptors go to ***mesencephalic nucleus***.
- Impulses then can go to sensorimotor cortex (conscious level) to produce VOLUNTARY changes in mandibular position or to motor nucleus of 5th N and then to mandibular ms (in a reflex arc) causing INVOLUNTARY movements of mandible.
- Due to loss of receptors in PDL in edentulous mouth causes loss of control of mandibular position.
- **Mastication**—is a programmed event residing in a CHEWING CENTRE located in brain-stem (in reticular formation of PONS).

CEREBELLUM

- Acts as feed back control.
- Does not initial mandibular movements.
- Compares information from outer cortex, etc. to the sensory information received form periphery.
- Sends signals back to motor cortex to excite antagonist ms and inhibit agonist ms—to generate a coordinated response from muscles.

Parallelogram of forces

- Direction of pull of posterior temporalis = upward and Backward.
- Direction of pull of anterior temporalis = more Upward and Forward.
- Direction of pull of superficial masseter and direction of pull of medial pterygoid = more Upward and Forward.
- Direction of pull of deep masseter m = more Upward and Backward.
- Direction of pull of resultant forces = exerted in line with long axes of teeth.

ENVELOPE OF MOTION IN SAGITTAL PLANE—i.e. maximum border movements. It is roughly **tear-drop shaped**.

- Tracing starts at most protruded position of mandible with teeth in contact.
- Dip in top line of tracing occurs as incisal edges of U and L anterior teeth pass across each other, when mandible is moved posteriorly.
- As CO is reached = U/L posterior teeth get maximally inter-cuspated.
- At CR = mandible is further retruded.
- Single restorations are generally made in harmony with CO; while multiple restorations and CD are made with their occlusion in harmony with CR.
- On opening mandible from CR, i.e. when mandible is most retruded position, opening can be done in this retruded position ***without any condylar translation*** till MHO (Maximum Hinge Opening) position.
- Any opening beyond MHO = condyle moves Downwards and Forwards; translation occurs.
- The track CR–MHO is know as ***posterior terminal hinge movements***. It is used to locate transverse hinge axis.
- At maximum opening—the jaws are separated maximally and condyles are in most anterior position in the mandibular fossa.
- Pathways of masticating cycle occur anterior to the line representing the terminal hinge movement.
- For edentulous patients, the teeth should contact evenly throughout the normal range of function.
- Mandibular rest position occurs somewhere downward and slightly forward from CR.
- At habitual rest position—the only ms activity is minimal tonic contraction required to support the mandible against the force of gravity.

Envelop of motion in FRONTAL PLANE

- Is **shield shaped.**
- Dip in upper line is seen = as U/L canines pass edge to edge.

♦ Masticatory cycle contacts the superior border of envelop at CO—it shows that opposing teeth penetrated the bolus and contacted each other.

BIOLOGICAL CONSIDERATIONS OF VERTICAL RELATIONS

VDR is assumed when ms of jaws are ***in a state of minimal contraction*** to maintain posture of mandible.

Physiological rest position—controlled by ms and force of gravity; posture of head should be upright and unsupported.

Physiological rest position = allows supporting tissues to take rest and so health is maintained, otherwise destruction/resorption of alveolar bone occurs due to continuous pressure.

Masseter, medial pterygoid and temporalis ms are closing ms to establish vertical jaw relations.

Opening ms are inframandibular and suprahyoid ms + Digastric + Platysma + GRAVITY = all help to control the TONIC BALANCE and rest position.

IOG is essential for closing ms, opening ms and gravity to be in balance when ms are in minimum tonic contraction.

Establishing VR

A. Excessive interarch distance (VD) should not be there, it causes:

- Premature contact of teeth.
- Clicking of CDs.
- Bone resorption/destruction.

B. Reduced VD

- Decreases biting forces.
- But facial expression are not good.
- Over closure of mouth; purse-string appearance may occur.
- Lips loose their fullness; decreased ms tone.
- Creases appear at corners of mouth and may lead to PRELECHE due to candidal infections.

- Leads to loss of CUBICLE space of oral cavity.
- Push tongue in the throat and may block EUSTACHIAN TUBE, so hearing and ear problems may appear.
- TMJ Trauma—may cause decreased VDO and its S/S are = clicking, headache, neuralgia, obscure pain and discomfort.
- **Rx denture**—VDO should be built/increased gradually, in successive sets of CDs.

METHODS TO DETERMINE VERTICAL RELATIONS

Mechanical methods

(a) Ridge relations

- Incisive papilla is a stable landmark.
- Incisive papillae is **4 mm** from incisal edge of lower anteriors, in normal natural dentition.
- Incisal edge of maxillary CI is **6 mm below** the incisive papilla.
- Average vertical overlap of U/L Central incisors = 2 mm.
- Correct amount of jaw separation = according to Sears, is paralleling of U/L ridges plus a 5° opening in posterior region.
- The residual ridges in the posterior region are parallel to each other.
- Crest of U/L residual ridges are parallel to each other at VDO, which provides ideal situation for denture stability.

(b) Physiological rest position tests

- Help to determine vertical relation of mandible to maxilla.
- Patient is asked to swallow and let the jaw relax.
- IOG should be 2–4 mm at rest position when seen in premolar region.

(c) PHONETICS/ESTHETICS as GUIDES

- **Ch, s, j, sounds** brings the U/L anterior teeth very close together, almost (but without) touching them.
- If teeth click = VDO is probably too great.

- Contour of lips depends on contour of labial surfaces of occlusion rims/AP position of teeth and contour of base of CD.

(d) **Esthetic guide** = selection of teeth the same size as natural teeth and estimation of amount of tissue loss from alveolar ridge.

(e) **SWALLOWING METHOD**

- On swallowing, the teeth come together with a very light contact at beginning of the swallowing cycle.

BIOLOGICAL CONSIDERATIONS OF HORIZONTAL JAW RELATIONS

♦ For best stability of CD, the opposing teeth should meet evenly on both sides within normal final range of mandibular movements. It is know as balanced occlusion.

Centric relation is a:

♦ ***Bone to bone relation***.

♦ Is a type of horizontal relation.

♦ **CR** is the most retruded unstrained position of condyles in glenoid fossa at a given degree of opening.

♦ Is the most posterior relation of the mandible to maxilla at established VR along the pathway of THM.

♦ Is a reference relation, which is **constant for each individual patient**.

♦ Is a mandibular position determined by the nm/neuromuscular reflex learned when primary teeth are in occlusion.

♦ Centres of vertical and lateral motion are in their posterior THP.

♦ Posterior and middle parts of temporalis and suprahyoid m (geniohyoid and digastric ms) move and fix the mandible in its most retruded relation to the maxilla.

♦ Masseter, medial pterygoid and temporalis ms/(MMT) ms elevate the mandible to a particular vertical relation with maxilla.

♦ Lateral pterygoid/LT m shows little activity when mandible is in its CR.

Centric occlusion/CO is a **tooth-to-tooth relation** of U and L teeth.

- Edentulous patients cannot control mandibular movements or avoid deflective occlusal contacts in CR due to loss of receptors in PDL.
- CR must be recorded for edentulous patients to establish CO in harmony.
- Upper cast is accurately oriented to the opening axis of articulator by location of a physiologic terminal hinge axis/THA and a face bow transfer.
- At THA—there is NO TRANSLATION movement occurs.
  - is within THM/terminal hinge movments.
  - mandible is most retruded i.r.t. maxillary.
  - THM are those posterior border movements, which occur without translation.
- A VDO should be established between 2 jaws to provide adequate inter occlusal gap/IOG and allow the mandibular ms to function at their optimal physiologic length.
- With face bow-casts should be mounted to a physiologic THA to correspond with THA of articulator.
- CR serves as a references relation for establishing an occlusion. CR is a HORIZONTAL relation used to orient the lower cast to the upper cast for CD patients.
- Edentulous patients use CR closures in mastication and in other functions, e.g. Swallowing.
- CR permits ***proper adjustments of CG***/condylar guidance for control of eccentric movements.
- CR orients the lower cast to the opening axis of articulator and orients CR to hinge axis of articulator and mandible.
- CR records can be made either by minimal closing pressures or under heavy closing pressures.
- If minimal closing pressures is used, the occlusion should be tested under heavy pressure.

- Minimal pressure teeth produces the BEST results for most patients.

REALEFF—is the tissue resiliency.

- Known as **phase resiliency and like effect**.
- Undue pressure in securing the relation must be avoided to eliminate the possibility of excessive displacement of soft tissues.
- Materials used for minimal pressure technique are—soft POP, ZOE or soft wax.
- Minimal pressure should be applied to avoid distortion of soft tissues and especially if the tissue depth is uneven and opposing ridge relation or size is not normal.
- Temporal m. shows reduced functions when the mandible is in a protruded position.

Recording CR

- **Static methods** = advantage is that it causes minimal displacement of recording bases on the basal seat.
- **Functional methods**—involve functional activity/movement of mandible at the time of recording. The disadvantage is that it causes lateral and AP displacement of recording bases.
- Swallowing procedure establishes both proper vertical and horizontal relation of mandible to maxilla.

Extra-oral tracings

Gothic arch tracing/arrow point tracings

- Are made ***in horizontal plane*** to record the relation of U/L jaws.
- To find out ***true retruded position of mandible, indicated by sharp apex*** of tracing.
- This centre point varies at different levels of VDO.
- Extra-oral tracings are preferred over intra-oral tracings, as I/O tracings are very small and not clear.
- Central bearing point should not be used when ridge relation is not normal or when there is excess soft tissue on the ridges.

- **Neutral zone** = given by Fish; is a portion of equilibrium of tongue, lips and cheek forces. It is occupied by the teeth and polished surface of CD.

Level of occlusal plane/OP

- Incisal plane is parallel to **interpupillary line**.
- Height should be adjusted to allow for the length of natural tooth and the amount of tissue resorption.
- **2 mm below** the border of upper lip.
- OP posteriorly should be parallel to the **ala-tragus line**.

- **Occlusal table** = i.e. mandibular occlusal surfaces; is an area bounded by cheek, tongue, pterygomandibular raphe and its overlying tissues posteriorly, and the contraction of corner of mouth anteriorly.
- **Modiolus = 8 muscles meet** at the corner of mouth; becomes fixed when buccinator contracts; presses corner of mouth at premolars to close the occlusal table in front/mesially; food can not escape at corner of mouth unless 7th damaged (e.g. Bell's Palsy).
- RMP are relatively **STABLE posterior landmarks** even in patients with advanced ridge resorption.
- Mandibular first molar = is at a level corresponding to ***two thirds of the way up*** the RMP.
- To test the correct VDO—the ***average speaking space*** or interocclusal/inter-rim space is observed on making **'S' sound** (e.g. sixty six).
- This speaking space between posterior teeth is not related to inter-occlusal space of rest position.
- This space is 1.5–3 mm for most of the patients.
- Patients with Class II m.o. have large space (3–6 mm).
- Patients with Class III m.o. have small space = 1 mm.

Arch form

- Natural teeth are in a zone of equilibrium/neutral zone, which is the resultant of all the forces acting on it [**Buccinator mechanism**].

- **Best guide** = consider pattern of bone resorption and use stable anatomic landmarks.

Mandibular Arch form

1. Pattern of Bone loss

- From labial side of anterior residual ridge.
- Equally on buccal and lingual sides of the ridge in PM region.
- Mainly on lingual side of ridge in MOLAR REGION, because mandible is wider at its inferior border than at ridge crest.
- Residual ridge becomes more lingually in anterior region and more bucally in posterior region.
- Lingual surfaces of posterior teeth should be placed on a line joining lingual side of RMP to a point just lingual to crest of ridge in PM region.
- Corners of mouth determine approx location for C and First PM.
- In cases of advanced anterior ridge reduction, when mentalis m migrates to the crest of ridge = surgical labial sulcus deepening is done.

Maxillary Arch form

Bone loss occurs at

- Labial and buccal areas of maxillary residual ridge.
- So ridge is usually PALATAL to the original location of the natural teeth.
- **Incisive papilla** is a very stable landmark on the palate.
- Incisal edges of max. CI are = **8–10 mm anterior** to the centre of incisive papilla.
- Tips of canines are ± 1 mm in front of the CENTRE of papilla.
- Canines should be located in a coronal **plane passing through posterior border of the papillae**.

Degenerative changes in skin appear if not proper lip support is there as:

- Deep vertical lines in body and margin of lips (**Purse-string appearance**).

- ♦ Shortening and thinning of lips.
- ♦ Tendency for lip margins to roll inwards.
- ♦ Nasolabial fold changes direction; becomes continuous with the groove at the corner of mouth.
- ♦ Cheek support is not affected as much as lip, because buccinator m is stretched between modiolus and pterygomandibular raphe.
- ♦ Anterior part of maxillary occlusal rim is gently caressed by the lower lip during pronunciation of the letter **'f'**.

4 jaw relations are transferred from the patient to the articulator— It helps to simulate jaw movements.

1. Relation of jaws to opening axis.
2. Vertical separation of jaws.
3. Horizontal relation of U/L jaws in CR.
4. Relation of lower jaw to upper jaw when incisors are edge to edge.

ARTICULATOR—is a mechanical device to which U/L casts may be attached, to represent TMJ and Jaw members.

Theories of occlusion—3:

1. BONWILL THEORY

- Teeth move i.r.t. each other as guided by condylar controls and incisal point.
- Also known as ***theory of equilateral triangle.***
- **4″ (10 cm)** inter-condylar distance and between each condyle and the mid-incisal point.
- Its articulator allows lateral movement also.
- But CG is not adjustable, so movement permitted were in horizontal plane.

2. CONICAL THEORY

- Lower teeth move over surfaces of upper teeth as over the surface of a cone, at a **generating angle of 45°**
- Central axis of cone is tipped at a 45° angle.
- Teeth with 45° cusps are necessary for making CD on Hall–articulator.

3. **SPIERICAL THEORY**—By Monson (1918).
   - Lower teeth move on the surface of upper teeth, as over the surface of a sphere with a **diameter of 8″** (20 cm).
   - Centre of sphere is located in the region of glabella.
   - Surface of sphere passes through the glenoid fossa along the ARTICULAR EMINENCES.
   - Based on relation of teeth with skull observed by von Spee.

TYPES OF RECORDS ON ARTICULATOR—3 classes of records for transferring maxillo-mandibular relations are taken:

1. **Inter occlusal record adjustment**
2. **Graphic record adjustment**
   - Graphic records consists of records of extreme border positions of mandibular movements, which are in CURVES.
   - Articulator must be capable of producing equivalent of these curved movements.
3. **Hinge axis location for adjusting articulators.**
   - H.A. of patients should be correctly located for correct adjustment of the articulators, e.g. transograph.

Selection of articulators

1. If occlusal contacts are to be perfected in CO only = A HINGE TYPE of articulator or one-dimensional instrument, without lateral/protrusive movement is enough.
2. If denture teeth are to have cross-arch and cross-tooth balanced occlusion/BO = A SEMI-ADJUSTABLE articulator is required, e.g. Hanau; whip-mix, etc.
3. If complete control of occlusion is required = A FULLY ADJUSTABLE articulator is required.
   - But these articulators are problematic because of RESILIENCY OF BASAL SOFT TISSUES.

HANAU—is semi-adjustable, arcon type articulator.

- Is a modified 2–D instrument.
- Hanau face bow = U shaped; 2–3″ away from face in front and wide enough not to touch side of the face.

- Condyle rods are placed 13 mm in front of external auditory meatus, on a lateral canthus tragus line.
- The condylar rods will be located with in 2 mm of true centre of opening axis of the jaws.
- Horizontal CG is adjusted by = inter-occlusal protrusive record.
- Lateral CG = adjusted by right and left lateral inter-occlusal records.
- IG table = to adjust lateral incisal guidance.
- Incisal pin on Hanau is adjustable and allows for vertical changes.
- Inter condylar distance is adjustable, though this adjustment is rarely done in CD construction, but is required in FPD construction.

RELATING patient to whip mix articulator.

- Is semi adjustable, arcon type articulator.
- Upper and lower members are not mechanically connected.
- Inter condylar distance is semi-adjustable to small (88 mm), medium (100 mm) and large (112 mm) (i.e. a difference of 12 mm b/w each type).
- Vertical axis of rotation of mandible can be approximated.
- Lateral plates of adjustable incisal guide table can be adjusted for later IG.
- Balancing condyle moves D/F/M and working condyle moves laterally (i.e. Bennett shift).
- Face bow is anteriorly located in the region of infra orbital notch.
- Nasion relator determines vertical position of face bow anteriorly and establishes axis-orbital plane on the patient.
- Metal rods of face bow are located = 6 mm posteriorly from actual transverse axis of articulator to compensate for the location of ear posts in auditory meatus, which are roughly the same distance posterior from mandibular THA of the patient.

OCCLUSAL RIM

- Size and form of rim represents the dental arch of natural teeth plus part of ridge resorbed.

- Occlusal rim may be slightly above the Vermillion border of the upper lip if the lip is long.
- In normal lip–U rim is 2 mm visible below the relaxed upper lip.
- OP is made parallel to ALA TRAGUS line.
- Lower occlusal rim anteriorly at the level of corner of mouth and posteriorly at the level of post. 1/3rd of RMP. This height approximates level of OP.

TEETH SELECTION

- Best way to find colour/form/size of teeth is = By trial in patients mouth.
- Diagnostic cast of the natural teeth are most RELIABLE guide in selection and arranging the anteriors.
- Photos = width of teeth and outline form can be seen.
- R/G images = slightly enlarged and distorted due to divergence of x-rays.
- Women's teeth are smaller than men's teeth, especially LI.
- Approximately canines are placed at the corners of the mouth.
- Apex of maxillary natural canine is found by extension of parallel lines from the lateral surfaces of the alae of nose on to middle of the labial surface of upper occlusal rim.
- Greatest bizygomatic width divided by 3.3 = overall width of upper 6 anteriors.
- Ratio of cranial circumference to the width of upper anteriors = 10:1.
- Av. width of upper anteriors = 48–52 mm

  < 48 mm = Small teeth.

  > 52 mm = Large teeth.

FORM OF ANTERIOR TEETH

- Should harmonize with the shape of patients face, e.g. square/tapering/ovoid.
- Shape of LABIAL surface is more important than the outline form.

- Grinding should be done on anteriors according to age of the patient.
- Labial face of tooth viewed from proximal aspect = should show PROFILE/CONTOUR OF FACE, i.e. convex/straight/concave.
- Labial surface of tooth as viewed from incisal edge = should be similar to contour of face as seen from under the chin.
- **LEON–WILLIAM'S RULE.**
- Broad contact areas look more natural, because long contact surfaces give a truer appearance of age.
- **SPA concept**—i.e. **dentogenic concept** is based on sex/personality/age of the patient.

♦ Squareness of tooth form = MUSCULANITY.

♦ Rounded incisal and proximal contours = femininity.

♦ LI smaller than CI feminine.

♦ LI almost equal to CI musculine.

COLOUR OF TEETH—colour of face and teeth came from the effects of reflected light on the rods and cones of retina.

♦ Colour of **most concern to dentists** is = **yellow band** in spectrum, because colours of face and teeth are primarily yellow.

4 qualities of colour are:

(a) Hue
(b) Saturation (chroma)
(c) Brilliance (value)
(d) Translucency

HUE—is the specific colour produced by a specific wavelength of light acting on retina.

♦ It is the COLOUR itself.

♦ Must be in harmony with face.

CHROMA

♦ Amount of colour per unit of area of an object, i.e. same colour but different shade/concentration.

VALUE—i.e. brilliance (Light or Dark).

- Is the lightness or darkness of an object.
- Variance is produced by **dilution of the colour** (i.e. hue) by black or white.
- It must correspond to the lightness/darkness of the patient's face.
- In fair people = teeth are of less colour; Colours are less saturated; teeth are lighter in colour.
- In dark people = darker teeth.

TRANSLUCENCY

- Property of an object which permits passage of light through it, but cannot give any distinguishing image. It is a characteristic of enamel.
- Translucency of teeth has the effect of mixing of various colours (hues) of porcelain in the teeth with changing colours within the oral cavity.
- Teeth appear darker when mouth is nearly closed than when it is open wide.
- ***Blue is the complementary colour of yellow.***
- So stare at blue cloth for 30 sec. before colour matching for better observation.
- Colour of face is the BASIC GUIDE to the colour of the teeth.

AGE—colour of natural teeth becomes progressively DARKER with age (especially incisal edges of lower anteriors).

- So darker teeth are better for older patients and lighter teeth in young patients.
- Extracted teeth are valuable for selection of size and form of teeth but not the colour, because of the loss of colour and H_2O from the extracted tooth.

COLOUR SELECTION OF ARTIFICIAL TEETH—is done in 3 positions:

1. Outside the mouth alongside of the nose = to establish basic hue, brilliance and saturation.

2. Under the lips with only incisal edges exposed = to reveal effect of tooth colour when patient's mouth is relaxed.
3. Under the lips with only cervical end covered and mouth open = to simulate tooth exposure during smiling, when light is reflected through the teeth from inside of mouth.
   - Colour of teeth should be selected on a bright day; patient sits close to natural light; should be observed in artificial light also (i.e. **2 sources of light** used).
   - **SQUINT TEST** = to correlate tooth colour with face colour. The colour which fades away from the view first is least conspicuous in comparison with colour of the face.

Most common error in selection of anterior teeth = is to select teeth which are too small in size and too light in colour. They create DENTURE–LOOK.

POSTERIOR TEETH SELECTION

- ♦ Occlusal surfaces of artificial teeth should be modified.
- ♦ 2 types of teeth—anatomic, non-anatomic.
- ♦ **Anatomic teeth**—used for those posterior teeth that more nearly resemble the teeth of a dentition.
- ♦ BL width of artificial teeth should be greatly reduced from the width of natural teeth they replace.
- ♦ Narrow posterior teeth enhance the development of correct form of polished surfaces of CD by allowing buccal and lingual flanges to slope away from occlusal surfaces.
- ♦ Helps denture stability on ridges.
- ♦ Also decreases stresses falling on basal seat.

MD lengths of posterior teeth

- Area available for artificial posterior teeth is = from distal surface of canine to the beginning of RMP.
- **Mold No.** = total MD width of four posterior teeth in mm.

- ♦ Posterior teeth should not be placed too close to the posterior border of maxillary denture = to avoid cheek biting.

- ♦ If mandibular ridge slopes up sharply at its distal end = DO NOT PLACE POSTERIOR TEETH on this slope, otherwise lower denture will SLIDE FORWARD during working.
- ♦ Posterior teeth SHOULD NOT BE placed on RMP; because soft tissue of RMP is easily displaced and hence, CD tips during function.

VERTICAL LENGTH OF POSTERIOR TEETH

- ♦ Should correlate with inter-arch space and to the length of anterior teeth.
- ♦ Length of maxillary first PM should be comparable to canine = for proper esthetic effect.
- ♦ Dental arch form should be as nearly same as possible to the NATURAL ARCH FORM; should be in neutral zone.

Types of posterior teeth

- **Resin teeth**, wear faster and stain easily than porcelain teeth, because they are softer.
- Resin teeth are used against natural teeth/resin teeth/gold covered teeth—to minimize abrasion of enamel/gold.
- Porcelain teeth should be used against porcelain only; so that no abrasion of natural teeth occurs.
- Porcelain teeth used against natural teeth/gold restoration leads to enamel/metal abrasion, because porcelain is harder than enamel.
- Resin teeth also required if inter arch space is less, as it can be decreased in height during set-up but porcelain cannot.
- Resin posterior teeth should not be used with porcelain anterior teeth on CD, because posterior teeth will wear more and will create excessive and destructive forces at anterior part of basal seat, which is least able to bear increased forces.
- Cuspal inclines of posterior teeth depend on plane of occlusion.
- IG = is in control of dentist.
- CG = is in control of anatomy.

- With deep overbite + low posterior teeth inclines = anterior teeth are set with increased overjet.
- With a flat/nearly horizontal IG the posterior tooth inclines should be SHALLOW.
- In CD, IG is determined by the Dr, so posterior tooth inclines are decided after settling the overjet.

Types of posterior teeth are:

1. Anatomic = 33° teeth.
2. Semi anatomic = 20° teeth.
3. Non anatomic = 0° teeth.
   - Cuspal inclination is the angle formed by incline of MB cusp of lower first molar with the horizontal plane.
   - 33° teeth = give maximum opportunity for fully BO (Best for BO).
   - But final effective height of the cusps is related to many factors, e.g. inclination of teeth, IG, height of OP and COS/COM/COW curves, i.e. curves of spee, Monsoon and Wilson.

Curves	Features
Curve of Spee	• Is the AP curve which begins at the tip of lower canines and follows cusp tips of premolars and molars follows an arc through condyle. • It may form a circle of 4 inches diameter if extended.
Curve of Monsoon	• It is formed by extending the curve of spee and curve of Wilson to all cusps and incisal edges.
Curve of Wilson	• It contacts the buccal and lingual cusp tips of the mandibular posterior teeth. • It is mediolateral on each side of arch. • It occurs due to inward inclination of the crowns of lower posterior teeth. • It helps to align the teeth parallel to the **direction of medial pterygoid ms**.

- **Shallow IG** and esthetics allow as **little cusp height** as possible of posterior teeth for BO and so lateral forces are reduced on residual ridge.
- Anatomic teeth are healthy to support tissues than other teeth.
- **20° teeth** = wider BL dimension than 33° teeth; they have less cusp height.
- **0° teeth** = used ONLY if CR record is set on articulator and no BO is to be established.

Or when it is impossible to record CR/ or in abnormal jaw relations.

TEETH SETTING: Use setting instructions; **Andrews keys**; Fenn-also.

According to Andrews, there are 6 keys to normal occlusion as given below:

Key	Features
I. molar relation	MB cusp of upper first molar falls in the MB groove of the lower first molar; the ML cusp of upper first molar falls in the central fossa of lower first molar; the distal surface of distal marginal ridge of upper first molar contacts and occludes with the mesial surface of MMR of lower second molar.
II. crown	The gingival portion of long axis of each crown angulation; MD tip is distal to the occlusal part of the axis.
III. crown inclination; torque	The angle b/w a line 90° to the OP and a line tangent to the middle of the labial or buccal surface of the clinical crown.
IV. rotations	Should not be there.
V.	Tight contacts.
VI.	Curve of spee; normal depth is 1.5 mm.

Guidelines

1. Amount of bone resorption is proportional to the time of teeth loss.
2. Amount of resorption and the time of edentulousness indicates the distance the teeth should be set from the residual ridge, (should replace natural positions).
3. If natural teeth oppose/occlude a CD then more bone loss occurs in the residual ridges; due to heavy forces.
4. OP of the CD should be in same position as occupied by natural teeth.

Incisive papilla

- Has a constant relation with natural CI.
- Acts as a guide for teeth setting.
- Present in lingual embrasure between CI in midline.
- Labial surfaces of CI = 8–10 mm in front of it.
- Papilla moves distally with severe vertical resorption of ridge.
- Distance of labial surfaces of teeth from papilla may become increased with much vertical bone loss.

Reflection of soft tissues

- Labial surfaces and incisal edges of teeth should be anterior to the tissues at the reflection, where the denture borders would be placed.
- There is an OBTUSE angle between labial surface of root of CI and the clinical crown of the tooth.
- A thin layer of bone exists over the labial surface of root of CI.
- Labial surface of ridge acts as a guide to determine the proper inclination of anterior teeth; but becomes LESS-ACCURATE with extreme resorption.

AP position of dental arch

- Governed by orbicularis oris, its supporting ms; and tone of skin of lips.

- Orbicularis ORIS is affected by 7 other ms at MODIOLUS which are

♦ Quadratus labii superioris.

♦ Caninus (levator anguli oris).

♦ Qudratus labii inferioris.

♦ Zygomaticus.

♦ Resorius.

♦ Triangularis (deeper anguli oris).

♦ Buccinator.

♦ Zone and action of these ms depends on AP support provided by teeth and denture base materials.

♦ MAXILLARY anterior alveolar process is at an angle to the labial face of maxillary incisors and its direction is Upward and Backward. So ridge CREST is more posterior than in recently extracted case.

♦ Imaginary roots of the teeth should extend into the residual ridge (before resorption).

♦ Position of teeth should resemble NATURAL TOOTH POSITION for best support and esthetics and health of tissues.

♦ If horizontal overlap of natural teeth is decreased to develop contacts in CO, unfavorable forces are applied on the anterior residual ridge.

♦ Relation of U/L anterior ridges has an influence on AP position of U/L anterior teeth.

♦ AP position of teeth should vary with AP relation of ridges, e.g. Class II, Class III.

♦ In Class III, i.e. prognathic mandible, the incisors can be placed end-to-end, but never labial to lower anteriors. Incisal edges of U/L teeth should cut at an angle, which have a seating action on maxillary denture.

♦ Insufficient space between ridges indicates that either artificial teeth are LONGER than natural teeth or the VD of face is too short.

- Fibrous tissues of maxillary tuberosity should be SURGICALLY removed for better stability.

MANDIBULAR ANTERIOR TEETH

- Roots of mandibular incisors should be seen to be coming out of mandibular alveolar process.
- Mandibular natural teeth are mostly LABIAL to the apices of their roots. It is because the pattern of bone resorption in mandibular anterior region is on labial side.
- The long axis of all natural mandibular teeth if extended apically seem to DIVERGE, while that of maxillary teeth seem to converge.
- Overbite of U/L incisors = 1.5 mm.
- Overjet of U/L incisors varies with sizes of U/L Jaws.
- Upper teeth should be related to the upper jaw and lower teeth to lower jaw, for BEST positioning and stability.

OCCLUSAL PLANE

- Posterior end of OP should be at the level of junction of middle and distal 3rd of RMP.
- This level is BEST familiar to the TONGUE, which then helps in the stability of denture and mastication.
- OP level is anterior region is influenced by—length of lips, ridge fullness, ridge height, maxillo-mandibular space, incisal guide angle.
- If OP is too low anteriorly and/or too high posteriorly, then the mandibular denture slides forward under biting pressure.
- Level of OP should be placed as nearly as possible to position of natural O.P.
- Most reliable guides for OP height are corners of mouth and RMPs.

Bucco-lingual position of posteriors

- Determined anteriorly by position/arch form of anterior teeth and posteriorly by the shape of the basal seat of MANDIBLE.

- Should be properly related to supporting bone and to the soft tissues which contact their buccal-lingual surfaces.
- Determined by NEUTRAL ZONE between cheeks and tongue, where these forces are in perfect balance.
- Forces provided by the tongue/cheeks and lips influence the alignment of teeth in dental arches. See forces from profit.
- Buccinator mechanism (Refer to orthodontics–section).
- Posterior teeth have most FAVORABLE LEVERAGE if set close to the residual ridge and LINGUAL to it.
- Amount of leverage exerted on OP depends on the distance the OP is above the ridge (i.e. Moment = Force × Distance).

Posterior Arch form

- Should conform the shape of residual ridge.
- Teeth should be placed so as to have erupted from the ridge.
- RULE = a perpendicular erected from buccal side of crest of ridge should bisect the buccal cusp of lower first molar.
- Form of each dental arch must be in harmony within itself and with its foundation.
- Posterior teeth are set between 2 lines extending posteriorly from the distal surface of canines to the buccal and lingual margins of RMP.
- 30° teeth are more effective for checking accuracy of jaw relations than 20° or 0° teeth.
- Most residual ridges are curved laterally between the position of canine and RMP.

Guidelines for CO

- Long axis of each upper tooth is DISTAL to long axis of corresponding lower tooth.
- Each tooth is opposed by 2 teeth except lower CI and upper LAST molar.
- Mandibular first molar is set such that it contacts both 2nd PMs and its buccal cusp would be bisected by a perpendicular on buccal side of crest of ridge.

- Alignment of lower buccal cusps should correspond with the curvature of arch form of the residual ridge.
- Distance between distal surface of lower canines and mesial end of RMP determines the total AP space, which may be covered by the teeth.
- Distal limit of posterior teeth is governed by incline of the lower ridge. If tooth is placed on this incline—the denture will slide forward if pressure is applied on that tooth.
- The BL width of posterior teeth should be narrower than natural teeth to decrease biting pressure and to increase tongue space.
- Anterior teeth play important role in 3 basic oral functions, i.e. ESTHETICS, INCISION, PHONETICS.
- So they should be of same size, shape, colour and position.
- They also help to regain TONE OF SKIN and lips and proper ms functions.
- Phonetics can serve as a guide to esthetics and to establish VR of the Jaws.

VERIFICATION OF JAW RELATIONS

- Patients should leave existing dentures out of the mouth for a minimum of 24 hrs before the jaw relation records are verified and try-in.
- It allows soft tissues of basal seat to take rest and come in the same form as they were at final impression.
- An error in CR will cause error in CO and produce contact of inclined planes of teeth. Amount of error is magnified by the effect of inclined plane contacts.
- Further closure causes teeth to slide in CO.
- Path of closure is an arc about posterior THA.
- There should be uniform and simultaneous contacts on both sides of mouth and in front and back, without any detectable touch and slide of teeth.
- SQUASH BITE is taken ST there are imprints of all posterior teeth, without perforation and penetration of wax.

- If perforation is there—it shows defective occlusal contacts and shifting of bases.
- Uniform contacts without pressure are less damaging to the tissues of basal seat, because the dentures do not get displaced.

FACIAL EXPRESSION AND HARMONY

- Appearance of lower half of face depends on

1. S/S of reduced VRO = thin, drooping, long upper lip; reduced vermilion border; so tense wrinkled lips show patient's efforts to hold in CD.
2. Premature aging appearance of lips is due to—lack of support for lips and cheeks; improper replacement.
3. Apparent extra fullness of lower lip = too broad mandibular arch. or elimination/reduction of mento-labial sulcus. It may also be due to lingual placement of lower anteriors or overextended/ thick labial flanges.

- **Nasolabial sulcus**/groove = from ALA of nose to just outside the level of rima-oris (corner of lip line).
- **Zygomaticus** m = origin from zygomatic bone, goes D and F; inserts in corner of mouth; produces nasolabial sulcus during smiling/laughing.
- Upper lip rests on labial surfaces of upper anteriors.
- Lower lip rests on labial surface of lower anteriors and incisal 3rd of the upper teeth.
- So edge of lower lip should extend upward and outward from mento labial sulcus.
- Clinical crowns of lower teeth are labial to the bone, which supports them.
- Many ms are inserted in modiolus and orbicularis oris m. at the corner of the mouth, and their functioning length depends on the function of orbicularis oris m.
- **8 ms** inserted in modiolus/orbicularis oris m are:
  - Mentalis
  - Zygomaticus

- Quadratus labii superioris
- Quadratus labii inferioris
- Levator anguli oris (caninus)
- Depressor anguli oris (triangularis)
- Buccinator
- Risorius

- If teeth are placed over the crest of ridge, it leads to the lack of lip support.
- Bone resorption in mandibular anterior region = moves the ridge first LINGUALLY and then LABIALLY, as resorption continues.
- **ORBICULARIS ORIS m** = is the m. of lips, attached by maxillary labial frenum to maxilla along the midline, and by mandibular labial frenum to the mandible.
- **Buccinator** = forms entire side-wall of cheek from the corner of mouth; reaches the lingual surface of ramus to join the superior constrictor of the pharynx at PTERYGOMANDIBULAR RAPHE.
- Buccinator ms and orbicularis oris form a FUNCTIONAL UNIT.
- If VDO is v. less and the teeth are placed far posteriorly, the ms sag at rest and are less effective on contraction. It is due to movement of INSERTION of THESE Ms closer to their ORIGIN. It gives senile appearances.
- If ridges are very much resorbed due to long-standing–the denture borders are made THICK to restore position of these ms.
- Position and expression of lips and face are BEST GUIDE = to determines proper AP position of teeth.
- Insufficient support of lips is characterized by drooping of corners of mouth, reduction of visible part of Vermillion border, drooping/ deepening of nasolabial grooves, reduction of prominence of philtrum, vertical lines above the vermilion border.
- AP position of teeth must correspond to the positions of ridges. e.g. in prognathic patients—the anterior teeth can be set end-to-end, with incisal edges producing a SEATING ACTION as upper CD.

- Imaginary roots of teeth should appear farther in front of the crest of the ridge, if there is greater amount of resorption.
- Imaginary transverse line between upper canines should cross the middle of incisive fossa for proper AP width and position of 6 anteriors.
- During normal smile, the incisal and middle 3rd of max anteriors are seen.
- Incisal 3rd of mandibular anteriors are visible.
- Mandibular anterior teeth are seen more than maxillary anteriors during SPEAKING and are seen more in men than in women.
- Lower lip is a better GUIDE for vertical position of anteriors than the upper lip.
- Incisal edges of natural lower canines and cusp tip of mand first PM are at the level of lower lip at corner of the mouth when mouth is slightly open.
- U/L natural teeth occupy approx the same amount of inter-arch space, and should be replicated in CD.

PHONETICS ("from fenn also)

Sound	Examples	Features
Labial	**B, p, m**	AP position of anterior teeth and thickness of labial flange of denture affect them.
Labio-dental, e.g. fifty five	**F, v**	• Made between upper incisors and labio-lingual centre to the posterior 1/3rd of lower lip. • Relation of incisal edges to lower lip should be observed. • If upper teeth touch labial side of lower lip. • During f, v speaking, it shows too far forward placed upper teeth. • If lower anterior are placed too far forward, then lower lip tends to raise the lower CD.

PHONETICS ("from fenn also) (*Contd.*)

Sound	Examples	Features
Dental	**Th**	• Tip of tongue comes slightly between U/L anteriors. • If about 3 mm of tip of tongue is not seen, implies anterior teeth are probably too far forward (except $C_2 D_1$ malocclusion) for increased overbite. • If > 6 mm tip seen, it implies teeth are placed too far lingually.
Alveolar	**T, d, n, s, z**	• Tongue–tip contacts with anterior most past of palate. • If teeth are set lingually, the t will come like d. • If teeth are placed anteriorly, the d will sound as t. • Thick acrylic in RUGAE AREA has same effect.
Sibilants	**S, z, sh, ch, zh, j**	Are alveolar sounds. U/L incisors come end-to-end, without touching. Produced between rest and occluding position. If incisors do not come exactly end-to-end, it implies overjet error, e.g. Class II, Class III.
S-sounds		• S-sound can be considered as dental and alveolar sound. • S-sound is made with tip of tongue against the alveolus in rugae area, with small space for escape of air between tongue and alveolus.

PHONETICS ("from fenn also) (*Contd.*)

Sound	Examples	Features
		• **Lisping** occurs if space is too broad and thin. • Frequent cause of undesired whistles with CD is. • A NARROW POSTERIOR DENTAL ARCH FORM, because tongue comes forward leaving a very small space for escape of air. • In 30% patients, S-sound occurs with tongue tip contacting lingual side of anterior part of lower CD, and arching against the palate to form desired size/slope of airway.
Palatal	**e.g. in year, vision; she; onion**	These do not present any problem in CD making.
Velar	**K, g, ng**	

Important points

- ♦ Sound of speech sounds is NOT A SAFE GUIDE for teeth setting.
- ♦ OBSERVING the position of lips and tongue to the teeth and CD bases when sounds are made is A SAFE GUIDE.
- ♦ Functional contouring of palatal surface of CD helps to attain a physiologic space for sounds.

INCLINATION OF ANTERIOR TEETH

- ♦ Roots of anterior teeth are parallel to and very close to the labial surface of the bone.
- ♦ An obtuse angle exists between bone and labial surfaces of the teeth.

- ♦ Profile of face also represents the inclination of anteriors, which is parallel to the profile line of face, e.g. in Class I, II, III malocclusion cases.

A. Harmony of arch form with residual ridge

- Anterior arch may be square/tapering/ovoid.
- CI in square arch form is more nearly on a line with canines; no rotations in incisors; harmonize with a BROAD-SQUARE FACE.
- In tapering arch form—CI are a greater distance forward from the canines; incisors are rotated/crowded due to less space in the arch; harmonize with a narrow-tapering face.
- In ovoid arch, CI are forward of the canines, in a position between square and tapering arch from; seldom rotated incisors; broader effect harmonious with ovoid face.

PALATAL VAULT

- ♦ If Broad and shallow = arch form SQUARE.
- ♦ If High and V-shaped = arch form TAPERING.
- ♦ If Rounded vault of average height = arch form OVOID.

BUCCAL CORRIDOR SIZE

- ♦ Is the space between buccal surfaces of upper teeth and corner of mouth, which is seen when patient smiles.
- ♦ It helps eliminate an appearance of too many teeth in the front of the mouth.

B. Harmony of long axes of CI and the face

- Incisal plane should be parallel to inter-pupillary line.
- Midline of arch should be at the centre of the face.
- Long axes of CI should be parallel to the long axis of the face.
- Midline position of CI is guided by position of incisive papilla.
- Lower CI, the imaginary line should pass between middle of lower denture and between lower CI.

C. Harmony of teeth with smiling line of lower lip

- Lower lip forms a pleasant curvature know as SMILING LINE, which is used to set upper anterior.
- Incisal edges of upper anteriors follow this smiling line during smiling.
- Vertical position of upper canines is mainly responsible for the shape of smiling line.
- When incisal edges of canines a slightly shorter than LI, the smiling line will tend to be parallel with the lower lip on smiling.

D. Harmony of opposing lines of labial and buccal surfaces

- There should be ASYMMETRICAL SYMMETRY in arrangement of the teeth to give NATURAL APPEARANCE.
- Long axes are the balanced opposing lines on either side of midline.
- Labial and buccal lines must have opposing equivalent angles.
- Labial and buccal lines of teeth and lines of the face should be harmonious.
- Square and ovoid faces should have teeth that have lines, which are more nearly perpendicular, and in tapering faces should have lines which are more divergent from the perpendicular.

E. Harmony of teeth and profile lines of the face

- Labial surfaces of maxillary CI are parallel to the profile line of the face.
- When maxillary CI are parallel to profile line, the LI should be set at an opposite angel to prevent parallelism from being dominant.
- Most predominant facial form can be helpful as a guide for teeth positioning.

F. Harmony of tooth wear and age

- Incisal edges and proximal surfaces wear with age, which should be incorporated in the artificial teeth.

- More lingually placed upper teeth or parts of teeth wear more than more labially placed upper teeth.
- Greatest amount of wear on lower anteriors occur on more labially placed lower teeth.
- Wear should be placed on teeth, where it would have occurred during function and also where it assists in mechanics of BO.

REFINEMENT OF INDIVIDUAL TOOTH POSITION

- ♦ Should be set with typical inclination and rotations for natural appearance.
- ♦ Labial surface of maxillary CI is parallel to profile line, which is approx perpendicular.
- ♦ Labial surface of LI is in at the cervical end more than adjacent teeth.
- ♦ Labial surface of canine is out at cervical end more than the other maxillary teeth.
- ♦ Degree to which cervical end of canine is out is in harmony with the lateral lines of the face.
- ♦ Labial surface of mandibular CI is in at cervical end more than LI or canine.
- ♦ Mandibular LI is out at cervical end more than CI such that it is almost perpendicular.
- ♦ MD inclination
  - CI is almost perpendicular.
  - LI is inclined distally at CEJ.
  - C is inclined distally at CEJ less than LI; more than CI.
- ♦ Mandibular canine is out at CEJ same as maxillary.

Location

- CI is slightly rotated from parallelism to a tangent of the line of arch contour.
- LI rotated to have its distal surface turned lingually at a larger angle to the tangent.

- Canine rotated to half its DISTAL half in the direction of posterior arch form.
- Mandibular incisor are generally parallel to tangent of arch contour.

VERTICAL POSITION

- ♦ Max LI and C are slightly above the level of the inclined plane.
- ♦ Mandibular 1, 2, 3 are at the same level.

HARMONY with SPA features of patients

- ♦ **Femininity** = curved surfaces/softness in form of dentition/ prominent smiling line.
- ♦ **Masculinity** = boldness/vigor and squareness of dentition/ straightness of incisal line of teeth.

Esthetics and IG = best plan for CD STABILITY is:

- With SHALLOW IG.
- If overbite is decreased, then increase overjet.
- Protrusive balance is less important than lateral balance.
- Angle of IG for lateral occlusion must be adjusted so that the posterior teeth contact at the same time the U/L canines are end-to-end.
- Also, U/L anterior teeth should not be in contact when posterior teeth are in CO to avoid excess pressure and bone resorption of anterior ridge.

REMOVABLE PARTIAL DENTURES

Kennedy classification

Classification	Features
I	Bilateral edentulous areas located posterior to remaining teeth.
II	A unilateral edentulous area located posterior to remaining teeth.
III	A unilateral edentulous area, with natural teeth remaining anterior and posterior to it.
IV	A single, bilateral, i.e. crossing the midline edentulous area, located anterior to remaining teeth.

Kennedy's classification of edentulous spaces

- Class I bilateral free end saddle.
- Class II unilateral free end saddle.
- Class III unilateral bounded saddle.
- Class IV anterior/across the midline.

Rules

- The most posterior edentulous area's determine the classification.
- There can be no modification areas in Class IV arch.
- Class I RPD—tooth and tissue supported. 3 features required for it are—adequate support for distal extension, flexible direct retainers; and some provision for indirect retention; mostly support is TISSUE–borne; FUNCTIONAL impression is required, relining required.

- Class III PD—entirely tooth borne RPD; no Indirect Retainer required; no functional impression required; total metallic; no relining required.
- Class II PD (with modification areas) is in between Class I and III and has design features of both Class I and III; combination of tooth bone and tissue borne PD; distal extension is made of acrylic.
- Modification spaces—are edentulous areas in the arch, other than the main area describing the classification.
- Maximum % age is of Kennedy Class I; Class II; Class I mod 2; Class II mod 1 = 72% and Kennedy Class III; Class III mod 1 (14%).

COMPONENTS OF RPD

1. Major connector.
2. Mino connector .
3. Rests.
4. Direct retainers.
5. Reciprocal/stabilising components.
6. Indirect retainers.
7. Bases.

Major Connectors

- Connects the part of prosthesis located on one side of arch with those of opposite side.
- All parts are directly/indirectly attached to it.
- Must be RIGID—for proper distribution of forces.
- **RIGIDITY**—important requirement; resists flexing and torque.
- Superior border of a lingual bar connector should be located at least 4 mm below gingival margins and its width should be at least 4 mm.
- It should be free from movable tissues.
- There should be minimal gap between MC and tissue in mandible to avoid overgrowth of tissues.

- There should be no gap in maxillary arch for wider force distribution.
- In upper arch-border of palatal connector should be 6 mm away from gingival margin and parallel to their mean curve.
- All MINOR connectors should connect the major connectors at RIGHT angle.
- Anterior border should avoid interference with tongue and should follow the valleys between rugae.
- Posterior border should be just anterior to the vibrating line.
- Most important property of an RPD esp of major connector is RIGIDITY.

Lingual Bar

- Half pear shaped with more bulk at lower border, above the moving tissues.
- **Continuous bar retainer** = located on or slightly above the cinguli of anterior teeth.
- **Linguoplate** = should be thin; should not extend above the middle 3rd of lingual surface.
- **Labial bar** = is used when there is extreme lingual inclination of lower incisors and PMs.

Maxillary major connectors–4:

1. **Single palatal strap**
   - Most widely used but least logical.
   - Must be rigid.
   - Bilateral tooth borne RPD of short spans especially posterior edentulous areas may be connected with broad palatal strap.
   - Used mostly in Class III type.

2. **U-shaped palatal connector**
   - Least desirable.
   - Used only if large torus or for replacing several anterior teeth.

- Lacks rigidity.
- Does not provide good support.

3. **Combination of Anterior and Posterior palatal strap–type connectors**
    - Most RIGID.
    - Posterior palatal bar should be half oval in shape and placed posteriorly to avoid interference with tongue and movable tissues.
    - Anterior strap should avoid Rugae coverage and tongue interferences.
    - Should cross midline at right angle.
    - Used mostly in Class II and IV types.

4. **Palatal plate type**
    - Used in Class I situations.
    - Located anterior to PPS; not on soft palate.

Release of inherent strains in resin base of CD requires some provision to maintain intimate contact of posterior part of denture and tissues. It is achieved by scoring the master cast to a depth of 1 × 1 mm as PPS.

- So beading (not more than 0.5 mm) is done to maintain the tissue contacts.

MINOR CONNECTORS

- Join the major connector with other parts of RPD.
- Also help to transfer functional stresses to the abutment teeth. It is ***prosthesis-to-abutment function***.
- It transfers effects of retainers; rests and stabilizing components to rest of the RPD. It is its ***abutment-to-prosthesis function***.
- Should be RIGID.
- Should be located in embrasure and so least irritating to the tongue.
- Should be thickest towards the lingual surface and tapering towards the contact area (V-shaped) (BUTT JOINT).

- Should be at right angle to major connectors.
- Contacts the guiding plane surfaces of abutment teeth and is 2/3rd the width b/w tips of buccal and lingual cusps.
- Extends from marginal ridge to 2/3rd the length of enamel crown, and is TRIANGULAR SHAPED when seen from above.
- Should not be located on convex axial surface of abutment.
- Minor connectors for mandibular distal extension base should extend posteriorly about 2/3rd the length of edentulous ridge and have elements on both lingual and buccal surfaces.
- Minor connector for maxillary distal extension should extend the ENTIRE length of the ridge and should be of a ladder like and loop design and extended to pterygomaxillary notch.

TISSUE STOPS

- Help in retention of acrylic resin bases.
- Prevent distortion of framework during resin processing.
- Should engage buccal and lingual slopes of the ridge for stability.
- Finishing index tissue stop = is located distal to the terminal abutment and is a continuation of minor connector contacting the guiding plane.
- Finishing lines should make an angle of less than 90° and should restore the natural palatal shape. It should minimize the bulk of acrylic resin attaching the artificial teeth.
- Junction of major and minor connectors at palatal finishing lines should be located 2 mm medial from an imaginary line, which would contact the lingual surfaces of missing posterior teeth.
- If OPD is not removed for a long period the mm may get changed in CT so the RPD should be removed at right s.t. tissues may rest.
- Most important property of RPD especially major connector is—RIGIDITY.

RESTS AND REST SEATS

- To provide VERTICAL SUPPORT.
- Prevents settling of denture and impingement of soft tissues.

- Direct forces along the long axis of abutment teeth.
- Must be RIGID.
- Rest seat should be rounded, triangular shape, with the apex towards the centre of the occlusal surface, inclined apically from marginal ridge.
- Base of the seat at MR should be at least 2.5 mm for bulk.
- MR is vertically decreased to 1.5 mm for bulk and to assist occlusal interference.
- Floor of seat should be **concave/spoon shaped**.
- Angle formed by occlusal rest and vertical minor connector from which it arises **should be less than 90°**—for avoiding slippage of RPD.
- Lingual extension of rest seat helps to provide strength.
- It is like a 'BALL and SOCKET JOINT'.

POSSIBLE MOVEMENT OF RPD—3 types:

1. Rotation about an axis through most posterior abutments. (i.e. **Fulcrum line**).
2. Rotation about a longitudinal axis as the distal extension base moves in a rotary direction about the residual ridge. It is resisted by RIGIDITY OF MAJOR CONNECTOR.
3. Rotation about an imaginary vertical axis located near the centre of dental arch. It is resisted by stabilizing components.
   - Occlusal rest should provide only OCCLUSAL SUPPORT; all movements of RPD other than in gingival direction should be resisted by other components.
   - In a tooth borne RPD, only HORIZONTAL rotation is of any significance, which is resisted by STABILISING components.
   - Canine is preferred over incisors for rest placement, because it is a strong tooth.
   - Lingual rest is preferred over incisal rests because of = ESTHETICS.
   - Lingual rest is also better, because it is placed near the horizontal axis of rotation (tipping) of abutment and so will have less tendency to tip the tooth.

- Rests seats in crowns and inlays are made deeper and larger than those in enamel.
- Incisal rests are placed at incisal angles of anterior teeth; it is least desirable. Used mainly as INDIRECT RETAINERS or auxiliary rests. It is more applicable to MANDIBULAR canine.
- It is better than 3/4 crown esthetically.
- Rest seat inclined s.t the deepest part should be apical to incisal edge = it helps to direct the forces along the long axis of teeth.
- Slight labial bevel is also given.

Functions of different components of the RPD

Components	Functions
Occlusal rest Residual ridge Denture base	Support Stability against horizontal movements
Rigid connectors IR Other stabilizing components	
Retaining elements Intimate relationship of denture bases and maxillary major connector with tissues	Retention against dislodging forces

Retention—depends on:

- ♦ Accuracy of impression.
- ♦ Accuracy of fit of denture bases.
- ♦ Total area of contact.

Retentive forces are:

1. **Adhesion** = saliva to denture and tissues.
2. Cohesion = saliva to saliva attraction.
3. Atmospheric pressure.
4. Tissues around the polished surfaces of denture.
5. Gravity.

- Adhesion and cohesion are effective if there is PERFECT APPOSITION of impression surface of denture to mucosal surfaces.
- Atmospheric pressure acts as rescue force when extreme dislodging forces are applied to the denture. It depends on perfect BORDER SEAL.
- These 3 factors are directly proportional to the AREA COVERED by denture.
- Plastic molding of tissues around the polished surfaces helps to perfect the BORDER SEAL and also provide MECHANICAL lock.

DIRECT RETAINER—is a unit of RPD, which engages an abutment to RESIST DISPLACEMENT of RPD away from the basal seat.

- ♦ **Intracoronal retainers** = depend on frictional resistance for RETENTION of RPD.
- ♦ **Extracoronal retainers** = the clasp type retainer engages external surface of abutment cervical to HOC. Here, no frictional resistance is used. A flexible arm or a spring device produces resistance to removal.
- ♦ **Internal attachments** are better from esthetic point of view.
- ♦ An internal attachment should not be used with tissue supported distal extension denture bases, unless a stress-breaker is used between them.

EXTRACORONAL DR

Component	**Function**	**Location**
Rest	Support	Occlusion, lingual, incisal
Minor Connectors	Stabilisation	Proximal surfaces, from MR to 2/3rd height of crown
Clasp Arms	Stabilisation	Apical part of middle 3rd of crown.
	Reciprocation	Apical part of middle 3rd of crown.
	Retention	Gingival 3rd of crown in measured undercut.

- **Angle of cervical convergence** = is the angle formed by tooth surface (at HOC) to the vertical blade of surveyor.
- Greater angle requires placement of clasp terminus nearer the HOC. Uniform clasp retention depends on the degree of tooth undercut, rather than on the distance below HOC, at which clasp terminal is placed.
- Area below HOC/infrabulge—for retentive arm; flexible component.
- Area above HOC/suprabulge = for reciprocating /stabilizing arms.
- Clasp retention is based on the **resistance of metal to deformation** (i.e. Proportional Limit), which is proportional to FLEXIBILITY of the clasp arm.
- **Guiding planes** = rigid parts of RPD contact these parallel tooth surfaces during path of insertion and removal; act as additional retention.
- Clasp should be PASSIVE with teeth except when a dislodging force is applied.
- Retention is provided mainly by FLEXIBLE PART of clasp assembly.
- It depends on retentive clasp arm as:
  - **(a) Length** = longer arm is more flexible; should be tapered uniformly; tip is 1/2 thick than base.
  - **(b) Diameter** = more diameter means less flexible.
  - **(c) Cross section form** = one–direction flexible is half round form. UNIVERSALLY FLEXIBLE form is the ROUND FORM.
  - **(d) Contour.**
- **Type of alloy.**
- **Location and depth of undercut** = is the most important single factor to select a clasp for use with DISTAL EXTENSION RPD.
- Should be tapered in 2–dimensions, i.e. (length and width wise).
- Cast gold alloy has greater resiliency than cast chromium alloys.
- Wrought wire clasp arm, i.e. drawn in wire, has more toughness than cast clasp arm, by at least 25%. So it may be used in smaller diameter.

- Greater rigidity with less bulk can be achieved with chromium alloys, as compared to gold.

Reciprocal stabilizing cast clasp arm

- Should be RIGID.
- Average diameter should be more than the average diameter of retentive arm.
- Tapered in OND Dimension only (only length wise); width remains the same
- **Circumferential clasp arm** = approaches the retentive undercut from an OCCLUSAL DIRECTION.
- **BAR clasp arm**—approaches from CERVICAL DIRECTION.

CLASP ASSEMBLY: Has following components

- One or more minor connectors.
- Principal rest.
- Retentive arm.
- Non-retentive arm = against horizontal movement, for stabilization and reciprocation.

Basic principle of clasp design

- **More than 180° of greatest circumference** of the crown of the tooth should be included.
- When bar clasp is used = at least 2 areas of tooth contact must embrace more than one half of tooth circumference.
- Occlusal rest should prevent cervical movement of clasp arm.
- Each retentive arm should be opposed by reciprocal arm.
- Retentive clasps should be BILATERALLY OPPOSED.
- Path of removal of retentive clasp end should not be parallel to the path of removal of RPD.
- Should not transmit forces to abutment.
- Reciprocal element should be located at the junction of gingival and middle 3rd of crown.
- Terminal end of retentive arm is placed in gingival 3rd.

- Reciprocal arm stabilizes the RPD against horizontal movement; should be RIGID.
- Reciprocal arm may act as indirect retainer if placed on supra-bulge area anterior to the fulcrum line.
- Retentive and reciprocal arms should be located nearer to the horizontal axis of rotation of abutment (which lies somewhere in its root) to avoid heavy forces on PDL.

BAR CLASP: Parts and functions.

- SUPPORT = by occlusal rest.
- STABILIZATION = by rest, Mesial and Distal minor connectors.
- RETENTION = by buccal I-bar.
- Reciprocation = by location of minor connectors.

CIRCUMFERENTIAL CLASP

- Most logical clasp.
- Approaches from occlusal direction.
- More tooth coverage (so unesthetic).
- True adjustment is IMPOSSIBLE with cast clasp—it only increases/decreases frictional resistance.
- Better/superior to BAR–CLASP.
- It has one retentive and one stabilizing/non-retentive arm.

RING CLASP

- Encircles nearly all of a tooth from its point of origin.
- Used when a proximal undercut cannot be approached by other means.
- Should always be used with a SUPPORTING STRUT on non-retentive side.
- Covers more tooth surface and is esthetically objectionable.
- It is used ONLY IF Disto-buccal or Disto-lingual undercut can't be approached from occlusal rest area.

BACK-ACTION CLASP

- Biologically and mechanically unsound.

EMBRASURE CLASP

- Used in unmodified Class II or III RPD.
- Should be used with DOUBLE OCCLUSAL RESTS to avoid food impaction and helps to shunt food.
- It has 2 retentive and 2 reciprocal clasp arms.

MULTIPLE CLASP

- 2 opposing C–clasps joined at terminal ends of 2 reciprocal arms.
- Used when PD replaces entire half of the dental arch.

HALF AND HALF CLASP

- Has a C-clasp retentive arm from one direction and a reciprocal arm from other.
- Used to provide **DUAL retention** only in UNILATERAL denture design.

Reverse action/hair pin clasp

- Engages proximal undercut from occlusal direction (below the point of origin).
- Its lower arm only is FLEXIBLE passing over HOC.

Bar clasp/roach clasp

- Approaches from GINGIVAL DIRECTION.
- RPI system = Rest, proximal plate and I–bar.
- It consists of a mesio-occlusal rest with minor connector placed in Mesiolingual embrasure, but not touching the adjacent tooth.
- I–bar should be located in gingival 3rd of buccal surface, in an 0.01 inch undercut and only 2 mm of its tip only should touch the tooth.

Combination clasp

- Has a WROUGHT wire retentive arm and a cast RECIPROCAL arm.
- Used when **maximum flexibility** is required.
- Being wrought—a **smaller diameter** can be used; so better esthetic.
- Round in form.
- Most common use = on an abutment adjacent to a distal extension base, where only a Mucogingival undercut exists.
- Advantages = flexibility/adjustability/esthetics/less fatigue failures/line contact with tooth/less tooth area covered.

INDIRECT RETAINERS

- Placed as far as possible from distal extension base, giving best possible leverage advantage against lifting of the distal extension base.
- Placed **on the opposite side** of the fulcrum line, in a REST SEAT.
- Most effective location of IR is incisors, but it is a weak tooth, so canine or 1st PM (mesio-occlusal) may be used.
- Most frequently used is an AUXILIARY OCCLUSAL REST, e.g. in Mandibular Class I arch = MMR of 1st PM is used.
- In Class II PD = MR of first PM on the opposite side of arch from the distal extension base.

DENTURE BASE

- Broader coverage helps in wider distribution of forces.
- Resin is attached to PD framework by MINOR CONNECTOR.
- Space (at least 20 gauge thick) should be there between metal and residual ridge for flow of resin.
- 1.5 mm thick RESIN must be there s.t. RELIEVING may be done if required.
- More ***open ladder like framework*** is preferred over a MESH-LIKE framework.

- Should be located both buccally and lingually.
- Ladder like pattern also prevent warping of resin after processing due to release of inherent strains.
- Metal is preferred as denture base than resin, because it provides stimulation to underlying tissues; intimate contact and good retention; accuracy of fit.
- Distortion of resin base in maxillary denture is manifested as a distortion away from palate in midline and towards the tuberosities.
- Temperature changes get transmitted through the metal bases to basal tissues and help to maintain the health of tissues.
- Metal being more rigid, is used in less BULK and so does not encroach the tongue space.
- Resin may be required if due to extreme tissue resorption, the fullness of tissues is to be achieved by bulk of resin and for contours of functional check and tongue and for esthetic reasons.

Acrylic teeth can be attached by

1. With acrylic resin.
2. Cemented.
3. Processed directly to metal.
4. Cast with the framework.

- **Porcelain teeth** = are mechanically retained, as they have a PIN on ridge lap area.
- **Diatoric teeth** = have holes on their ridge lap in which resin flows.
- **Resin teeth** = retained by chemical union with the resin.
- Pressing on a resin tooth = i.e. attaching a ready-made resin tooth to the metal base, with acrylic resin of same shade.
- **Metal tooth** = is cast in framework, where only a small space is present.
- Occlusal adjustment on **gold tooth** is easier than chrome alloy teeth.

RELINING

- Base should be made of material, which can be relined/ribased especially distal extension.
- Loss of support of distal extension bases occur from changes in residual ridge and loss of occlusal contact between artificial teeth.
- To check the occlusion—***Wax strip is better*** than articulating paper. The indentation in wax strip are QUANTITATIVE, But in articulating paper are only QUALITATIVE.
- If IR lifts from their rest seat, it also implies need of relining.

STRESS BREAKER

All parts or RPD are rigid except—Retentive arm of DR wrought wire retentive clasp acts as a STRESS BREAKER between denture base and abutment, because of its flexibility.

They allow some movement b/w denture bases and DR and so prevents transfer of forces to the abutments.

2 types

1. Having a movable joint between Denture Base and Direct Retainer, e.g. hinge; sleeve and cylinder; Ball and socket. It permits both vertical and hinge action of distal extension base.
2. Having a FLEXIBLE connection between DB and DR. It is made by DUAL CASTING technique.

PRINCIPLES OF RPD

Simple machines–are of 6 types, i.e.

- Lever, wedge, pulley, screw, wheel and axle; inclined plane.
- Lever and incline plane design should be AVOIDED in RPD.

If effort arm of a lever is larger than the resistance arm, the mechanical advantage is in favour of effort arm.

$$\text{Mechanical advantage} = \frac{\text{Effort arm}}{\text{Resistance arm}}$$

CANTILEVER

- Beam supported at one end only; acts as a first class lever; it should be avoided.
- A tooth can withstand vertical forces better than oblique/ horizontal forces. It is because more PDL fibers are activated to resist the application of vertical forces to teeth than are activated to resist off-vertical forces.
- Flat ridge provide good support but poor stability.

Differences b/w different types of RPDs

Class I **Class II with distal extension**	**Class III**
Support derived from tissues under Denture Base, i.e. tissue supported	All support derived from the abutment teeth, i.e. tooth supported
Impression = Dual impression technique is used; functional impression required.	No functional impression required.
Indirect retainer required in Distal Extension Base	Not required
DB material used should be able to be RELINED/REBASED to compensate for tissue changes.	No relieving required
Made of Acrylic/Resin	Metallic
Retentive arm should lie in mesial undercut and should be able to flex to dissipate stresses. Wrought wire retentive arm can flex in all directions.	DR is a clasp at each abutment/end. Retentive arm should be passive and should flex only while removal.

IMPRESSION MAKING

1. **Anatomic form** = recorded s.t. no pressure is exerted on soft tissues beyond their PHYSIOLOGIC LIMITS, s.t. its retentive and stabilizing components may be properly placed, e.g. by Agar, alginate, rubber base materials.
2. **Supporting form** = of soft tissues under the distal extension of RPD should be recorded s.t. FIRM areas are used as PRIMARY SUPPROT BEARING AREAS and easily displaceable tissues are not overloaded, e.g. by ZOE, rubber base impression materials.
   - Denture made in functional form is generally less irregular and has great cover area than the denture made to anatomic or resting form.
   - Denture made on anatomic form exhibits less stability under rotating forces than on functional form and fails to maintain occlusal relation.
   - It also fails to distribute occlusal loads and so damages to abutments.

GUIDING PLANES

- 2 or more parallel vertical surfaces of abutment teeth, which help to direct RPD during placement or removal.
- Provide one path of placement or removal of RPD.
- It should be 2/3rd as wide as the distance between buccal.
- 1/3rd the buccolingual width of tooth.
- 2/3rd the length of crown from Marginal Ridge cervically.
- Should be located on abutment surface adjacent to an edentulous area.
- Avoid to create buccolingual line angles on the tooth.

SURVEYING

SURVEYOR is an instrument to determine the relative parallelism of 2 or more surfaces of teeth or other parts of cast of dental Arch.

For a clasp to be retentive, its path of escaping must be other than parallel to the path of removal of RPD, otherwise it will not flex.

Retentive arm tip should engage on undercut of 0.01″ (0.25 mm); but wrought-wire clasp can engage 0.02″ provided arm is long enough (at least 8 mm).

Retentive clasp should be placed at a more disto-gingival area for esthetic purpose.

BLOCK OUT OF THE CAST

1. ***Shaped block out***
   - Done on buccolingual surfaces to locate clasp patterns.
   - Ledges or shelves are blocked out.
2. ***Parallel block out***
   - Done cervical to guiding plane surfaces and overall undercut areas, which will be crossed by major or minor connectors.
3. ***Arbitrary block out***
   - All gingival crevices.
   - Undercuts distal to cast framework.
   - Labial and buccal tooth and tissue undercuts not involved in denture design.

Relief

- Areas in which major connector will contact the tissues, e.g. mid-palatal raphe.
- Beneath the framework extensions on the ridge areas for attachment of resin bases.
- Relief is not used below palatal major connectors except if TORI are present.

STERILISATION (Ref. to section of microbiology for details.)

- Cleaning = scrub with detergent solution and wiping with I_2/Cl_2 solution (dil. Household bleach).
- O clothes = 140°–160°F wash cycle with normal bleach conc. and machine drying (at 212°F/100°C).
- Disinfection by—, 2% glutraldehyde at 10 min.
- Heat sensitive items by ethylene oxide gas.
- Impressions, relines, face bow forks, etc. should be disinfected with IODOPHORES.

Some important points about bones

- Changes in bone calcification upto 25% can't be seen by R/G..
- Trabecular space size tends to decrease slightly from root apex towards the coronal part.
- **Index areas** = are those areas of alveolar support that disclose the reaction of bone to additional stresses.
  - **Positive bone factor**—means there is an ability of building additional support.
  - **Negative bone factor**—i.e. inability to respond favorably to stresses.

LAMINA DURA—is a **R/G feature:**

- Is the **thin layer of hard cortical bone,** which normally lines the sockets of all teeth.
- Gives **attachment to PDL** fibers.
- Withstands mechanical strain.
- **Cortical** in nature.
- Seen as **Radiopaque** line around the teeth.
- During tipping, C rot. of tooth is in apical 3rd of root.
- Bone resorption occurs in pressure zone and deposition in tension zone.
- DURING TIPPING—LD is seen UNEVEN in the R/G.
- If a tooth tips in edentulous area—the LD on that side becomes HEAVIER, which is nature's reinforcement against abnormal stresses. The TRABECULAE are arranged at right angle to heavier LD.
- Bone is 30% organic and mostly PROTEIN.
- Teeth with multiple and divergent roots resists forces BETTER, as forces are distributed to a LARGER AREA.

ALLOYS (Also refer to dental materials section.)

- Gold alloy (type IV) or chrome-cobalt alloy are used.
- Recontouring of abutments depends on MOE (STIFFNESS) of the alloy being used.

- Cr-Co alloy—low density/wt; high MOE, low cost, tarnish resistant.
- Wrought wire components can be soldered to Au or Cr–Co.
- Cr-Co has low yield strength/YS than Au.
- YS is the greatest STRESS applied within elastic limits.
- MOE—STIFFNESS of Au is 1/2 that of Cr-Co alloy.
  - So it is more RIGID in less bulk.
  - Can be good if undercut is very small.
- A high YS and low MOE—HIGHER flexibility.
- Au is 2 times flexible than Cr-Co.
- Greater flexibility of Au allows placement of retentive arm tips in GINGIVAL 3rd of abutment.
- Grain size of Cr-Co is LARGER and associated with low proportional limit/PL and so it may get fractured.
- Cr-Co gets work HARDENED RAPIDLY and so facture. So adjustment should be done with extreme caution.
- Cr-Co = has 1ow density than Au and so 1/2 as heavy as Au.
- Attrition of enamel is more with Cr-Co than with Au.
- Au more prone to GALVANIC SHOCK to teeth restored with Ag.
- Many mechanical properties of wrought structure are better than cast structure.
- A min YS of 60,000 psi is required for retentive arm.
- If electric soldering of wrought wire is done, the higher heat evolved may cause RECRYSTALLIZATION of grain growth, by changing FIBROUS microstructure of wrought wire to the crystalline structure. It should be avoided by controlling the TEMPERATURE.
- 650 fine gold solder is used.
- Electric soldering is better than torch soldering, because of the localization of heat.
- Flux prevents OXIDATION of parts being joined.
- **Borax flux** = for Au to Au soldering.
- **F-flux** = Cr-Co alloy soldered to alloys having Cr.

- **F-flux** = Au soldered to Cr-Co.
- Au alloy WROUGHT wires are given HARDENING HEAT Rx to increase PL, tensile strength/TS and hardness. It is done at placing at.
  - 840° F × 5 min and then.
  - Coding to 480° F in 30 min.
  - Then quenching in water.

Hydroxyapatite

- Used for bone augmentation.
- No toxicity; non-inflammatory or foreign body response.
- Not resorbable.
- Stops further bone resorption.

Tissue conditioners—are elasto-polymers, which continue to flow for an extended period of time, permitting distorted tissues to rebound and assume their normal form.

Changes seen in an unopposed tooth:

- Loss of orientation of PDL fibers.
- Loss of supporting bone.
- Narrowing of PDL space.

All abutment surfaces facing edentulous areas should be made parallel to the path of placement.

Proximal surfaces are prepared parallel to the path of placement to create guiding planes.

HOC should be lowered till the junction of middle and gingival 3rd.

Mandibular molars are WEAKEST of posterior abutment.

Impression materials

(A) RIGID – POP, ZOE.

(B) Thermoplastic – modeling plastic; Impression waxes and natural resins.

(C) Elastic – Reversible HC (Agar, Agar).
– Irreversible hydrocolloids (Alginate).
– Merceptan rubber base (Thiokol).
– Silicone.
– Polyethers.

- Difference between impression wax and modeling plastic—impression wax has the ability to flow as long as they are in mouth and so permit equalization of pressure and prevent displacement.
- Most commonly used modeling plastic is red material in cake form —it softens at 132°F and should never be softened at higher temperature.
- Reversible and irreversible HC impressions cannot be stored for any length of time and should be POURED immediately.
- Used for orthodontic impressions, etc.

  For accuracy, Thiokol impression materials should have uniform thickness of 3 mm. Cast made in thikol is SMOOTHER and harder than in HC.
- Used for RPD impressions.

Silicone impression materials.

- Used for FPD impression.
- Addition reaction type is more dimensionally stable and has excellent detail reproduction.

Polyether impression materials:

- Flow characteristics are very low.
- Flow is lowest of any rubber impression materials.
- Stiffness is high.
- Used in FPD, but less in RPD impression.

♦ Agar changes from sol to gel under heat by ***a physical change*** which is reversible.

♦ Alginate changes to gel by ***an irreversible chemical change***.

♦ Syneresis is associated with release of a mucinous exudate, which has a retarding effect on gypsum, and so chalky surface of the cast occurs. It can be prevented by using chemical accelerators, e.g. K_2SO_4.

- So agar impression is placed in 2% K_2SO_4 for 5–10 min before making the cast.

OCCLUSION

Occlusal harmony between RPD and natural teeth is a major factor in the preservation of health of supporting structures.

Simultaneous Bilateral contacts of posterior teeth must occur in CO.

BO is required if RPD is opposed by Maxillary CD.

Working side contacts should be there for mandibular distal extension denture. These should occur simultaneously with working side contacts of natural teeth to widely distribute the stresses.

Simultaneous balancing and working side contacts should be formulated for maxillary bilateral distal extension RPD.

Only working side contacts required for maxillary or mandibular unilateral distal extension RPD.

In Class IV RPD, opposite anterior teeth should contact in ICP so as to prevent continuous eruption of opposing natural incisors.

Contact of opposing incisors in eccentric positions should not be developed.

Contact of opposite posteriors in protrusion is NOT DESIRABLE in any situation, except when an opposing CD is placed.

SPRUE

- Should be large s.t. molten metal will not solidify until the metal in casting is frozen.
- 8–12 gauge ROUND wax is used as sprue.
- Should induce minimum amount of turbulence.
- Should be attached at the bulkier sections of the patterns.
- Should be lightly curved, i.e. no acute angles should be there which can lead to entrapment of gases and turbulence.
- Point of attachment to the patterns should be FLARED OUT, and so shrinkage porosity will be avoided in casting—due to continuous feeding of molten metal.

- Multiple spruing is done for RPDs.
- Main sprue hole = 3/8″.
- Investment for casting gold alloys = plastics (gypsum) bound silica material.
- Casting shrinkage of gold = 1–1.74%.
- Higher the % age of Au in the alloy, the greater is the casting shrinkage.
- Casting shrinkage of Cr-Co alloy is 2.3%, and so silica-bounded investment is used. (Ethyl silicate or sodium silicate as binder); thermal expansion occurs.
- Occlusal adjustment of distal extension RPD is better done on articulator than intra–orally.

CLEFT LIP AND PALATE

VEAU'S classification:

Class	Features
I	Involves soft palate.
II	Involves soft palate and hard palate but not alveolus.
III	Involves SP + HP + Alveolus; UNILATERAL.
IV	Involves SP + HP + Alveolus of both sides leaving free premaxilla.

- CP III, IV are associated with CL also.
- CL closed surgically at = 6–12 weeks.
- CP closed surgically at = 18 months.
- Gag reflex of CP patient is markedly decreased.
- Sounds like /puh/ and /kuk/ are practically impossible.
- Vowel sounds, e.g. a, e and sibilants 'S' aid in assessing palato pharyngeal competence.
- Palato–pharyngeal closure = closing off the nasal cavity by the action of ms attached to soft palate.
- Main problems appear in pronouncing B, D, K, P, T sounds.

Levator veli palatini m

- Origin = petrous part of termporal bone and cartilage of eustachiun tube.
- Runs D and F.
- Inserts in palatine aponeurosis.
- Action-pulls soft palate upwards and backwards.
- **Makes a SLING** with other side m.

Tensor veli palatine

- Origin = scaphoid fossa, spheroid spine, eustachian cartilage.
- Runs = D and F to lateral aspects of hamulus (used as pulley).
- Insert = in soft palate.
- Action = effects tension on SP in U and B direction.

Pharynx = comes forward and medially by 3 ms:

1. Pterygo-pharyngeal portion of superior constrictor m = it contracts to pull the posterior pharyngeal wall forward to meet the soft palate.
2. Palatopharyngeus m = seen as posterior pillars of tonsils. Pharyngopalatal part produces a ridge or bunching up of posterior pharyngeal m. known as PASAVANT'S PAD, which approximates soft palate and pharynx. This ***compensatory structure is USUALLY seen in patients of CP***.
3. Salpingopharyngeus m. = closes lateral pharyngeal wall with soft palate.
   - Helps in producing PLOSIVE sounds.

These close the nasal cavity from oral cavity and pharynx.

Closure of oral cavity

1. By contraction of thyropalatal portion of palato-pharyngeus m.
   - Pulls soft palate down towards the tongue.
2. Tensor m. flattens the dome of soft palate.

3. Tongue is forced U and B.
4. Palatoglossus m helps to complete the closure.

SPEECH—Is a function of:

- Respiration = lungs/exchange of air.
- Phonation = vocal cords/change pitch.
- Resonation = nasal/oral/pharynx cavities.
- Articulation = teeth, tongue, lip, palate.
- Integration = brain.

Obturator = serves not to close the soft palate, but rather to fill the space between palatal remnants.

3 types of obturators, viz.

1. Hinge type.
2. Fixed types = most commonly used; fixed type is at the level of palato pharyngeal m/PP.
3. Meatus type.

13

MCQs in Prosthodontics

Part I

1. **The masticatory loads with complete dentures are in the range of**
   A. 1 to 2 kg
   B. 6 to 8 kg
   C. 18 to 20 kg
   D. 30 to 40 kg

2. **The ratio of the periodontal membrane of natural teeth to the denture bearing area of maxilla is approx.**
   A. 2:1
   B. 2.5:1
   C. 1:2
   D. 4:1

3. **In a complete denture which area is capable of carrying maximum masticatory load ?**
   A. Canine region
   B. Premolar region
   C. Molar region
   D. anterior region

4. **The morphological changes associated with edentulous state include all of the following except**
   A. Prognathic appearance

B. Increase in columella-philtral angle
C. Widening of lips
D. Deepening of nasolabial groove

5. A common problem associated with the use of suction discs in maxillary denture is
A. Epulis fissuratum
B. Denture stomatitis
C. Papillary hyperplasia
D. Candida infection

6. In patients planned for a complete denture, torus mandibularis should be
A. Relieved in the final denture
B. Removed before the impressions are made
C. Torus lie deep in the floor of the mouth, so do not affect the denture
D. Relieved in the preliminary impression

7. The ideal form of ridge for a complete denture has
A. Parallel sides with broad top
B. Converging sides with broad top
C. Parallel sides with a narrow top
D. Converging sides with narrow top

8. The maxillary denture is supported by
A. Palatine process of maxilla only
B. Maxilla and sphenoid bone
C. Maxilla and palatine bone
D. Maxilla and palatal process of nasal bone

9. The glandular region of the hard plate
A. Provides support but not retention
B. Provides support and retention
C. Provides retention but not support
D. Provides neither support nor retention

10. The muscle present in labial frenum is
A. Orbicularis oris
B. Levator anguli oris
C. Buccinator
D. None of the above

11. The muscles influencing the action of buccal frenum include
A. Buccinator, massèter, depressor anguli oris
B. Buccinator, orbicularis oris, depressor anguli oris
C. Buccinator, orbicularis oris, levator anguli oris
D. Masseter, orbicularis oris, levator anguli oris.

12. About posterior palatal seal, which of the following is not correct?
A. It is about 1mm high and 1.5mm wide at its base
B. It is made over the vibrating line.
C. It is always located on soft palate
D. Stress cannot be placed in area of PPS

13. Which of the following statement is incorrect?
A. The buccal shelf functions as a primary stress- bearing area in mandible.
B. The buccal shelf area is covered with cortical bone, which is usually at right angles to the occlusal plane.
C. Buccinator muscle fibers attached in the area of buccal shelf tend to displace the lower denture.
D. Buccal flange is bordered anteriorly by buccal frenum and posteriorly by masseter muscle.

14. The space available for distobuccal border of mandibular denture is influenced by
A. Contraction of masseter and buccinator
B. Contraction of masseter pusning against buccinator and buccal pad of fat
C. Contraction of buccinator pushing against masseter and buccal pad of fat
D. None of the above

15. The distal ends of the lingual flange of mandibular denture is governed by
A. Superior constrictor and mylohyoid
B. Superior constrictor only.
C. Superior constrictor, glossopalatine and medial pterygoid.
D. Superior constrictor and glossopalatine muscle

16. Mylohyoid muscle directly influences the lingual border anatomy of mandibular denture except in
A. Incisor region
B. Canine region
C. Premolar region
D. Molar region

17. For boxing the impression, the vertical walls of the boxing are formed by
A. Modeling wax
B. Beeswax
C. Carnuba wax
D. Inlay wax

18. The kinematic face-bow is attached to
A. Maxillary occlusal rim
B. Mandibular occlusal rim
C. Either maxillary or mandibular occlusal rims
D. None of the above

19. The face-bow record is a
A. Maxillo-mandibular relation
B. Record of the orientation of the casts to the articulator
C. Record of centric occlusion
D. Record of interocclusal distance

20. The antero-posterior translation of the condyle is approximately
A. 9 mmm
B. 12 mm
C. 18 mm
D. 24 mm

21. The bennet movement in TMJ is seen on
A. working side only
B. Balancing side only
C. Either working or balancing side
D. None of the above

22. A reduced interarch space may cause all of the following except

A. Closure or occlusion of the opening of the Eustachian tube
B. Trauma to TMJ
C. Reduces soreness in knife-edged ridges.
D. Increased cubicle space of the oral cavity.

23. The muscles involved in holding the mandible in centric relation are

A. Lateral pterygoid and temporalis
B. Middle and posterior parts of temporalis and digastric
C. Anterior part of temporalis and masseter
D. Massetter and temporalis

24. The average speaking space in Class II occlusion is

A. Less than class i occlusion
B. Greater than class i occclusion
C. Equal to class i occlusion
D. Same as in class i and iii

25. The posterior occlusal plane in maxillary occlusal rim is established at

A. Ala-tragus line
B. Ala to the centre of the auditory meatus
C. Frankfort horizontal plane
D. Palatal plane

26. The concept of "neutral zone" in complete denture construction was given by

A. Wright
B. Boos
C. Hanau
D. Fish

27. The height of the distal end of the occlusal plane for mandibular denture is established at

A. Posterior end of the retromolar pad
B. 1/3 length of retromolar pad from the anterior border
C. 2/3 length of retromolar pad from the anterior border
D. 2/3 3 length of retromolar pad from the posterior border

28. If a mandibular denture is to oppose natural teeth restored with gold in maxillary arch, the artificial teeth of choice would be
A. Porcelain teeth
B. Acrylic resin teeth
C. Acombination of acrylic resin and metal occlusal surface
D. Both b) and c)

29. The cuspal inclination of artificial teeth that offers the maximum opportunity for a fully balanced occlusion in a majority of cases is
A. 0 degree
B. 20 degree
C. 33 degree
D. 45 degree

30. The use of acrylic resin posterior teeth in combination with porcelain anterior teeth in complete denture is
A. Used only in patients with high aesthetic concern
B. Not justified
C. Routinely used
D. Done in cases with steep incisal guidance

31. Nonanatomic teeth are advisable when
A. Only a centric relation record is transferred to the articulator
B. Difficulty in recording precise centric relation
C. In cases of abnormal jaw relationships
D. All of the above

32. A set of acrylic resin denture teeth is marked as 32M. The number 32 signifies
A. The combined width of maxillary anterior teeth
B. The combined width of mandibular anterior teeth
C. The combined width of posterior teeth
D. The shade of the teeth

33. At the stage of trial of maxillary anterior teeth in complete denture fabrication, the alphabet "f" sounds like "v". This means
A. Maxillary anteriors are set far down

B. Maxillary anteriors are set too high up
C. Maxillary anteriors are too labially
D. Maxillary anteriors are set too far lingually.

34. The sounds which have no effect on the dentures are
A. Labiodental sounds
B. Palatal sounds
C. Velar sounds
D. Sibilants

35. The sounds which are produced between the physiologic rest position and the occluding position is
A. Labial sounds
B. Palatal sounds
C. Velar sounds
D. Sibilant sounds

36. In complete denture fabrication which of the following factors is not controlled by the dentist?
A. Incisal guidance
B. Condylar guidance
C. Orientation of occlusal plane
D. Cuspal inclination

37. Occlusion of complete dentures should be perfected
A. Before the dentures are first delivered to the patient
B. At the time of first post- insertion appointment
C. After a waiting period of 2 weeks when the patient gets accustomed to the new dentures
D. As and when patient complains

38. The correction of errors in occlusion of complete dentures should be done in
A. Articulator
B. Mouth using articulating paper
C. Mouth utilizing the tactile ability of fingers
D. Either in mouth or on articulator

39. The occlusal errors in centric occlusion are corrected on the articulator by
A. Reducing cusps leaving fossae intact

B. Reducing fossae leaving cusps intact
C. Reducing both cusps and fossae
D. Reducing cusps on maxillary teeth and fossae on mandibular teeth

40. A patient who has recently had a complete denture complains, "My dentures are tight when I place them in my mouth, but they seem to loosen after several hours." This problem indicates
A. Ill-fitting dentures
B. Overextended borders
C. Occlusal errors
D. Insufficient relief of frenums

41. A complete denture patient complains of soreness while swallowing. It indicates
A. Excessive pressure in the region of retromylohyoid fossa
B. Over-extended denture flange in retromylohyoid fossa
C. Irritation in the region of mylohyoid ridges
D. All of the above

42. A complete denture patient complains that his denture causes him to gag. The problem may be related to
A. Psychologic component
B. Improper extension of maxillary denture
C. Problems with the lower denture
D. All of the above

43. The gagging reflex in complete denture patient indicates
A. Making and breaking of the posterior palatal seal
B. Underextended upper denture
C. Too deep posterior palatal seal
D. Underextended distolingual flange of lower denture

44. A person with periodontally compromised dentition is scheduled for both upper and lower immediate complete dentures. He should go in for
A. Construction of maxillary denture first
B. Construction of mandibular denture first
C. Both to be constructed simultaneously
D. Either may be constructed first

45. In cases of immediate complete dentures, occlusal perfection is done

A. Before the dentures are first delivered
B. At the time of first post-insertion appointment at 24 hours
C. By the end of 48-hour period
D. Occlusal perfection is usually not required for immediate complete dentures

46. A patient with edentulous maxilla wants a maxillary denture to be fabricated against remaining mandibular teeth. But the problem is compounded by bilateral loss mandibular first molars resulting in mesial migration of second and third molars bilaterally. In such a case

A. Maxillary artificial teeth should be arranged in tight intercuspal position with lower teeth
B. Maxillary artificial teeth should be arranged to contact only the highest parts of natural teeth
C. The vertical height of the maxillary bite rim should be slightly reduced
D. Use of porcelain teeth for maxillary denture is a must

47. The use of a tooth with grade III mobility as an abutment for fixed partial denture

A. Is not indicated
B. Is done by splinting the mobile tooth
C. Is done by involving an extra tooth as abutment
D. Can de done in short span bridges

48. A mandibular II premolar and I molar are prepared for a metal ceramic crown. The axial height and taper are kept same for both the teeth. The preparation that is more retentive is

A. Mandibular premolar
B. Mandibular molar
C. Both are equally retentive
D. Retention is not dependent on either axial height or taper

49. During tooth preparation for a fixed partial denture, the line angles are rounded to

A. Reduce stress concentration at the corners when occlusal forces are applied

B. Reduce the possibility of trappi.g air bubbles during pouring of impression
C. Reduces the likelihood of air trappment during investment of wax pattern
D. All of the above

50. The preferred finishing line on the mesial surface of a mesially tipped second molar is
A. shoulder
B. Chamfer
C. beveled shoulder
D. knife-edge

Answer Key to MCQs in Prosthodontics Part I

1. (B) With natural teeth, the masticatory loads are around 20 kg while with complete dentures maximium forces recorded are just 6 to 8 kg.
2. (A) The mean denture bearing area of maxilla is 22.96 cm^2 while that of mandible is 12.25 cm^2. The area of periodontal membrane is 45 cm^2 approx. foe each jaw.
3. (B) Although chewing occurs bilaterally in premolar and molar region , but if the consistency of the food is tough there is a greater preference for using the premolar region.
4. (C) Besides a, b and d, it also causes loss of labiodental angle, decrease in horizontal labial angle along with narrowing of lips.
5. (C) Papillary hyperplasis is a granular type of palatal inflammation associated with the presence of suction discs. Denture stomatitis is the inflammation of the denture bearing mucosa. Epulis fissuratum is a fibrous growth around the denture borders confined to the alveolar mucosa.
6. (B) Tori are usually removed long before the impressions are made. Since tori lie too close to the floor of the mouth, relieving the tori would break the border seal.
7. (A)

8. (C)
9. (C) Coverage of the glandular region provides retention but not support because pressure on the glands interferes with their function
10. (D) Labial frenum is just a fold of mucous membrane devoid of any muscular attachment
11. (C) Orbicularis oris muscle pulls the buccal frenum forward, buccinator backwards and levator anguli oris downwards.
12. (D) The posterior palatal seal area is slightly elevated to slightly displace the soft tissue at the distal end of the denture to enhance the posterior border seal.
13. (C) The action of buccinator muscle occurs in horizontal direction and so it cannot lift the lower denture, even though the buccal flange of a properly extended denture will rest on its inferior attachment.
14. (B) When the masscter muscle contracts, it pushes against the buccinator muscle and buccal pad of fat.
15. (C)
16. (C) In the second premolar region, although the mylohyoid muscle extends nearly to the inferior border of the mandible but the presence of sublingual gland above it does not let it directly influence the denture border
17. (A) Beeswax or boxing wax is used for boxing the impression.
18. (B) The kinematic face bow is attached to the mandibular occlusal rim while the arbitary face-bow is attached to the maxillary occlusal rim.
19. (B) The face bow record is not a maxillo-mandibular relation. It is used to record the relationship of the jaws to the TMJ or the opening axis of the jaws and also helps to orient the casts in the same relationship on the articulator
20. (C) The TMJ is divided into 2 compartments by the articular disc-superior and inferior. The superior compartment promotes translation of the condyle while the lower compartment promotes rotational movement.

21. (B) During a lateral excursion, the mandible shifts bodily towards the lateral side on the working side. This direct lateral shift is called Bennet Movement and is a result of mesial movement of the balancing condyle, with a corresponding lateral movement of the working condyle.
22. (D) The reduced interarch space results in loss of cubicle space of the oral cavity. This pushes the tongue towards the throat resulting in displacement and encroachment of the adjacent tissues. It may cause closure or obstruction of the opening of the Eustachian tube resulting in ear pain. Also reduced interarch distance decreases the biting force thereby reducing soreness in patients with knife–edged ridges.
23. (B) The lateral pterygoid muscle shows little activity when the mandible is in centric relation
24. (B) The average speaking space is the space that exists between posterior teeth when the patient is enunciating s sound. It is not related to interocclusal space of rest position. This space is about 1.5 to 3 mm for Class I occlusion. For class II, it is about 3 to 6 mm while class III have a small space of about 1mm.
25. (A)
26. (D)
27. (C) The distal end of the occlusal plane for mandibular rim is established at 2/3 the length of retrolmolar pad from it's anterior border.
28. (D) Using either acrylic resin teeth or a combination of resin teeth with metal occlusal surface reduces the possibility of the artificial teeth causing unnecessary abrasion and destruction of metallic occlusal surfaces of the opposing teeth.
29. (C)
30. (B) Acrylic resin teeth wear more rapidly than porcelain anterior teeth and eventually create excessive and destructive occlusal forces in the anterior part of the mouth.
31. (D) Non-anatomic teeth are those that have a flat occlusal surface.
32. (C) While 32 relates to the combined width of posterior teeth, M signifies medium occluso-cervical length. (Also available are S-small and L-large moulds)

33. (A) The alphabets f and v are labiodental sounds. If the upper anterior teeth are set too high up, v will sound like f. If they are set too far down, f will sound like v.

    Similarly, during the pronunciation of sibilants (s, z, sh, zh, ch and j) the upper and lower incisors approach each other end to end but they should not touch.

34. (C) The velar sounds such as k, g and ng have no effect on dentures.
35. (D) During the production of sibilant sounds the upper and lower incisors come close to each other but do not touch each other i.e. mandible is in between rest and occluding position.
36. (B) All factors except condylar guidance are controlled by the dentist
37. (A) Occlusion of all complete dentures should be perfected before the patient is allowed to wear them.
38. (A) The occlusal errors should be corrected on articulator. If corrections are attempted in the mouth, it is difficult to see the errors because the soft tissue will be distorted and obscure the errors. In fact, much of the selective grinding done according to the articulating paper marks made in the mouth actually increases the amount of error in the occlusion.
39. (B) Whenever occlusal adjustment is done in centric relation on the articulator, grinding is to be done only in fossae and not on cusps.
40. (C) The dentures become loose because the deflective occlusal contacts cause a continual shifting of the denture bases on the basal seat.
41. (D) Any of these problems can lead to the patient feeling soreness while swallowing.
42. (D) The problem of gagging may be related to the denture themselves (maxillary and mandibular) or there may be a psychologic component or both.
43. (A) The gagging is caused by a making and breaking of the posterior palatal sealas the tissue posterior to the vibrating line move upwards and downwards during function. However,

occlusion may also be a factor, since shifting of the denture bases may cause the making and breaking of the posterior palatal seal and hence gagging.

44. (C) When both maxillary and mandibular immediate complete dentures are proposed, it is advisable to construct them simultaneously. This ensures that cosmetic or occlusal irregularities in the remaining dentulous arch will not interfere with tooth positioning in the immediate prosthesis.
45. (C) Occlusion may be perfected at the end of 48-hour period because by that time most of the swelling has disappeared and the denture can be frequently removed without too much discomfort.
46. (B) The use of maxillary artificial teeth arranged in tight intercuspal position will cause a forward thrust to be exerted whenever teeth are brought into contact. This will cause rotation of maxillary denrure and retention will be lost. Similarly, use of porcelain teeth is not indicated as they will cause wearing of opposing natural teeth in a very short time. Maxillary teeth arranged to contact only the highest parts of natural teeth will help in the stability of the denture. Alternatively, the occlusal plane of the remaining natural teeth may be leveled.
47. (A) A tooth with grade III mobility is not suitable as an abutment. A mobility value of two requires assessment of the cause and the consideration of the number of teeth to be replaces. If the mobility is due to deflective occlusal contacts, that can be eliminated and a short span bridge is involved, the tooth can be used as an abutment. If however, mobility is due to considerable bone loss and more than one tooth is to be replaced, the tooth is not suitable for use as an abutment, unless it can be splinted to another sound tooth.
48. (A) It is often a common mistake to assume that a larger diameter tooth will yield a more retentive preparation. If axial height and taper are kept same for both, the smaller diameter tooth interferes more effectively with the arc of rotation because the smaller radius of curvature allows the preparation to better resist dislodgement.
49. (D)

50. (D) On a mesially inclined molar, a knife-edged finishing line on the mesial surface provides adequate thickness of material for strength in the final preparation and keeps the axial reduction further from the pulp than if a shoulder or chamfer is used.

Part II

1. **The size of posterior teeth for a removable partial denture is determined primarily by which two of the following?**
   A. The useful posterior tooth space
   B. The lip line of the patient
   C. The age of the patient
   D. The characteristics of the denture-supporting tissues
   E. The facebow transfer

2. **A device that relieves the abutment teeth, to which a fixed or removable partial denture is attached, of all or part of the forces generated by occlusal function is called a:**
   A. Pontic
   B. Stressbreaker
   C. Major connector
   D. Minor connector

3. **Custom trays are an important part of rubber base impression technique since elastomers are**
   A. More accurate in uniform, thin layers 0.5 to 1.0 mm thick
   B. More accurate in uniform, thin layers 1.0 to 1.5 mm thick
   C. More accurate in uniform, thin layers 2.0 to 4.0 mm thick
   D. More accurate in uniform, thin layers 5.0 to 6.0 mm thick

4. **Which of the following are functions of the reciprocal clasp arm of a removable partial denture?**
   A. Reciprocation
   B. Stabilization
   C. Auxiliary indirect retention (bracing)
   D. All of the above

5. **Inflammatory papillary hyperplasia frequently is observed**
   A. On the dorsum of the tongue
   B. Under ill-fitting maxillary dentures, especially those having a relief chamber
   C. On the gingiva of a pregnant patient

D. About the anterior part of a complete maxillary denture when a patient has natural anterior mandibular teeth but no posterior replacement.

6. After taking an alginate impression you notice that the impression material appears grainy. Which of the following could be the cause?

A. Improper mixing
B. Prolonged mixing
C. Water/powder ratio too low
D. All of the above

7. The periodontium remains much healthier when crown margins are placed

A. Above the gingival crest
B. At the gingival crest
C. Below the gingival crest
D. Anywhere

8. A bony extension of the medical pterygoid plate of the sphenoid bone is called the:

A. Hamulus
B. Hamular notch
C. Maxillary tuberosity
D. Fovea palatini

9. The finish line of choice when fabricating either a porcelain jacket crown or an all - ceramic crown is:

A. Shoulder
B. Bevel
C. Chamfer
D. Shoulder with a bevel

10. The absolute maximum number of posterior teeth, which can be safely replaced with a fixed bridge is:

A. One
B. Two
C. Three
D. Four

11. How would you classify a removable partial denture in which a portion of the functional load is carried by the ridge at one end of the denture base segment while the other end of the base segment is supported by natural teeth?

A. A tooth borne removable partial denture
B. A bilateral distal extension removable partial denture
C. A unilateral distal extension removable partial denture
D. None of the above

12. Which of the following marginal designs is theoretically the best finishing margin for cast gold restorations, allowing burnishing and adaptation of the gold to the tooth?

A. Shoulder
B. Shoulder with a bevel
C. Chamfer
D. Bevel or feathered edge

13. A good temporary restoration for a tooth prepared for a crown should

A. Provide pulpal protection
B. Be able to be easily cleaned
C. Have non-impinging margins
D. All of the above

14. Paget's disease is often discovered in the dental office because:

A. These patients will have rampant caries due to xerostomia
B. The patient's dentures do not fit due to widening of the alveolar ridges
C. These patients will have multiple fractured restorations due to bruxims
D. These patients often have a sore tongue

15. The principal difference between dental plaster and dental stone powders is:

A. Color
B. Shelf life
C. Particle size and shape
D. Chemical formula

16. Dental stone is produced by:
A. Heating gypsum in an open kettle
B. Heating gypsum under pressure with water vapor in an autoclave
C. Heating gypsum in a 30% solution of calcium chloride
D. None of the above

17. Which of the following are indications for porcelain veneers?
A. Coverage of labial surface defects, e.g. hypoplasia of the enamel
B. Masking of discolored teeth, e.g. tetracycline staining, discoloration following loss of vitality
C. Repair of structural damage, e.g. fractured incisal edges
D. Reduction of spacing in cases when orthodontics would be inappropriate
E. All of the above

18. High-gold noble alloys, which are used in fabricating metal-ceramic restorations, are:
A. 50% gold, platinum
B. 75% gold, platinum, and palladium
C. 98% gold, platinum, and palladium
D. 100% gold, platinum, and palladium

19. A wrought-wire clasp
A. Is less flexible than a cast clasp
B. Is not as tough as cast clasp
C. Has a tensile strength that is at least 25% greater than that of the cast alloy from which it was made
D. Is not as adjustable as cast clasp

20. In the early stages of lateral movements, the condyle appears to rotate with a slight lateral Shift in the direction of the movement. This movement is called the Bennett movement. This Bennett movement refers to the
A. Nonworking side condyle only
B. Working side condyle only
C. Both the nonworking and working side condyles
D. None of the above

21 Which muscle listed below moves the disc of the TMJ forward (protrusion of mandible) ?

A. Masseter
B. Medial pterygoid
C. Lateral pterygoid
D. Temporalis

22. Which of the following is not an advantage of using polysulfide rubber impression materials?

A. Superior strength in a deep sulcus
B. Dimensionally stable after one pour
C. Have a short setting time
D. Pouring may be delayed for one hour if necessary
E. The finish line can be easily read
F. Have a good tear resistance
G. Compatible with all die materials and may be electroplated
H. Long working time and shelf life

23. Which of the following are considered to be the basic principles for occlusal adjustment?

A. The maximum distribution of occlusal stresses in centric relation
B. The forces of occlusion should be borne as much as possible by the long axis of the teeth
C. When there is surface-to-surface contact of flat cusps, it should be changed to a point-to-surface contact
D. Once centric occlusion is established, never take the teeth out of centric occlusion
E. All of the above

24. All of the following are considered to be standard components used to describe color except:

A. Chroma
B. Hue
C. Intensity
D. Value

25. Which of the following is not associated with diabetes?

A. Delayed healing
B. Rapidly periodontal disease with marked alveolar bone loss
C. Mucosal bleeding

D. Increased calculus formation
E. A predilection for periapical abscesses

26. The compensating curve is defined as:

A. The amount of separation between the mandible and maxilla when the mandible and its supporting muscles are in a resting position
B. The anteroposterior and lateral curvature in a alignment of the occluding surfaces and incisal edges of artificial teeth which is used to develop a balanced occlusion
C. The angle made by the slopes of a cusp with a perpendicular line bisecting the cusp, measured Mesiodistally or buccolingually
D. None of the above

27. Which of the following constituents of alginate power (irreversible hydrocolloid) functions as a plasticizer?

A. Trisodium phosphate
B. Zinc oxide
C. Calcium sulfate
D. Potassium titanium fluoride

28. All of the following statements concerning pontics are true except:

A. With regard to the ease of cleaning and good tissue health proper pontic design is more important than the choice of material used in fabricating the pontic
B. The contour and nature of the pontic contact with the ridge is very important
C. The area of contact between the pontic and the ridge should be small
D. The portion of the pontic approximating the ridge should be as concave as possible
E. The pontic should exert no pressure on the ridge (passive contact with no blanching of the tissue)

29. Soldering flux is composed of:

A. Chromium, graphite and silica
B. Boric acid, silica and chromium

C. Graphite sodium pyroborate and boric acid
D. Sodium pyroborate, boric aid and silica

30. Which of the following statements concerning centric relation are true ?

A. The mandible cannot be forced into centric relation from the rest position because the patient reflex neuromuscular defense would resist the applied force
B. The mandible should be relaxed and gently guided into centric relation
C. In fixed and removable prosthodontics, centric relation should be established prior to designing the frame works
D. All of the above statements are true

31. All of the following are advantage of reversible hydrocolloid impression materials except

A. No custom trays required
B. Some moisture can be tolerated in the sulcus
C. Clean and easy placement
D. Easy to pour
E. Can be poured whenever you want
F. Inexpensive
G. Excellent shelf life *(3.5 years)*

32. When treatment planning for fixed prosthodontics, all of the following information can be obtained by studying diagnostic casts *except*

A. The length of the abutment teeth can be accurately gauged
B. The true inclination of the abutment teeth will be evident
C. The presence of periodontal pockets and the crown-to-root ratio of potential abutment teeth
D. Mesiodistal drifting rotation and faciolingual displacement of potential abutment teeth can be clearly seen

33. The partially edentulous arch which is bilateral without any distal abutments would be classified as :

A. Kennedy Class I
B. Kennedy Class II
C. Kennedy Class III
D. Kennedy Class IV

34. Which of the following is not a characteristic of polyether impression material

A. Have a clean, pleasant taste and odor
B. Slow setting
C. Dimensionally stable if more than one cast is poured
D. Excellent dimensionally stability when dry

35. Prior to fabricating removable partial denture for a patient surveying the diagnostic casts will enable the dentist to determine

A. Areas that can be used for support
B. A path of travel for insertion and removal of the denture
C. The crown to root ratio of potential abutment teeth
D. The periodontal health of potential abutment teeth

36. A wrought-wire of a given composition is:

A. Generally inferior in mechanical properties to a casting of the same composition
B. Generally has the same mechanical properties as a casting of the same composition
C. Generally superior in mechanical properties to a casting of the same composition
D. None of the above

37. Anterior guidance is the result of :

A. Horizontal overlap
B. Vertical overlap
C. Horizontal and vertical overlap
D. Cusp heights

38. Conventional feldspathic porcelain is composed of :

A. Silica
B. Alumina
C. Potash and soda
D. All of the above

39. Which of the following are function of the posterior palatal seal ?

A. Completes the border seal of the maxillary denture
B. Prevents impaction of food beneath the tissue surface of the denture

C. Improves the physiologic retention of the denture
D. Compensates for shrinkage of the denture resin during processing
E. All of the above

40. "T" and "D" sounds are formed by:
A. The tongue protruding slightly between the maxillary and mandibular anterior teeth
B. Contact of the tip of the tongue with the anterior palate and lingual surfaces of the maxillary anterior teeth
C. The lips only
D. None of the above

41. The ease and accuracy in border molding depends on which of the following
A. An accurately fitting custom tray
B. Control of bulk and temperature of the modeling compound
C. The tray being thoroughly cured
D. All of the above

42. Which of the following are indications for fixed bridgework or important considerations to think about when contemplating the fabrication of fixed bridge work for a patient?
A. A limited number of edentulous areas which would not otherwise be more satisfactorily restored with removable partial denture
B. The need to prevent the over-eruption of opposing teeth and the drifting of teeth neighboring the edentulous space
C. The presence of suitable abutment teeth, favorable crown/ root ratio, adequate alveolar support, absence of apical pathology etc.
D. Esthetics
E. Patient motivation including time availability
F. Clinical and technical ability
G. All of the above

43. Which of the following elastomeric impression materials has the longest working and setting times?
A. Polyester
B. Polysulfide

C. Condensation silicone
D. Addition silicone

44. Which of the following elastomeric impression materials has very poor dimensional stability?
A. Polyether
B. Polysulfide
C. Condensation silicone
D. Addition silicone

45. The preparation for a full gold crown involves circumferential and occlusal reduction of between:
A. 0.5 and 1.0 mm
B. 2.0 and 2.5 mm
C. 3.0 and 3.5 mm
D. 4.0 and 4.5 mm

46. In casting the metal substructure for a metal-ceramic crown it is necessary to use which type of investment?
A. Gypsum-bonded investment
B. Phosphate-bonded investment
C. Silica-bonded investment
D. Any of the above

47. The principal component of dental plaster is:
A. Alpha hemihydrates
B. Beta-hemihydrates
C. Delta-hemihydrates
D. None of the above

48. Which of the following statements is correct in reference to polysulfide rubber base impression materials?
A. A decrease in temperature or humidity will accelerate the setting time of this material
B. An increase in temperature or humidity will accelerate the setting time of this material
C. Temperature and humidity have no effect the setting time of this material
D. All of the above

49. As the width of a claps increases, its flexibility

A. Increases

B. Decreases

C. Stays the same

D. First increases and then decreases

50. Claps that originated from above the survey line usually form an occlusal rest and angle downward across the clinical crown until the tip is located in a prescribed amount of undercut are:

A. Suprabulge retainers

B. Infrabulge retainers

C. Bar clasps

D. Roach clasps

51. Decreased vertical dimension of occlusion refers to an occluding vertical dimension that results in

A. A loss of interocclusal distance when the mandible is in the rest position *(decreased freeway space)*

B. An excessive interocclusal distance when the mandible is in the rest position (Increased freeway space)

C. An increase in leeway space

D. None of the above

52. Which of the following statements concerning the altered cast technique are true ?

A. The purpose of this technique is two fold :

To record the form of the edentulous segment without tissue displacement

To accurately relate the edentulous segment to the teeth via the framework

B. The technique helps to obtain soft tissue support to aid abutments in resisting functional streses

C. This technique is a secondary impression system which utilizes the metal framework to hold customized impression trays for the edentulous areas

D. All of the above statements are true

53. All of the following are advantages of dental porcelain restorations except:

A. Excellent color and translucency

B. Low thermal and electrical conductivity
C. Low plastic deformation
D. High hardness

54. During typical empty mouth swallowing, the mandible is braced in:
A. The intercuspal position (IP)
B. The retruded contact position (RCP)
C. The protruded contact position (PCP)
D. Centric relation (CR)

55. Which teeth on a maxillary complete denture are the most important when considering esthetics?
A. Maxillary laterals
B. Maxillary centrals
C. Maxillary canines
D. Maxillary first premolars

56. Which of the following are the primary requirements for making a centric relation record when fabricating a removable partial denture?
A. To record the correct horizontal relation of the mandible to the maxilla
B. To stabilize the lower record base with equalized vertical pressure
C. To retain the record in an undistorted condition until the casts have been accurately mounted on the articulator or until a previous record can be verified
D. All of the above

57. Remounting and equilibration of complete dentures is carried out to:
A. Compensate for slight errors which may have occurred during the mounting of the casts
B. Correct for minor deficiencies in the setting of the denture teeth
C. Correct for tooth movement which may have occurred during processing of the dentures
D. All of the above

58. All of the following are disadvantages to immediate denture therapy. Which one is considered to be the major disadvantages to immediate denture therapy?

A. Increased post-insertion care
B. Increased post-insertion soreness
C. Not being able to have an anterior tooth try in to evaluate esthetics
D. Greater complexity of clinical procedures
E. A higher cost of treatment

59. An articulator which has the condylar elements on the lower member of the articulator and the condylar path elements on the upper member is called the

A. Arcon articulator
B. Non-arcon articulator
C. Hinge articulator
D. Free plane articulator

60. The first step in the treatment of abused tissues in a patient with existing dentures is to:

A. Fabricate a new set of dentures
B. Reline the dentures
C. Educate the patient
D. Excise the abused tissues

61. The primary reason for choosing a ¾ crown over a full cast crown is:

A. The preparation is easier
B. Tooth structure is spared
C. Less anesthesia is required
D. It's cheaper to make

62. Which of the following best describes the term "quenching"?

A. A metal is elevated to a temperature above room temperature and held there for a length of time
B. A metal is rapidly cooled from an elevated temperature to room temperature or below
C. Softening a metal by controlled heating and cooling
D. None of the above

63. Which of the following indirect retainers will provide the best leverage against lifting of the denture base?

A. To one located the closest to the clasp tips which is located furthest from the edentulous area

B. The one located the farthest from the clasp tips which is located nearest to the edentulous area

C. The one located the furthest from the clasp tips which is located furthest from the edentulous area

D. It doesn't matter

64. Clasps are:

A. Intracoronal retainers

B. Extracoronal retainers

C. May be both

D. Subgingival retainers

65. Condylar guidance is a factor which:

A. Is totally controlled by the dentist

B. Is totally dictated by the patient

C. Is partially dictated by the patient but can be adjusted by the dentist if necessary

D. Can be adjusted by the laboratory technician

66. Frequently overextended areas of the acrylic denture base include:

A. Frenal attachments

B. Distobuccal flange

C. Distolingual flange

D. In the vestibules (mucobuccal area)

E. All of the above

67. Which of the following statements concerning the functionally generated pathway technique are true:

A. A prerequisite for the use of this technique for the restoration of a single tocth is the presence of an optimal occlusion

B. This technique allows the cuspal movements of the dentition to be recorded in wax intra-orally and transferred to the articulator in the form of a static plaster cast

C. This static plaster cast is also called the functional index

D. By registering the pathways of the opposing tooth surfaces during mandibular movements, the technique allows a laboratory technician to provide a restoration with an occlusal surface less likely to incorporate occlusal interferences.
E. All of the above statements concerning the functionally generated pathway are true

68. Posterior teeth that are set edge to edge may cause:
A. Gagging
B. Cheek biting
C. Reduced taste
D. Speech aberrations

69. Bite registration material used to make an accurate interocclusal record should have what important characteristic listed below?
A. Offer a maximum resistance to the patient's jaw closure and have high flow at mixing
B. Offer a maximum resistance to the patient's jaw closure and have low flow at mixing
C. Offer a minimum resistance to the patient's jaw closure and have low flow at mixing
D. Offer a minimum resistance to the patient's jaw closure and have high flow at mixing

70. All of the following statements are true concerning a facebow or a facebow transfer except:
A. The face bow is a caliper like device used to record the patient's maxilla/hinge axis relationship (opening and closing axis)
B. If the transfer is done properly, the arc of closure on the articulator should duplicate that exhibited by the patient
C. The facebow transfer is a maxillo-mandibular record
D. The facebow transfer is used to transfer the maxilla/hinge axis relationship to the articulator during the mounting of the maxillary cast.

71 Factors that may contribute to porosities in a denture include:
A. Insufficient pressure on the flask during processing
B. Insufficient material in the mold

C. A rapid elevation in temperature to 212°F causing vaporization of the liquid
D. All of the above

72. An edentulous patient has slight undercuts in both tuberosities and also in the facial of the anterior maxilla. To construct a satisfactory maxillary complete denture, you should reduce which of the following:
A. All undercuts
B. The anterior undercut only
C. Both tuberosity undercuts
D. None of them

73. The treatment plan for a patient indicates that both mandibular and maxillary immediate dentures are to be fabricated. The ideal way to do this is:
A. Fabricate the maxillary immediate denture first
B. Fabricate the mandibular immediate denture first
C. Fabricate the maxillary and mandibular Immediate dentures at the same time
D. None of the above

74. Balancing side (nonworking side) interferences generally occur on the inner aspects of the:
A. Facial cusps of mandibular molars
B. Facial cusps of maxillary premolars
C. Lingual of mandibular molars
D. Facial cusps of maxillary molars

75. Which of the following elastomeric impression materials has the shortest working and setting times?
A. Polyether
B. Polysulfide
C. Condensation silicone
D. Addition silicone

76. The ideal crown-to-root ratio of a tooth to be utilized as a bridge abutment is
A. 3:1
B. 2:1

C. 1:2
D. 1:1

77. Which of the following is defined as "the vertical distance or space between the incisal and occlusal surfaces of the maxillary and mandibular teeth with the mandible in the physiological test position?
A. Vertical dimension of occlusal (VDO)
B. Vertical dimension of rest (VDR)
C. Interocclusal distance (freeway space)
D. None of the above

78. The setting time of a zinc oxide-eugenol impression paste may be accelerated by
A. Adding a drop of alcohol to the mix
B. Using the frozen-stab method of mixing
C. Adding a drop of water to the mix
D. Decreasing the amount of eugenol

79. The path of insertion for an anterior ¾ crown should:
A. Be perpendicular to the incisal one-half of the labial surface rather than the long axis of the tooth
B. Be parallel to the incisal one-half to two-thirds of the labial surface rather than the long axis of the tooth
C. Be parallel to the long axis of the tooth
D. Be parallel to the cervical one-third of the labial surface rather than the long axis of the tooth

80. Which of the following Kennedy classes of removable partial dentures are tooth borne?
A. Class I
B. Class II
C. Class III
D. Class IV

81. An increase in the temperature of the water used in mixing alginate impression materials will:
A. Shorten the setting time
B. Lengthen the setting time
C. Prevent setting
D. Not effect on the setting time at all

82. All of the following advantages of precision attachment restorations except:

A. They provide retention without an unsightly display of metal

B. They are easy to repair

C. The functional load is dispersed down the long axis of the abutments by virtue of the low central loading at the base of the attachments

D. The restorations permit the patient access to all areas of the tissues when the denture is not in place

E. If both sides of the dental arch have this type of restoration and are joined by a rigid major connector excellent bilateral stabilization is provided to the abutments.

83. All of the following are indications for using a lingucplate as a mandibular major connector except:

A. To avoid a high lingual frenum or when there is no space in the floor of the mouth

B. Mandibular tori that cannot be removed

C. To support periodontically weakened teeth

D. Severe anterior crowding

E. To serve as retention for lower anterior denture teeth when the prognosis for the natural teeth is guarded

84. All of the following statements concerning supporting cusps are true, except:

A. They contact the opposing tooth in the intercuspal position

B. They support the vertical dimension of the face

C. They are nearer the faciolingual center of the tooth than the non-supporting cusps

D. The outer incline has a potential for contact

E. They have narrower and sharper cusp ridges than non-supporting cusps

85. The process by which investment ring is heated in a porcelain furnace to a temperature of 980°C to burn off any remaining impurities prior to adding porcelain is called:

A. Quenching

B. Pickling

C. Degassing
D. Investing

86. All of the following are the theoretical determinants needed for restoring a complete and functional occlusal surface of a tooth, except:
A. The amount of vertical overlap of the anterior teeth
B. The contour of the articular eminence
C. The height of the pulp horn of that particular tooth
D. The amount and direction of lateral shift in the working side condyle
E. The position of the tooth in the arch

87. The first layer of porcelain applied to the metal coping is called the:
A. Opaque porcelain
B. Body porcelain
C. Incisal porcelain
D. None of the above

88. Which of the following statements is true concerning the posterior palatal seal?
A. The outline and depth of the posterior seal is the same for every patient
B. The posterior palatal seal will vary in outline and depth according to the palatal form of the patient
C. A posterior palatal seal is not necessary when fabricating a complete denture on a patient with a flat palate
D. Once the complete denture fits properly, it is okay to remove the posterior palatal seal.

89. The most important benefit of an over denture (root-retained denture) is:
A. The psychological comfort of avoiding the loss of all teeth
B. The continuous functional feedback for the neuromuscular system from proprioceptors in the PDL
C. The preservation of the alveolar ridge
D. The improved support and stability for the denture
E. The increased retention of the denture

90. Which of the following changes are usually evident on the maxillary arch in a patient who wears a complete maxillary denture and lacs posterior occlusion

A. Excessive amount of hyperplasic tissue present on the anterior portion of the maxillary ridge
B. Poor bone structure in the anterior part of the maxilla
C. Fibrous tuberosities
D. All of the above

91. The process of the joining of two metals by the use of a filler material which has a substantially lower fusion temperature than that of the metal parts being joined is called

A. Pickling
B. Soldering
C. Fluxing
D. Casting

92. A patient comes to your office one week after delivery of new dentures She has developed a dispersed pattern of traumatic ulcers over the crest of the mandibular residual ridge. What is the most likely cause of these ulcers?

A. Acrylic resin spicules
B. An inaccurate denture base
C. Premature occlusal contacts
D. Particles of food trapped under the denture base

93. Before an accurate facebow transfer record can be made on a patient, which of the following must be determined?

A. Location of the hinge axis point
B. The inclination of each condyle
C. Vertical dimension of occlusal
D. Centric relation

94. The temporomandibular joint is a:

A. Hinge joint
B. Gliding *(Sliding)* joint
C. Combined hinge and gliding joint
D. Ball and socket joint

95. All new dentures should be evaluated:

A. 3 hours after delivery

B. 12 hours after delivery
C. 24 hours after delivery
D. 48 hours after delivery

96. Where do the occlusal contact possibility occur during protrusive movement

A. On the maxillary mesial inclines and mandibular distal inclines
B. On the maxillary mesial inclines and mandibular mesial inclines
C. On the maxillary distal inclines and mandibular mesial inclines
D. On the maxillary distal inclines and mandibular distal inclines

97. Your are about to take alginate impressions on a patient. What can you do to help prevent the patient from gagging during this procedure?

A. Take your time
B. Work quickly
C. Use warm water to mix the alginate
D. Use cold water to mix the alginate
E. Have the patient breathe through his/her nose
F. Have the patient breathe his/her mouth
G. Recline the patient
H. Seat the patient in an upright position

98. The determinants of occlusion include:

A. The right temporomandibular joint and its suspensor ligaments
B. The left temporomandibular joint and its suspensor ligaments
C. The occlusal surface of the teeth
D. The neuromuscular system
E. All of the above

99. The major weakness of all-ceramic crowns is:

A. Poor esthetics
B. Their inability to flex
C. Their lack of translucency
D. Their high compressive strength

100. In an ideal intercuspal position the mesio buccal cusp of the permanent maxillary second molars oppose what?

A. The distobuccal groove of the mandibular first molar
B. The buccal groove of the mandibular second molar
C. The mesio buccal groove of the mandibular second molar
D. The development groove between the distobuccal and the distal cusp of the mandibular first molar

101. Teeth that appear to be color matched under one type of light appear very different under light source. This phenomenon is called what?

A. Fluorescence
B. Metamerism
C. Opaqueness
D. None of the above

102. In metal-ceramic restorations, where does the failure or fractures usually occur?

A. In the porcelain
B. At the porcelain metal interface
C. In the metal
D. None of the above

103. The primary role of anterior teeth on denture is :

A. To incise food
B. Occlusion
C. Esthetics
D. Stability of the denture

104. The primary dentures support area for a mandibular complete denture is :

A. The labial vestibule
B. The buccal shelf
C. The palatopharyngeal fold
D. The frenulum

105. Endodontically treated teeth that have been restored with a cast and core and crown are subjected to the high incidence of :

A. Periodontal disease
B. Recurrent caries

C. Vertical root fracture
D. The need for an apicoectomy

106. Which of the following best describes Camper's line *(plane)*

A. It is a line *(plane)* which is determined by the occlusal surfaces of the teeth
B. It is a line *(plane)* which extends from the outer canthus of eye to the superior border of the tragus of the ear
C. It is the line *(plane)* running from the inferior border of the ala of the nose to the superior border of the tragus of the ear
D. None of the above

107. Alginate impressions were placed in a bowl of water so that they would not dry up before pouring them up in dental stone. Which of the following was the result of leaving these impressions immersed in water for a few hours?

A. Gelatin
B. Adsorption
C. Syneresis
D. Imbibition

108. Which of the following pontics is primarily used in the nonappearance zone ?

A. The saddle pontic
B. The sanitary pontic
C. The modified ridge lap pontic
D. Ridge lap pontics

109. Which of the following statements concerning selective grinding in complete denture fabrication for centric relation are true?

A. Ideally, selective grinding should result in harmonious cusp-fossa contacts of all upper and lower fossa (and marginal ridges of bicuspids)
B. Only grind cusp tips that interfere in centric, lateral and protrusive movements
C. Neither of the above statements are true
D. Both of the above statements are true

110. What is the recommended treatment for a patient that has lost her four maxillary incisors some time ago and suffered excessive ridge resorption?

A. A conventional six- unit fixed bridge
B. No treatment
C. A removable partial denture
D. A Maryland bridge

111. Which of the following impressions material are very accurate if the model is poured immediately but are dimensionally unstable on storage because they shrink due to the evaporation of ethanol, a by-product of the polymerization process ?

A. Polysulfide
B. Silicones
C. Polyvinyl siloxanes
D. Polyethers

112. All of the following are considered to be the basic rules for occlusal rest design when fabricating a removable partial denture except:

A. The rest should minimize the tilting action of the appliance
B. The rest must be placed so that it will prevent movement of the appliance in an occlusal direction
C. The rest should be placed so that it will prevent movement of the appliance in a cervical direction
D. The rest must have sharp angles to permit maximum retention

113. The function of an indirect retainer is:

A. To prevent horizontal dislodgement of the distal extension base of a removable partial denture
B. To connect the parts of the prosthesis located on one side of the arch with those on the opposite side
C. To prevent vertical dislodgement of the distal extension base of a removable partial denture
D. To link the major connector and other parts of the prosthesis together

114. The fixed vegetable or mineral oil present in a tube of zinc oxide performs what function when it is mixed with eugenol to form ZOE impression paste?
A. Accelerator
B. Plasticizer
C. Filler
D. All of the above

115. Which of the following elastic impression materials have very limited dimensional stability?
A. Irreversible (alginate) & Reversible hydrocolloid (agar-agar)
B. Silicones
C. Polyethers
D. Polyvinyl siloxanes

116. You are ready to place packing cord around a tooth that was prepared for a crown on a patient with hypertension. It is recommended to use a cord impregnated with:
A. Epinephrine
B. Alum (aluminum potassium sulfate)
C. Zinc chloride
D. None of the above

117. Which of the following is the most important reason for treatment of hyperplastic tissue before construction of a complete or removable partial denture?
A. It will make the patient feel better
B. It will make the facebow transfer easier to perform
C. To provide a firm, stable base for the denture
D. The final impression material will flow better

118. A nonrigid connector is comprised of:
A. A key
B. A keyway
C. A key and a keyway
D. None of the above

119. Which of the following cements is indicated when maximum retention is required or when the pulp is of no concern?
A. Zinc polycarboxylate cement
B. Glass ionomer cement

C. Zinc phosphate cement
D. ZOE cement

120. The most rigid palatal major connector is the:
A. Single palatal bar
B. Palatal horseshoe-shaped connector
C. Palatal plate
D. Anterior posterior palatal bar connector

121. The glaze firing:
A. Is the first firing and produces a rough surface
B. Is performed prior to adding body porcelain to ensure a rough surface
C. Is a separate firing and produces a smooth, translucent surface
D. Is performed on the metal coping to clean the surface of any impurities

122. The "Glossary of Prosthodontic Terms" defines balanced occlusion as:
A. An occlusion of the teeth which presents a harmonious relation of the occluding surfaces in centric position within the functional range
B. An occlusion of the teeth which presents a harmonious relation of the occluding surfaces in eccentric positions only within the functional range
C. An occlusion of the teeth which presents a harmonious relation of the occluding surfaces in centric and eccentric positions within the functional range
D. An occlusion of teeth of maximum intercuspation of teeth

123. In the inter cuspal position, the mesiolingual cusp of a permanent maxillary second molar occludes where?
A. Central fossa of the mandibular first molar
B. Central fossa of the mandibular second molar
C. The interproximal marginal ridge areas between the mandibular first and second molars
D. The interproximal marginal ridge areas between the mandibular second and third molars

124. The powder (polymer) used in self-cured or heat-cured acrylic resins is usually

A. Benzoyl peroxide
B. Polymethyl methacrylate (PMMA)
C. Hydroquinone
D. Methyl methacrylate (MMA)

125. When establishing a balanced occlusion, the lingual cusps of maxillary posterior teeth on the balancing side should contact:

A. The central fossae of mandibular posterior teeth
B. The lingual inclines of facial cusps of mandibular posterior teeth
C. The lingual inclines of lingual cusps of mandibular posterior teeth
D. The facial inclines of lingual cusps of mandibular posterior teeth

126. Which method below is the preferred method to preserve the facebow transfer?

A. Taking a plaster index
B. Using 10 X wax
C. Hand mount
D. None of the above

127. An overextended distobuccal corner of a mandibular denture will push against which muscle during function?

A. Zygomaticus
B. Orbicularis oris
C. Temporalis
D. Masseter

128. How will the alveolar ridge respond to a mandibular complete denture base that terminates short of the retromolar pad?

A. Marked ridge resorption will occur
B. The apposition of bone on the ridge will occur
C. The alveolar ridge will not be affected at all
D. It has no concern with bone

129. Which of the following impressions are not elastomers?
A. Alginate
B. Polysulfide
C. Silicones
D. Polyether
E. All of the above

130. Which of the following best describes "strain hardening" or work hardening"?
A. Hardening (or deformation) of a metal at room temperature
B. Hardening (or deformation) of a metal at a very high temperature
C. Softening a metal by controlled heating and cooling
D. Softening a metal at room temperature

131. Epulis fissuratum is caused by:
A. Poor oral hygiene
B. Denture cleaners
C. An ill-fitting denture flange
D. An incorrectly placed posterior palatal seal

132. Dental plaster and stone is vibrated after mixing to:
A. Minimize distortion
B. Reduce setting time
C. Eliminate air bubbles
D. Increase the setting time

133. All surfaces of the metal coping or substructure in a metal-ceramic crown should be:
A. Smooth
B. Well-rounded
C. Convex
D. All of the above

134. All of the following are advantages of using a cast chromium-cobalt alloy for removable partial dentures except:
A. Corrosion resistance
B. High strength
C. High flexibility
D. Low specific gravity

135. Die Stone is classified as which type of gypsum product?
A. Type I
B. Type II
C. Type III
D. Type IV

136. Which of the following is defined as "the quality of a restoration to be firm, steady, constant and not subject to change of position when forces are applied"?
A. Retention
B. Stability
C. Adhesion
D. Reciprocation

137. All of the following are advantages of infrabulge retainers as compared to suprabulge retainers except:
A. More efficient retention
B. Less distortion of coronal contours
C. Less tooth contact
D. Cleaner
E. Less bothersome to vestibular tissues
F. Less prone to caries
G. Esthetically superior in most cases
H. Greater adjustability

138. In a protrusive movement, the condyles of the mandible have moved in a:
A. Backward and upward direction
B. Downward and forward direction
C. Backward and downward direction
D. Forward and backward direction one by one

139. In a posterior fixed bridge, a pontic:
A. Should be in contact in centric occlusion
B. May or may not be in contact in working-side movements
C. Should not be in contact in nonworking side movements
D. All of the above

140. When the mandible is in its physiologic rest or postural position, the contact of teeth is:
A. Maximum

B. Not present
C. Premature
D. Slight

141. Centric occlusion (CO) is a:
A. "Muscle-guided" position
B. "Ligament-guided" position
C. "Tooth-guided" position
D. Bone guided position

142. Occlusion rims are used to:
A. Determine and establish the vertical dimension of occlusion
B. Make maxillo-mandibular jaw records
C. Establish and locate the future position of the artificial teeth
D. All of the above

143. An excessive vertical dimension of occlusion is the usual cause of:
A. Cheek biting
B. Gagging
C. Clicking
D. Reduced taste

144. A patient who wears a complete maxillary denture complains of a burning sensation in the palatal area of his/her mouth. This is indicative of too much pressure being exerted by the denture on the:
A. Incisive foramen
B. Palatal mucosa
C. Hamular notch
D. Posterior palatal seal

145. All of the following are benefits that a patient usually realizes from immediate dentures except:
A. Continuously acceptable esthetics
B. Improved speech adaptation
C. Protection of the extraction sites from trauma
D. Decreased post-delivery soreness
E. Continuously acceptable masticatory function
F. Prevention of tongue enlargement

146. Which component of zinc oxide-eugenol impression paste functions as an accelerator of the setting time?

A. Oil of cloves
B. Resinous balsam
C. Rosin
D. Calcium chloride

147. All of the following statements concerning elastomeric impression materials are true except:

A. All elastomeric impression materials expand slightly during setting
B. Elastomeric impression materials are unable to displace both oral fluids and gingival tissues
C. The prepared teeth should be free of surface moisture but not bone dry prior to taking an impression with elastomeric impression materials.
D. Compared to hydrocolloids, elastomeric impression materials are easier to prepare, are much more resistant to tearing on removal and have a superior dimensional stability.

148. Xerostomia can be caused by:

A. Medications (i.e. antihypertensives and antidepressants)
B. Cancer therapy (i.e. chemotherapeutic drugs and radiation treatment)
C. Sjogren's syndrome
D. Trauma to the head and neck causing nerve damage
E. Conditions such as bone marrow transplants, endocrine, disorders, stress, anxiety, depression and nutritional deficiencies
F. All of the above

149. Surgical removal of a maxillary torus is indicated when?

A. The torus impinges on the soft palate
B. The torus is so large that it fills the vault and prevents the formation of an adequate denture base
C. The torus is undercut
D. The torus extends so far posteriorly that it interferes with the posterior palatal seal

E. When it is psychologically disturbing to the patient who suffers from cancerphobia
F. All of the above

150. A reverse ¾ crown is most frequently fabricated for a:
A. Maxillary premolar
B. Mandibular premolar
C. Mandibular molar
D. Maxillary molar

151. When casting conventional gold alloys, which type of dental investment should be used?
A. Phosphate-bonded investment
B. Gypsum-bonded investment
C. Silica-bonded investment
D. None of the above

152. All of the following are indications for electrosurgery except:
A. To remove hyperplastic gingival tissue where it has proliferated into preparations or over crown margins
B. In place of gingival retraction cord where substantial attached gingiva is present
C. Where attached gingival tissues are thin or where an underlying dehiscence is suspected
D. For crown lengthening procedures prior to fabricating a provisional crown

153. What is the general rule for sprue pin diameter when using a centrifugal type of casting machine?
A. The diameter of the sprue pin should be equal to or greater than the thickest portion of the pattern
B. The diameter of the sprue pin should be equal to or smaller than the thickest portion of the pattern
C. The diameter of the sprue pin should be equal to or greater than the thinnest portion of the pattern
D. The diameter of the sprue pin should be equal to or smaller than the thinnest portion of the pattern

154. The major connector is:
A. The connecting tong between the denture and other units of the prosthesis

B. The part of the denture base which extends from the necks of the teeth to the border of the denture
C. The unit of a partial denture that connects the parts of the prosthesis located on one side of the arch with those on the opposite side
D. None of the above

155. Which component of the chromium alloys used to fabricate the framework for removable partial dentures increases the ductility of the alloy?
A. Chromium
B. Cobalt
C. Nickel
D. Copper

156. A definitive evaluation of existing occlusal disharmonies can only be made after:
A. Evaluating the full mouth radiographs
B. A periodontal evaluation
C. Mounting diagnostic casts
D. A full mouth scaling and polishing

157. The cingulum rest is usually confined to preparation on:
A. Maxillary lateral incisors
B. Maxillary canines
C. Mandibular lateral incisors
D. Mandibular canines

158. Prolonged sensitivity to heat, cold, and pressure after cementation of a crown or a fixed bridge is usually related to:
A. Recurrent decay
B. A periodontal problem
C. Occlusal trauma
D. An open margin

159. Which teeth listed below should ideally provide the predominant guidance through the full range of movement in lateral mandibular excursions?
A. Premolars
B. First molars

C. Incisors
D. Canines

160. When border molding a mandibular custom tray that will be used for a final denture impression:
A. The distofacial extension is determined by the position and action of the temporalis muscle and the distolingual extension is limited by the action of the superior constrictor muscle
B. The distofacial extension is determined by the position and action of the masseter muscle and the distolingual extension is limited by the action of the superior constrictor muscle
C. The distofacial extension is determined by the position and action of the mylohyoid muscle and the distolingual extension is limited by the action of the inferior constrictor muscle
D. The distofacial extension is determined by the position and action of the genioglossus muscle and the distolingual extension is limited by action of the inferior constrictor muscle

161. In the intercuspal position, the distobuccal cusp of a permanent mandibular first molar occludes where?
A. The interproximal marginal ridge area between the maxillary second bicuspid and first molar
B. Central fossa of the maxillary first molar
C. Central fossa of the maxillary second molar
D. The interproximal marginal ridge area between the maxillary first molar and second molar.

162. In the mesial rest, guide plane and 1-bar design, reciprocation is achieved by:
A. Rigid plating
B. Minor connectors
C. Guide planes extended around the vertical line of abutments
D. Contact areas of proximal teeth
E. Reciprocal clasp arms
F. All of the above

163. Which mandibular major connector listed below is more popular?
A. Lingual bar
B. Labial bar

C. Lingual plate
D. All of the above

164. In an ideal intercuspal position, the mesiolingual cusps of permanent mandibular molars oppose:
A. The opposing central fossae
B. The lingual embrasure between their class counterpart and the tooth distal to it
C. The opposing distal marginal ridge
D. The lingual embrasure between their class counterpart and the tooth mesial to it

165. When posterior teeth are in a normal ideal relationship, which of the following cusps are considered to be supporting cusps?
A. Maxillary lingual cusps
B. Maxillary buccal cusps
C. Mandibular lingual cusps
D. Mandibular buccal cusps

166. In an ideal intercuspal position, the facial cusps tips of permanent maxillary premolars oppose:
A. The facial embrasure between their class counterpart and the tooth mesial to it
B. The facial embrasure between their class counterpart and the tooth distal to it
C. The opposing central fossae
D. The opposing mesial marginal ridge

167. Reducing occlusal interferences (selective grinding) should usually be done:
A. After a fixed bridge or a partial denture is delivered to a patient
B. Before constructing a fixed bridge or a partial denture for a patient
C. After a fixed bridge but before a partial denture is delivered to a patient
D. After a partial denture but before a fixed bridge is delivered to a patient

168. After border molding the mandibular custom tray, it is important to check for dislodgement in order to detect areas of:
A. Underextension of the tray
B. Overextension of the tray
C. Thickness of the tray
D. None of the above

169. In dentistry, the most frequently used polymer system is:
A. Bis-GMA
B. Polyether
C. Methyl methacrylate
D. Polyvinyl

170. Immediate dentures should be scheduled for relines at:
A. 1 month and 3 months post extraction
B. 4 months and 7 months post extraction
C. 5 months and 10 months post extraction
D. 1 year and 2 years post extraction

171. A generalized speech difficulty with complete dentures is usually caused by which two of the following?
A. Faulty tooth position
B. Excess vertical dimension of occlusion
C. Faulty palatal contours
D. Faulty occlusion

172. Which of the following components found in alginate powder controls the setting time of alginate?
A. Sodium alginate
B. Sodium phosphate
C. Calcium ions
D. Calcium alginate

173. Latex gloves should not be worn when mixing which of the following elastomeric impression materials by hand?
A. Polyether
B. Polysulfide
C. Condensation silicone
D. Addition silicone

174. Overbite is:

A. The horizontal projection of the maxillary anterior teeth beyond the mandibular anterior teeth

B. The vertical overlapping of the maxillary anterior teeth over the mandibular anterior teeth

C. A malocclusion in which the anterior teeth do not close or come together

D. A malocclusion where some of the maxillary teeth are inside of the mandibular teeth.

Answer Key to MCQs in Prosthodontics Part II

1	A, D	2	B	3	C	4	D
5	B	6	D	7	A	8	A
9	A	10	C	11	C	12	D
13	D	14	B	15	C	16	B
17	E	18	C	19	C	20	B
21	C	22	C	23	E	24	C
25	C	26	B	27	B	28	D
29	D	30	D	31	E	32	C
33	A	34	B	35	B	36	C
37	C	38	D	39	E	40	B
41	D	42	G	43	B	44	C
45	A	46	B	47	B	48	B
49	B	50	A	51	B	52	D
53	C	54	A	55	B	56	D
57	D	58	C	59	A	60	C
61	B	62	B	63	B	64	B
65	B	66	E	67	E	68	B
69	C	70	C	71	D	72	C
73	C	74	A	75	A	76	C
77	C	78	C	79	B	80	C, D
81	A	82	B	83	D	84	E
85	C	86	C	87	A	88	B
89	C	90	D	91	B	92	C
93	A	94	C	95	C	96	C
97	B, C, E, H	98	E	99	B	100	B
101	B	102	A	103	C	104	B

105	C	106	C	107	D	108	B
109	D	110	C	111	B	112	D
113	C	114	B	115	A	116	B
117	C	118	C	119	C	120	D
121	C	122	C	123	B	124	B
125	B	126	A	127	D	128	A
129	A	130	A	131	C	132	C
133	D	134	C	135	D	136	B
137	E	138	B	139	D	140	B
141	C	142	D	143	C	144	A
145	D	146	D	147	A	148	F
149	F	150	C	151	B	152	C
153	A	154	C	155	C	156	C
157	B	158	C	159	D	160	B
161	B	162	F	163	A	164	D
165	A, D	166	B	167	B	168	B
169	C	170	C	171	A, C	172	B
173	D	174	B				

14

Basic Radiology

- 3 inherent characters of R/G = density, contrast, definition
- mA = controls no./ quantity of electrons / density of film
- **half value layer** = is an indication of quality of an x-ray
- Temp of filament = controls no. of H^+ (protons)
- Kv = quality / wavelength
- Caries diagnosis = high contrast/low grey scale required
- PD disease diagnosis = low contrast, high grey scale required
- Density = is function of mA, kV; inversely proportional to TFD dis., collimation and filtration; directly proportional to exposure time;
- Increased kVp = decreased patient exposure
- Silver halide = increases speed of film without loss of sharpness
- Lymphocytes = most sensitive of all blood cells
- **Vertical angulations:** while taking IOPA

Maxillary	Teeth	Mandibular
+ 60	I	- 30
+ 50	C	- 20
+ 40	P	- 10
+ 30	M	0

- **Horizontal angulations**

Maxillary	Teeth	Mandibular
0	I	0
60–75	C	45
70–80	P	70–80
80–90	M	80–90

- **Exposure time** = is directly proportional to square of anode-film distance; and inversely proportional to mA, kvp.
- **Intensity** = inversely proportional to square of distance.
- Increased kvp = increased density of film, decreased contrast; safe to the patients;
- **Collimation** = lead diaphragm, 2.75" in size at skin; decreases penumbra
- **Intensifying screens** = decrease exposure time and contrast
- **Grid** = decreases film fog; increases sharpness. But increases patient's radiation dose.
- **G2 phase** = most sensitive to radiations
- **S phase** = least sensitive to rays
- **Magnifications** = SFD/ OF distance
- **Miller's technique** = 2 R/G perpendicular to each other
- 30-40 % mineral loss / 13 % cortical bone loss should be present for R/G evidence.
- **Intensifying screens** = has a coating of calcium tungstate; TiO_2 and $MgCO_3$ as reflecting layers.
- **Filters** = made of Pb
- **Collimators** = made of Pb
- Image sharpness of an x-ray is increased by = using small focal spot size
- **Aluminium filters**; high speed films and increased TFD = decrease the amount of radiations to the patients

- Dental x-ray film has = a coating of cellulose acetate base coated with a silver bromide emulsion
- **Fixer** = is sodium thiosulphate, i.e. hypo.
- A pale x-ray is due to = low temp of developing solution
- Maximum permissible dose to a radiographer is = 5 R / yr.
- Complete intraoral R/G examination requires = 5 R.
- Diameter of pri beam = 2.75" ; rectangular
- To increase contrast = decrease kvp; increase mA.
- Decrease TOD = increased density of a R/G
- A low KV technique is most advantageous for demonstrating = early/ small caries lesions
- **Cervical burnout / adumbration** = CEJ resembling the caries.
- 1 RAD = 100 ergs/ gm
- **Buccal object rule** = when IOPA is taken at two different horizontal/vertical angulations of the same area, then the buccal image moves in the direction opposite to the direction of the movement of the x-ray tube. Also called CLARK's RULE/SLOB technique, i.e. Same side-LINGUAL, Opposite side-BUCCAL.

X-RAY RADIATIONS

Electromagnetic radiations = from long electrical and radiowaves, IR, visible light, UV, x-rays and gamma rays.

Particle radiations = generated through spontaneous decay of various radioactive substances and by accelerating devices, e.g. cyclotrons.

- Radium, thorium = give gamma rays + alpha + beta particles
- Alpha = are helium nuclei; little ability to penetrate tissues; give up their energy in a very short distance.
- Beta = are electrons; rapid motion; greater penetrating power; and loose their energy in a few mm of the tissues.
- Alpha, beta = have little value in medical fields.
- Radioactive isotopes = mainly produce beta particles only
- Ionizing radiations = i.e. rays which produce ionisation in materials which absorb them.

- **Roentgen** = is most commonly used unit of measure of x-rays and gamma-rays. It is the amount of rays which on passing through 1 CC of dry atm. air at 0 C and 760 mm Hg, causes emission of electrons which, when they give up all their energy produce 2.095×10^9 ions pairs (1 ESU).
- **RAD** = radiation absorbed dose = is a unit of absorbed dose rather than exposure, is the energy imparted to matter by ionising radiations per unit mass of irradiated material and is 100 ergs/gm.
- 1 R and 1 RAD are roughly equivalent.
- **Radiosensitivity** of cells = embryonic, immature or poorly differentiated cells are more easily injured than differentiated cells of the same type.
- Vulnerability increases during mitosis;
- **Latent tissue injury** = i.e. residual tissue damage after the initial radiation reaction has subsided.
- Radiosensitive tissues = lymphocytes; bone marrow; epithelial of intestine and stomach; germ cells.
- Radioresistant = mature bone; cartilage; muscles; brain and nervous tissues;
- Side effect on Oral mucosa = whitening of oral mucosa-due to impaired mitotic activity and prolonged retention of superficial epithelial cells and keratinisation.
- **Co-60 has a skin and bone sparing effect.**

Effect on Skin

Is the earliest visible reaction, may cause permanent pigmentation.

Later effects are mainly brought by changes in vascular bed and the intercellular material; dry skin due to decreased sebaceous secretions; epilation, etc.

Effects on Oral Mucosa

Loss of taste sensations due to damage to microvilli and outer surface of the taste cells.

Effects on Salivary Glands

Xerostomia = by damage to acinar cells and decreased no. of secretory granules and edema and inflammatory cells infiltration; saliva becomes thicker and more tenacious; but no change in ducts of salivary glands.

Postradiation sialoadenitis = increase in serum and **urinary amylase**, amylase comes from salivary glands only.

Effects on Teeth

Radiation caries = begins at cervical area of the teeth; lesions resemble demineralisation more than the true caries. It is due to altered saliva due to xerostomia and shift to cariogenic bacteria.

Its pattern of spread is that it sweeps across the tooth often causing amputation of crown.

It can be prevented by one daily application of 1% NaF gel for 5 mins. containing a plaque-disclosing dye and then brushing to remove the plaque. It is called as **Daly and Drane protocol 1972.**

Developing teeth are especially sensitive to x-rays = disorganisation of odontoblasts and formation of atypical dentin. Ameloblasts are more resistant to x-rays than odontoblasts.

Effects on Bones

Bone is resistant but osteoblasts are sensitive. There is inability to react normally to infections due to damage to vascular bed, may lead to **osteoradionecrosis**; ORN effects mandible more than maxilla; is due to difference in blood supply and density; causes intense pain; If doses of radiation is < 6500 rads, the risk of ORN of jaw is minimal; but increases if > 7500 rads.

RADIOLOGY

Filter	Aluminium disc	1.5-2.5 mm thick
Collimator	Lead, Pb	>= 1 / 16 inches
Grid	Lead, Pb	

Radiology (*Contd.*)

Intensifying Screen	Calcium tungstate	
Absorber	Aluminium	2 mm Al as HVL (half value layer)
Film	Silver bromide with base of cellulose acetate	

1. **Recommended beam size** for intra oral R/G should be ≤ 2. 75 inches at patient's skin
2. **Processing time** = 5 min. at 68 F
3. **Fixing time** = 2 × the developing time
4. **3 inherent characteristics** of a R/G = density, contrast, and definition (DCD)
5. **Maximum permissible dose** to a radiographer = 5 R / yr
6. Complete intraoral R/G examination requires = 5 R
7. **Diameter of primary beam** is 2.75 inches in circular ; and 1.5 × 2 inches, if rectangular
8. **POTTER-BUCKEY DIAPHRAGM** = ka moving grid
9. **Grid** is placed between object and film
10. **Photo electric effect** = when x-rays strike an electron of atom and gets completely absorbed then electro- magnetic radiations are produced.
11. **Compton effect** = x-rays hit an electron of atoms and give only a part of its energy, so x-ray photons of secondary type are produced.
12. In x-ray production, the part played by both the effects is 50-50%.
13. **Half value layer** is an indication of quality of an x-ray.
14. 1 RAD = 100 ergs /gm.; 1 ESU = 2.08×10^9 ion pairs.
15. **Speed** depends directly on the size of Ag –Br crystals. It refers to sensitivity of film to radiations.

16. **Density** is degree of blackness in the processed film. Its range is = 0.25-2
17. **Detail** is the ability of a film to produce sharp outlines of an object. It is mainly influenced **by size of focal spot.**
18. **Contrast** is the gradation of differences in film density in different areas of a R/G.
19. **Penumbra** it is the area of partial shadow and the unsharpness of image. It is the part of shadow of an object which is larger than a point and yet presents a single point on the object.
20. **Umbra** is the area of total shadow.
21. For **good R/G**
    a. Source of x-rays = as small as possible
    b. Target-object distance = as large as possible
    c. Object-film distance = as small as possible
22. Main damage by x-rays is due to = ionisation
23. Radio-density to tissues = depends of the degree of reproduction
24. In paralleling technique = long cone is used
25. In bisecting technique = short / long cone is used.
26. **Developer** = hydroquinone; at 68 F for 5 min., pH = 10 –11.5, alkaline, soapy feel to touch.
27. **Fixer** = hypo; sodium thiosulfate, for 10 –15 min., acidic, pH = 4-5, removes unexposed AgBr crystals;
28. Anterior bite-wing is not required, so to confirm proximal caries in anterior teeth-IOPA is the best choice.
29. For the **Rx of surface lesions** = decrease the TFD, i.e. target-film distance
30. For the **Rx of deeper lesions** = increase the TFD, i.e. target-film distance
31. Larger scale / low scale of contrast = means more shades of grey b/w black and white areas. Long grey scale is by **increased kvp.**
32. For destruction of interdental cancellous bone **to be recorded on a R/G,** the cortical bone thickness must have been reduced by at least 0.5-1.0 mm , i.e. 30 %.

33. Shortest wavelength is of **cosmic rays** and longest wavelength is of **radio waves**.
34. Cosmic rays, super voltage x-rays, gamma rays, x rays, grenz, UV, visible rays, IR, radio waves are in the order of increasing wavelengths.
35. For long grey scale contrast, the kvp sh be > 70
36. For early/ small caries lesions, the kvp sh be < 70
37. Long cone = helps to avoid magnification. It is 16 inches long for intraoral R/G.
38. **RAD, i.e. radiation absorbed dose** = amount of x-rays or dose the patient absorbs in body during dental x-ray procedure. 1 RAD = 100 ergs / gm of tissue.
39. **Roentgen equivalent man, i.e. REM** = amount of any ionising radiations that has same biologic effect in man as one R of x - rays.
40. A low kvp, i.e. < 70, is most advantageous for demonstrating = early or small carious lesions.
41. **Adumbration** = **cervical burn- out,** i.e. CEJ resembling a carious lesion. It is normal feature in IOPA. And should not be confused with a lesion.
42. A pale x-ray is due to = low temperature of developer.
43. For cephalogram, use 75–80 kvp, 7–8 mA, 0.8 sec, 5 feet distance. It is a standardised R/G.
44. Light R/G mostly is due to = use of an exhausted developer.
45. Cause of yellowish R/G = improper washing and so oxidation gives yellow color.
46. **Herring bone pattern** is due to = wrong side of film is exposed. The film is covered by lead sheath on the back side to avoid the passage of x-rays beyond the film after exposure.
47. For complete mouth R/G survey = at least 14 IOPAs and 4 bite-wings are required. Otherwise 14–17 IOPAs and 2-4 bite wings posterior are required.
48. **Buccal object rule** = when horizontal angle of central ray is changed, the object on buccal side moves on the R/G in the opposite direction to that of the central ray.

Radiolucent materials	**Radio-opaque materials**
Acrylic and resins	Gold, silver
Silicate	ZnO, zinc phosphate
Calcium hydroxide	Gutta percha
Porcelain	Wires
Cotton	Bands and crowns

Angulations required during IOPAs: vertical angulation is more important than horizontal.

Angulations	Maxillary				Mandibular			
Horizontal	0,	60–75	70–80	80–90	0	45	70–80	80–90
teeth	**I**	**C**	**PM**	**M**	**I**	**C**	**PM**	**M**
Vertical	+ 60	+ 50	+ 40	+ 30	– 30	– 20	– 10	0

Important Points

- Intensity is inversely proportional to = square of the TFD, i.e. I = 1 / R^2.
- Exposure time T is inversely proportional to = intensity, i.e. T = 1/ I
- Density is inversely proportional to target-object distance, i.e. D = 1 / TOD
- mA controls number of x-ray photons
- kvp controls energy/ quality of x-rays and speed of electrons
- T is directly proportional to density, i.e. T = D

Types of Radiations

1. Corpuscular/particulate radiations = have alpha, beta and gamma radiations. Radium and radioisotopes are corpuscular in nature

2. Electromagnetic radiations = no particles but only energy waves; e.g. x-rays
3. X-rays of wavelength of 0.8–0.1 A are used in dentistry as it has high penetrating-power.

Herring bone pattern = if during the exposure, the IOPA film is wrongly placed as reversed, i.e. apex of the punched point placed away from the rays, then there are metallic lines seen on the developed film. These lines are due to the image of the metallic sheet, covering the film on the back side to avoid the rays to cross the film.

Lane's pattern = is formed by, as beside the main beam, there are weak beams emerging in many directions which form symmetrically arranged spots on the film around the central spot.

Coolidge tube

- **Cathode** = **molybdenum**; current controls the quantity of electrons.
- **Anode** = **tungsten** target in a copper stem.
- **Focus** = area where the electrons strike
- Sharpness of image increases as the size of the focal spot target is placed at an angle of 45 degrees wrt the central beam.
- **Radiator** = for dissipating heat
- Intensity = controlled by adjusting the current through' the filament
- Energy of electrons = by voltage across the tube; high energy rays have high penetrating power.
- **Diaphragm** = absorbs the secondary rays; gives good contrast to the film.
- **Intensifying screens** = intensifies the photographic effect of rays and decreases the exposure time. Material used in them possess the florescence, e.g. calcium tungstate. It is used in all extraoral R/G and mounted in pairs in the cassette.
- Increased exposure time (ET) produces more x-rays; but of same intensity.
- As ET is increased; the density increases.
- **Contrast** = is the difference b/w objects of varying intensities. It increases with increased film exposure.

- Increased current = more no. of electrons; more energy and penetrating power.
- More kvp = more penetrating power, more energy; less ET is required; an increase of 15 kvp requires halving the ET. Also less the skin dose and more depth dose of rays.
- TFD = **inverse square law** = i.e. intensity is inversely proportional to square of the distance.
- ET = proportional to square of the TF distance.
- **Therapeutic R/G** = long distances are used for Rx of deep lesions; short distances for surface lesions.
- **Collimation** = Pb; decreases the fog and exposed area; decreases the scattered rays; and patient's exposure;

Radiography: Important Points

Increase exposure time	♦ more x-rays but of same intensity; ♦ density = increased ♦ contrast = increased
Increase mA/ current	Increased number of electrons
Increased kvP	Increased energy; decrease contrast; Increased penetrating power; less skin dose; increase depth Less exposure time required
Decreased kvP	Increased contrast
TFD	Intensity is inversely proportional to square of the distance; ka inverse square law
Exposure time	Directly proportional to square of the distance
Long TFD	Use for deep lesions during the radiation Rx
Short TFD	Use for surface lesions during the radiation Rx

Radiography Important Points (*Contd.*)

Collimation, Pb. Lead	♦ decreases the scattered rays ♦ decreases the patient exposure ♦ increases the film quality ♦ decreases the fog; ♦ decreases the exposure time
Filteration; aluminium; Al; 2 mm, HVL	Removes the less penetrating photons; HVL is thickness of an absorber required to decrease the number of x-rays photons passing through it to one half;
Filter	♦ increases the contrast and quality; ♦ decreases the density ♦ increases the exposure time
Quality	Mean energy of x-ray beam
Thicker object	If Increased kvp = so decrease the exposure time; decrease dose; decrease the blurring; High mA; Increase exposure time
Grid; Pb; lead	♦ placed b/w object and film ♦ disadv = production of dull white lines ♦ ET has to be increased.
Secondary radiations	Produce fog on R/G
Grid ratio	Is the distance of lead strips over the base
Quality of film	Depends on grain size of emulsion; Thicker the emulsion = lesser ET is required
Speed	Faster the speed = less the amount of x-rays required to expose it; less ET required; less radiation hazards; but less sharp image.
Intensifying screens	Decreases the ET; contrast is greater;

Radiography Important Points (*Contd.*)

Processing	Optimum temp = 65-70 F; / 4-5 min; At higher temp = greater contrast than at the lower temp. Excessive developing = increases the fog. Less developing = discoloration Longer fixation = less intensity
Latent period	Is the difference b/w time b/w exposure and the appearance of clinical signs and symptoms.
Tissues in order of susceptibility to x-rays are :	It depends on the **mitogenic activity of the tissues** ♦ Blood forming cells; ♦ Reproductive organs ♦ Bones and glandular tissues ♦ Epithelium of GIT ♦ Skin and muscles ♦ Nervous tissues
Lethal dose; LD 50/30	The whole body actual dose required to kill 50 % of exposed organism with in 30 days after irradiations; it is 400-600 rem for man.
Maximum permissible dose MPD	0.3 R / wk
Total accumulated dose	Should be less than 5 R/ yr
Protection of patient and operator	♦ > 6 feet distance ♦ 135 degree angle to the source of rays; behind it. ♦ Pb shields and apron; thyroid sheet
Paralleling technique/ long cone tech	♦ Longer the distance = less is the divergence; ♦ 16 inches distance

Radiography Important Points (*Contd.*)

	♦ increased SFD = prevents magnification of image; prevents the blurring of image;
Le Master's tech	♦ a cotton role is placed b/w film and tissues to make film parallel to long axis of the teeth.
With increased SFD Penumbra	♦ also increase the OFD ♦ it is the amount of unsharpness of the image. ♦ increases with decreased SOD ♦ decrease with decrease FOD ♦ increase with increased source size
Umbra	♦ part of object when all the light is absorbed
Hanging drop appearance	♦ is typical feature of orbital blow out fracture
Focal trough	♦ is the 3D area in which structures are reasonably defined in an OPG; i.e. images are clearer.
Noise	♦ those R/G structures which do not contain diagnostic informations of interest; ♦ in subtraction R/Graphy = noise is decreased to increase the detectability changes in R/G pattern.
Xero R/G	♦ image is recorded in an *aluminium* plate with a *selenium* coating; ♦ latent image is formed due to discharge of Se-particles due to x-rays.
Cervical burnout	♦ is an artefact or a non- pathological feature on an IOPA; the neck of a

Radiography Important Points (*Contd.*)

	tooth, i.e. area b/w root and crown absorbs less x-rays and appear R/L; and gives appearance of caries;
Cemental caries	♦ appears as saucer-shaped lesion; and mesial surfaces are more prone.
PDL thickening	♦ OTM ♦ Scleroderma ♦ PA pathology ♦ Apical periodontitis

Film

Base	Cellulose acetate; 0.2 mm thick	Supports Ag-halides	
Emulsion	Ag Br; 0.7 mm		
Protective coat	Gelatin		
Speed of film	Larger size of the Ag-halide particle; more is the speed and sensitive; But with increase in grain size = image sharpness decreases;		

Developer

Developer	For reduction of AgBr to Ag	31 C; **hydroquinone**
Activator	Alkalinity	KOH; K_2CO_3; NaOH
Restrainer	**Anti fog**	KBr + benzotriazole
Preservative		Na / K sulphate
Solvent		Water
Replenisher		NaOH

Fixer: to remove unexposed / under developed silver halides;

Fixing agent	Hypo/**sodium thio sulfate**	
Acid stabiliser/buffer	Acetic acid	
Hardener	K-alum; Al-chloride	
Solvent	Water	
Others, e.g. anti-sludging agents	Boric acid	

SYNONYMS

1. JUG HANDLE VIEW = oblique axial view / SM VIEW = for zygoma
2. Keyhole view = transpharyngeal / infracranial / Parma / McQueen projection view = TMJ
3. Water's view = occipitomental view; OM VIEW = PNS
4. Caldwell Luc view = PA view = frontal sinus
5. Rheese view = oblique / optic foramen view =
6. Towne's view = occipitofrontal view = TMJ space
7. Reverse Towne's = fronto-occipital view =
8. Transcranial view = posterior auricular approach of Lindblom = TMJ
9. Transorbital view = Zimmer projection = TMJ
10. PA at -10 degrees = Caldwell view

R/G VIEWS BEST FOR

Subcondylar fracture; condylar neck	Towne's view
Medially displaced condylar neck fracture	PA view
Ramus/body of mandible	LO at 15 degrees
Horizontal favorable/unfavorable mand fracture	LO at 30 degrees

R/G VIews Best For (*Contd.*)

Fracture body mand., base of skull, zygomatic arch	SMV view
Max sinus	Water's / PNS view.
Rim/floor of orbit	30 degree OM VIEW
Coronoid	PA skull
Base of skull	Towne's and SMV
Zygoma; fracture of maxilla zygomatic complex	OMV
Sialolith of submand gland	Cross-sectional occlusal view
Impacted mand 3 rd molar	Occlusal and IOPA
Zygomatic arch; base of skull	SMV/jug-handle view
Herniation and perforation of TMJ disk	Arthrography
Stenson's and Wharton's duct sialoliths	OPG
Condyle neck fracture in TMJ view	Infracranial/ transpharyngeal view
Internal derangement of TMJ	MRI
Difference b/w CSF and blood	CT scan
Middle face fracture	Water's view
Fracture of mand condylar neck	Fronto-occipital; OPG
Medial wall, orbital roof	OM; lateral skull
Coronoid process	OM, PA view
Palate	Oblique upper occlusal
Frontal sinus	Caldwell's view
Middle face fracture ; BEST view	Water's view
TMJ space;	Reverse towne's view; frontooccipital.

15

MCQs in Radiology

1. Which of the following is not a disadvantage of the bisecting technique?

A. Image on x-ray film may be dimensionally distorted (amount may vary)
B. Increased exposure time
C. Due to the use of a short cone (which results in divergent ray), the image is not a true reproduction of the object
D. May not be able to judge the correct alveolar bone height

2. Your dental hygienist has a patient that says she needs bite - wing x-ray because it has been six months since the last films were taken. Your hygienist should respond in which manner listed below?

A. Agree with the patient
B. Tell the patient that bite-wing x-ray should be taken once a year
C. Tell the patient that dental x-ray are taken only when needed as judged by each patient's needs
D. None of the above

3. Which of the following positioning errors is the most likely cause of a reverse occlusal plane curve on a panorex (panoramic radiograph?

A. Chin tilted too far upward
B. Chin tilted too far downward
C. Head turned slightly
D. None of the above

4. The period between radiation exposure and the onset of symptoms is called the:

A. Latent period
B. Period of cell injury
C. Recovery period
D. None of the above

5. All of the following are advantages of a panoramic radiograph except:

A. It shows areas that may not be visible on a full mouth series
B. It shows both arches on the same film
C. It gives better detail and definition than periapical radiographs
D. It is more comfortable for the patient (eliminates gagging)
E. It requires less time than a full mouth series

6. Which type of structure inhibits the passage of x-rays?

A. Radiopaque
B. Radiolucent
C. Translucent
D. All of the above

7. Kilovoltage controls the speed of:

A. Photons
B. Electrons
C. Anodes
D. Cathodes

8. The number of x-ray produced is controlled by:

A. Kilovoltage (kVp)
B. Milliamperage (mA)
C. Exposure time
D. All of the above

9. Which of the fallowing errors in radiographic technique is the most likely reason that an image on a radiograph would appear elongated?

A. Too much vertical angulation
B. Too little vertical angulation
C. Incorrect horizontal angulation
D. Beam not aimed at center of film

10. Which of the following is a major disadvantage of the paralleling technique?
   A. The image formed in the film will not have dimensional accuracy
   B. Due to the amount of distortion, periodontal bone height cannot be accurately diagnosed
   C. An increase in exposure time is necessary due to the use of a long cone
   D. An increase in exposure time is necessary due to the use of a short cone

11. One of the films in a full mouth series of dental radiographs has crescent shaped marks on it. What is the most likely cause of these marks?
   A. Overbent films / cracked emulsions
   B. Patient had glasses on
   C. Exposure to secondary radiation
   D. Cone cutting
   E. X-ray arm drifted

12. Suppose that in a periapical examination of the mandibular incisor region, an exposure time of 1/4 second and focus-film distance of 8 inches were used. If you increase the focus-film distances to 16 inches, what would be the new exposure time required to produce the same density in the radiograph?
   A. 1/2 second
   B. 1 second
   C. 2 second
   D. 4 second

13. Which of the following is the name of the bony projection that arises from the sphenoid bone and extends downward and slightly posteriorly?
   A. The lingula
   B. The hamular process
   C. Sella turcica
   D. Pubic symphysis

14. Which x-ray is designed for diagnosis of basilar skull fractures?
   A. Water's view
   B. Submental-vertical / submento-vertex view

C. Towne's view
D. Panorex view

15. **Image magnification may be minimized by :**
A. Using a short cone
B. Placing the film as far from the tooth as possible
C. Using a long cone
D. Shortening the exposure time

16. **X-ray fixer contains all of the following except:**
A. A clearing agent
B. An antioxidant preservative
C. An accelerator
D. An acidifier
E. A hardener

17. **The most effective means in reducing the time of exposure, the amount of radiation reaching the patient and the amount of radiation scattered to the dentist is:**
A. A lead apron
B. Ultra-speed film
C. Lead diaphragms
D. Increasing target-film distance

18. **It is recommended that the operator stand at least how many feet away from the patient when taking radiographs:**
A. Two feet
B. Four feet
C. Six feet
D. Eight feet

19. **Osteoradionecrosis is more common:**
A. In the mandible
B. In the maxilla
C. Equally in both
D. Zygoma

20. **Which of the following is a measure of the energy imparted by any type of ionizing radiation to a mass of any type of matter:**
A. Absorbed dose
B. Exposure
C. Equivalent dose
D. Effective dose

21. The area from which x-rays emanate is called the:
A. Target
B. Focal spot
C. Intensifying screen
D. Cone

22. Which of the following is the best film for visualizing the condyles and neck of the mandible from an A-P projection?
A. Water's view
B. Caldwell's view
C. Towne's view
D. Panorex

23. Increasing the kilovoltage (kVp) causes the resultant x-ray to have
A. Decreased density
B. More latitude
C. A shorter scale of contrast
D. A longer scale of contrast

24. The image of the coronoid process of the mandible often appears in periapical x-ray of
A. The incisor region of the mandible
B. The molar region of the mandible
C. The incisor region of the maxilla
D. The molar region of the maxilla

25. All of the following are radioresistant cells except:
A. Muscle
B. Nerve
C. Mature bone
D. Lymphocytes

26. It is best to retain dental radiographs for how many years?
A. 2 years
B. 4 years
C. 6 years
D. Indefinitely

27. An assistant has taken three panoramic x-ray films today. During the day as she developed each film, she noticed the

films getting lighter and lighter. What needs to be done so that this problem can be corrected?

A. Decrease the temperature of the developing solution
B. Increase the temperature of the developing solution
C. Replenish the developing solution
D. Increase the mA setting
E. Increase the kVp setting

28. Which of the following are the uses of cephalometrics in orthodontics?

A. Diagnosis
B. Analysis of treatment results
C. Longitudinal study of growth
D. All of the above

29. Foreshortening and elongation are produced by:

A. Incorrect horizontal angulation
B. Incorrect vertical angulation
C. Either of the above
D. None of the above

30. The screening x-ray for pathology of the jaws is:

A. A panorex
B. A cephalogram
C. A periapical x-ray
D. An occlusal x-ray

31. All of the following are true concerning collimation except:

A. It prevents overexposure to patients
B. It increases the area of patient exposure
C. It reduces secondary radiation to the film
D. It reduces secondary radiation to the patient

32. Which of the following is the standard radiograph of choice for showing an anterior view of the paranasal sinuses and of the mid-face and orbits?

A. Panorex
B. Towne's view
C. Water's view
D. Cephalogram

33. Which of the following types of intraoral radiographs are most useful in detecting inter proximal caries?
A. Periapical radiograph
B. Bitewing radiographs
C. Occlusal radiographs
D. Cephalogram

34. The radiographs were taken with the buccal object rule in mind. In film # 2, the x-ray tube was directed from a mesial angulation. The object also moved mesially. What is the special position of the object in these radiograph?
A. The object lies lingual to the first molar
B. The object lies buccal to the first molar
C. The object lies between the second premolar and the first molar
D. The object lies directly apical to the first molar

35. After processing film, you notice that it appears brown in color. What is the most likely cause of this?
A. Solutions are too strong
B. Solutions are too weak
C. Fixing time was not long enough
D. Fixing time was too long
E. Film was under developed

36. X-ray developer contains all of the following except:
A. A developing agent
B. An antioxidant preservative
C. A clearing agent
D. An accelerator
E. A restrainer

Answer Key to MCQs in Radiology

1	B	2	C	3	A	4	A
5	C	6	A	7	B	8	B
9	B	10	C	11	A	12	B
13	B	14	B	15	C	16	C
17	B	18	C	19	A	20	A
21	B	22	C	23	D	24	D
25	D	26	D	27	C	28	D
29	B	30	A	31	B	32	C
33	B	34	A	35	C	36	C

Self-Assessment Paper

1. **Shunting Effect Occurs in Complete Dentures.**
   A. If occlusal plane is lower in molar area
   B. If the occlusal plane is lower in incisor area
   C. It occlusal plane is lower in molar as well as incisor area
   D. When patient has poor muscular co-ordination.

2. **Training groove is placed in the lower denture.**
   A. To train the patients tongue position
   B. In cases of mandibulectomy
   C. To train the orbicularis oris muscle.
   D. To train tognetic patients

3. **Which of the following agent is used as a die hardner?**
   A. Cynoacrylate
   B. Nail polish
   C. Volatile relief agents
   D. Composite Resin

4. **A gnathodynameter is used to record.**
   A. Biting force
   B. Centric relation
   C. Vertical Dimensions
   D. FH plane

5. **Important diagnostic tool for achieving accurate implant angulation:**
   A. Diagnostic template
   B. Wax-up

C. Mounted diagnostic cast
D. Surgical template

6. Cavosuface margin angulation in chamfer finish line is:
A. Always 90º
B. 90º or less than 90º
C. 90º or more than 90º
D. 120º

7. To increase resistance form of an excessively tapered preparation:
A. Reduce height of preparation to shorten arc of rotation.
B. Increase cervical reduction to taper
C. Add groove
D. Use adhesive cement

8. Face bow is used to transfer:
A. Axis-orbital plane
B. Frankfort horizontal plane
C. Camper's plane
D. Occlusal plane

9. For A patient with missing canine what type of prosthesis we will prefer:
A. Three unit FPD
B. Resin Retained FPD
C. Implant Retained Crown
D. It will depend on patient choice

10. A Pier abutment is:
A. Periodontal weak abutment
B. With an edentulous space on both side of the abutment
C. Edentulous space on one side of the abutment
D. Abutment adjacent to edentulous space

11. In case, if maxillary canine is missing and we have to make a tooth supported FPD Abutments will be:
A. Central incisor, lateral incisor and 1st pre- molar.
B. Lateral incisor, 1st premolar and 2nd premolar
C. Lateral incisor and 1st premolar
D. It depends upon periodontal status of remaining teeth.

12. Pivoting movement better resisted by a tooth preparation if:
A. Diameter is smaller
B. Diameter is large
C. Diameter is large and length is small
D. Do not depend on diameter of tooth

13. Denture stability refers to resistance of a denture
A. To move in a vertical direction away from basal seat
B. To move in vertical dimension towards basal seat
C. To movement of its tissue foundation especially to lateral forces
D. Against any kind of movement more the 25 µm in any direction

14. Most recent type of denture adhesive is:
A. Salts of Gontrez
B. Natural gums
C. Cellulose based slats
D. Acrylic adhesives

15. Ideal site for implant placement in a completely edentulous mandible:
A. 1st Molar region bilaterally
B. Retromolar pad area because it is resistant to resorption
C. Buccal shelf area because it is most ideally suited for loading
D. Interforaminal region

16. Beyron point is located at:
A. 13 mm anterior to posterior margin of tragus on a line from center of tragus to outer canthus
B. 11 mm anterior to posterior margin of tragus on a line from parallel to and 7 mm below FHP
C. 10 mm anterior to posterior margin of tragus on a line from center of tragus to outer canthus
D. 13 mm anterior to tragus on a line from base of tragus to outer canthus

17. Pontic design not indicated in anterior region:
A. Ovate pontic
B. Modified ridge lap pontic

C. Stein pontic
D. Spheroidal pontic

18. Cavity preparation on which location of tooth will give rise to blank class I cavity (spot the location of caries to make blank Class I cavity preparation):
A. 1
B. 2
C. 3
D. 4

19. Find out the correct contoured buccal surface for food deflection:
A. 1
B. 2
C. 3
D. 4

20. Which of the following is not true about lubricant for rubber dam placement?
A. Should have water-miscible vehicle
B. Vaseline is an ideal choice
C. Should be easy to remove
D. Should not interfere with bonding procedures

21. The average diameter of coronal dentinal tubules near the pulp is:
A. 0.2–0.5 microns
B. 2–3 microns
C. 0.2–0.3 microns
D. 4 –7 microns

22. Ecologic Determinants of plaque depend on all except:
A. Sugar content of diet
B. Host resistance
C. Age and sex of the patient
D. Status of dentition

23. Salivary pellicle is composed of the following except:
A. Immunoglobulin G
B. Immunoglobulin A

C. Amylase
D. Albumin

24. Caries detection dye can stain the following except:
A. Granular necrotic tissue
B. Dry, leathery dentin
C. Reversibly denatured collage
D. Irreversibly denatured collagen

25. Torsional Force is:
A. Compression
B. Tensile force
C. Shear
D. Transverse bending force

26. All of the following are true for traditional solution liner except:
A. It is not necessary in moderately deep cavities under glass ionomer restoration
B. Have film thickness of 1–50 micron
C. Do not provide thermal or electric insulation
D. Protect the pulp from reaction products leaching out o restoration

27. One of the following is not true about treatment of den al hypersensitivity with dentin bonding agents:
A. It denatures protein
B. It forms a hybrid layer
C. It does not alter dentin permeability
D. It forms resin tags into dentinal tubule

28. Which of the following is not true about hand instruments used in operative dentistry?
A. They are generally made of stainless steel
B. Nickel-Cobalt-chromium is never used in its fabrication
C. Carbon steel is more efficient than stainless steel
D. It can be made with stainless steel with carbide inserts

29. Which one of the following does not commonly survive in a peri-apical lesion?
A. Pseudomonas

B. Streeptococcus
C. Porphyromonas
D. Actinomyces

30. In endodontic surgery, which of the following about chromic gut suture is not true?
A. Its properties are inferior to plain gut suture
B. It is coated with chromium tri-oxide
C. It is less bio compatible than plain gut suture
D. Its absorption is faster than the plain gut sutures

31. 1 PPM fluoride implies.
A. 1 mg of fluoride in 1 liter of water
B. 1gm of fluoride in 1 liter of water
C. 0.1 gm of florideín 1 liter of water
D. 1 mg of fluoride in 100 ml of water

32. Caries activity test that gives a quantitative determination of the acidogenic microorganism in the oral cavity.
A. Fasdick test
B. Synder test
C. Abans test
D. Blawary red

33. Class II cavity preparation for amalgam restoration in deciduous teeth requires:
A. More buccolingual extension
B. More mesiodistal extension
C. More Gingival
D. More cervical

34. Amalgam achieves 70% of the strength by:
A. 2 hours
B. 4 hours
C. 8 hours
D. 16 hours

35. Hand over mouth technique was first described by:
A. Dr. Evengeline Jordan
B. Addelson and Gold Fried

C. Dr. G.V. Black
D. Dr. Goldman

36. Nitrous Oxide is a colorless, sweet smelling gas with a density of:
A. 1.5
B. 0.5
C. 2.5
D. 3.5

37. Oral Screen:
A. Causes the child to breathe through the nose
B. Allows for the passage of air through mouth
C. Prevents passage of air through nares
D. Allows the passage of air through mouth and nose

38. Ormocers are:
A. Organically modified ceramics
B. Inorganically modified composites
C. Organically modified glass inomer cement
D. Inorganically modified Glass inomer cement

39. Nanofillers are in the range of:
A. 10–100 microns
B. 0.1–1 microns
C. 0.01–0.1 microns
D. 0.005–0.01 microns

40. Speech retardation may be considered if the child does not talk by:
A. 12 months
B. 18 months
C. 24 months
D. 36 months

41. Which of the following dentitions shows the highest frequency of occurrence of supernumerary teeth?
A. Maxillary deciduous dentition
B. Maxillary permanent dentition
C. Mandibular deciduous dentition
D. Mandibular permanent dentition

42. What is the thickness of the layer of prismless enamel found in primary teeth?

A. 25 um
B. 50 um
C. 75 um
D. 100 um

43. When is the first evidence of calcification of primary teeth?

A. 4 months in utero
B. 4 and ½ months in- utero
C. 5 months in- utero
D. 6 months in- utero

44. By what age does the startle and grasp reflex disappear?

A. 1 year
B. 1 ½ year
C. 2 year
D. 3 year

45. Who proposed the operant conditioning theory of child psychology:

A. Pavlov
B. Skinner
C. Jean Piaget
D. Sigmond Freud

46. The longest acting local anaesthetic is

A. Prilocaine
B. Lingnocine
C. Bupivacaine
D. Ropivacaine

47. The first drug of choice to be administered for anaphylaxis is:

A. Hydrocortisone
B. Adernaline
C. Atropine
D. Chlorpheneramine maleate

48. In gillies temporal approach for reduction of Zygomatic arch fracture Rowes Zygomatic Elevator is placed between:

A. Superficial fascia and the temporal fascia

B. Between the temporal bone and the temporalis muscle
C. Between the temporal fascia and the temporalis muscle
D. Skin and superficial fascia

49. The most lethal of complications due to blood transfusion is:
A. Jaundice
B. Antigen antibody reaction
C. Hepatitis B transmission
D. HIV transmission

50. In cardio pulmonary resuscitation chest compressions is done:
A. On the upper part of sternum
B. On the Xiphisterum
C. On the middle of the lower part of the sternum
D. On the left side of the chest

51. Which of the following statement is tri with reference to the Glasgow Coma Scale?
A. In the first 24 hrs following a head injury an overall score of 11 indicates a good prognosis
B. An overall score of less than 9 indicated poor prognosis
C. Gives an accurate impression of the neurological status
D. Cannot be assessed in an unconscious patient

52. Musoperiosteal flaps:
A. When raised do not cause post operative swelling and pain
B. Are raised whenever bone removal is desired to facilitate ectraction
C. Are routinely raised during extraction
D. When raised will cause trauma and injury to underlying osseous tissues

53. A dermatome is used:
A. To remove scar tissue
B. To harvest skin grafts
C. To abrade skin which is pigmented
D. For pairing of lacerated soft tissue

54. In Treacher Collin's Syndrome there is:
A. Upward sloping of the palpebral fissure

B. Poorly developed or absent malar bones
C. Progeina mandibular prognathism
D. No loss of hearing

55. Pierre Robin Syndrome is associated with:
A. Micrognathia
B. Cleft of the lip and palate
C. Tetrology of fallot
D. Syndactally

56. Vitamin A:
A. Is water soluble
B. Deficiency causes impaired cision
C. Maintains normal plasma calcium lavels
D. Is required for formation of clotting factors

57. Which of the following is used to show the base of the skull, sphenoid sinus, position and orientation of the condyles, and fractures of the zygomatic arch:
A. The TMJ surgery
B. Submobtovertex projection
C. Reverse-towne projection
D. The facial profile survey

58. Which survey has the purpose of examining fractures of the condular neck of the mandible?
A. Lateral Jaw projection
B. Lateral skull projection
C. Waters projection
D. Reverse-Townes view

59. In patients infected with HIV will have:
A. Elevated blastogenesis
B. Depressed serum globulim levels
C. High T4-T8 Ratio
D. Thrombocytopenia

60. Conditional gingival enlargements is usually not:
A. Hormonal
B. Luekemic

C. Granuloma pyogenicum
D. Drug induced

61. Hypercementosis of the entire dentition is a feature of:
A. Alber Schonberg disease
B. Paget's disease
C. Lathyrism
D. Low grade periapical inflammation

62. Desmodont is another name for:
A. The tooth with one wall pocket
B. Tooth with three walled pocket
C. Periodontal ligament
D. Degiscence

63. The oxygen consumption of normal gingival is:
A. 1.6 ± 0.37
B. 0.9 ± 0.22
C. 2.7 ± 0.41
D. 1.9 ± 0.21

64. Glucose levels in gingival crevicular fluid (GCF) are:
A. Equal to glucose level in serum
B. Zero
C. 3–4 times greater than serum levels
D. More than 10 times the serum levels

65. A black line on the gingival which follows the contour of the margin is due to:
A. Lead
B. Argyria
C. Iron
D. Mercury

66. Gracey curette No. 11–12 are used for:
A. Anterior teeth
B. Posterior teeth mesial
C. Posterior teeth distal
D. Posterior teeth facial and lingual

67. The brushing technique recommended for patients with periodontal disease is:
A. Scrub technique
B. Sulcular technique
C. Roll technique
D. Circular technique

68. Embrasure characterized by a slight to moderate recession of interdental papilla are:
A. Type I
B. Type II
C. Type III
D. Type IV

69. Malocclusion characterized by retroclined central and proclined lateral incisor is:
A. Class II division I
B. Class II Division II
C. Class III
D. Class I

70. Six keys to normal occlusion were given by:
A. Andrews
B. Angle
C. Tweed
D. Steiner

71. The permanent anterior tooth that most often shows variation in size is the:
A. Mandibular canine
B. Mandibular central incisor
C. Maxillary canine
D. Maxillary lateral incisor

72. Relative to primary mandibular incisor permanent mandibular incisors erupt:
A. Lingually
B. Facially
C. Distally
D. Mesially

73. In cephalometrics, the Frankfort plane is constrected:
A. Horizontally from nasion through porion
B. Horizontally from nasion to the superior aspect of external auditory meatus
C. Vertically from orbitale through the maxillary canine
D. Horizontally from orbitale to the superior aspect of the external auditory meatus

74. The last primary tooth to be replaced by a permanent tooth is usually
A. Maxillary canine
B. Mandibular canine
C. Maxillary first molar
D. Mandibular second molar

75. Which is the predominant factor in the formation of the alveolar process:
A. Eruption of teeth
B. Normal process of growth
C. Lengthening of the condyle
D. Overall growth of the bodies of the maxilla and the mandible

76. Resistance units of equal size pulling against each is an example of which form of anchorage:
A. Cortical anchorage
B. Reciprocal anchorage
C. Reinforced anchorage
D. Stationary anchorage

77. A single force applied at which point of a tooth will allow complete translation of the tooth:
A. At the apex
B. At the incisal edge
C. At the center of resistance
D. At the center of rotation

78. Which of the fibers attached to cementum are most likely to contribute to relapse of tooth rotation:
A. Apical fibers
B. Gingival group of fibers

C. Horizontal fibers
D. Oblique fibers

79. What is the average amount of Leeway space available in the upper arch?
A. 0.9 mm
B. 1.8 mm
C. 3.5 mm
D. 5.0 mm

80. As age advances, the human profile generally:
A. Remain the same
B. Increase in convexity
C. Decreases in convexity
D. Decreases in concavity

81. Which position is the most important in diagnosis of anterior or posterior crossbite?
A. Habitual position
B. Lateral Shift
C. Maximum intercupation
D. The point of first contact at centric relation

82. Which of the following forces best accomplish orthodontic tooth movement?
A. Heavy and continuous
B. Heavy and intermittent
C. Light and continuous
D. Light and intermittent

83. Which of the following is the least stable orthodontic correction?
A. Maxillary expansion
B. Rotations
C. Overbite
D. Overjet

84. Hyperplasia with regard to tissue growth refer to:
A. An increase in the number of cells
B. An increase in the size of cells

C. Cellular maturation
D. Cellular differentiation from stem cells

85. The midpalatal suture is most lokely to open at which following ages of expansion?
A. 18 years old
B. 13 years old
C. 25 years old
D. 55 years old

86. Functional appliances:
A. Only move teeth
B. Can change the direction of growth
C. Are fabrication in the original
D. Correct malocclusion rapidly

87. According to Wolff's law
A. Human teeth drift mesially as interproximal wear occurs
B. Pressure causes bone resorption
C. The optimal level of force for moving teeth is 10 to 200 grams.
D. Bone trabeculae line up in response to mechanical stresses

88. Which of the following teeth is most likely to be congenitally missing?
A. Maxillary central incisor
B. Mandibular canine
C. Mandibular second premolar
D. Maxillary first premolar

89. The term refers to a type of fusion in which the formed teeth are joined only along the line of cementum:
A. Gemination
B. Fusion
C. Concrescence
D. Dilacerations

90. Which is a degeneration disorder characterized by trophic changes of the deeper structures (e.g. fat muscle, cartilage and bone) involving one side of the face.
A. Sclerderma
B. Parry Romberg syndrome

C. Miescher's syndrome
D. Peutz-jeghers syndrome

91. Hodgkin's disease is diagnosed by finding which cells in the biopsy from lymph glands:
A. Recquet cell
B. Tzanck cell
C. Reed Sternberg cell
D. Lecunal cell

92. The best laboratory test to use in the diagnosis of Lupus vulgaris in the oral cavity is:
A. Bacterial smear
B. Blood studies
C. Biopsy
D. Blood chemistry

93. The most common benign tumor occurring in oral cavity is:
A. Papilloma
B. Fibroma
C. Adenoma
D. Epulis

94. Name the lesion which is not a radiolucent lesion of the jaws:
A. Ameloblastoma
B. Cherubism
C. Focal periapical osteopertrosis
D. Odontogenic cyst

95. Name the lesion where cotton wool. Multifocal radiodense conglomerates is not seen usually:
A. Gardner's syndrome
B. Cemento-osseous dysplasia
C. Peget's disease
D. Fibrous dysplasia

96. What is non characteristic of eagle's syndrome:
A. Excessive lacrimation
B. Pain during mandibular movement
C. Stabbing type pain originate in the tonsillar regions
D. When the jaws are closed the pain subsided.

97. The posterior tooth that gives a better support is:
A. With concergant roots
B. Divergant roots
C. Conical roots
D. Corved roots

98. According to the Freudian psychosexual stages of development the stage which corresponds with development of mixed dentition and character formation is:
A. Concrete operational
B. Latency
C. Phallic
D. Genital

99. The range of wavelength of visible light curing system is:
A. 400–700 mm
B. 410–500 mm
C. 365–400 mm
D. 700–900 mm

100. The commonest teeth involved transposition are:
A. Maxillary central incisor and lateral incisor
B. Maxillary canine and first premolar
C. Maxillary 1st premolar and 2nd premolar
D. Maxillary canine and lateral incisor

101. In which part of oral cavity mucosa membrane is the thinnest?
A. Soft palate
B. Labial mucosa
C. Floor of mouth
D. Buccal mucosa

102. Which of the following is the normal arrangement of lingual nerve and vessels in the tongue from medial to lateral?
A. Nerve, Artery and vein
B. Artery, Nerve and vein
C. Vein, artery and nerve
D. Nerve, Artery

103. Palatine aponeururosis is:
A. Tendon of levator veil palatine
B. Tendon of Tensor veil palatine
C. A part of musculus uvuale
D. A modification of palatal periosteum

104. The tactile threshold of the natural teeth during axial loading is:
A. 0.001–0.01 N
B. 0.01–0.10 N
C. 0.10–0.50 N
D. 1–2 N

105. During Bennett movement of shift of mandible:
A. Condyle of working side exhibit bodily forward movement
B. Condyle of non working side exhibit bodily lateral movement
C. Condyle of working side exhibit bodily lateral movement
D. Condyle of working side exhibit bodily lateral and forward movement

106. Amide- type local anesthetics are metabolized in the:
A. Serum
B. Liver
C. Spleen
D. Kidneys

107. Reduced salivary flow following irradiation is dose dependent. At what dose the flow reach essentially zero?
A. 4000 rads
B. 5000 rads
C. 6000 rads
D. 7000 rads

108. The cell component that is genetically continuous from one cell generation of the next to:
A. Nuclear membrane
B. Golgi complex
C. Central bodies
D. Chromatin

109. Golgi bodies are responsible for:
A. Synthesis of polpeptides
B. Formation of glycorproteins only
C. Modification and sorting of glycoproteins
D. Lipid and steroid synthesis

110. Deficiency of all the three components of coagulation factor VIII result in:
A. Von willebrand's disease
B. Haemophilia-A
C. Parahaemophilia
D. Haemophilia-A

111. Ectodermal dysplasia is:
A. Autosomal recessive
B. Autosomal dominant
C. X-linked dominant
D. X linked recessive

112. The normal depth of the gingival cervice in an adult does not exceed:
A. 0.5–1 mm
B. 1–2 mm
C. 1–3 mm
D. 2–3 mm

113. The characteristic lesion of scute necrotizing gingivitis is the necrosis of the gingival mainly of the:
A. Interdental papilla
B. Marginal gingiva
C. Attached gingiva
D. Free gingiva.

114. Cavity formation in a tooth due to dental caries is due to:
A. Destructive potential of streptococcus mutans
B. Destructive poternital of lactobacillus Acedophilus
C. Lateral spread of cavies along DE junction and weaking of the ourlying enamel
D. Mastectomy force and unrelated to the extent of carious precess.

115. Enamel hypoplasia is not a feature of:
A. Ostepetrosis
B. Downs syndrome
C. Some types of epidermolsis bullosa
D. Cleidocranial

116. Café an lait sports are seen in:
A. Pagets disease of bone
B. Cherubism
C. Von reckilghausen disease
D. Von willebrand disease

117. The durg of choice in management of a patient with an acute allergic reaction involving bronchospasm and hypotension is:
A. Epinephrine
B. Aminophyline
C. Dexmethesone
D. Diphenhudramine

118. The agent of choice to reverse status epolepticus induced by local anesthetic overdose is:
A. Oxgen
B. Diazepam
C. Epinephrine
D. Phenbarbital

119. A person with glaucoma should not receive.
A. Sedatives
B. Vasoconstrictors
C. Antisialogogues
D. Local anaesthetic

120. Prolonged administration of streptomycin may result in damage to the:
A. Optic nerve
B. Facial nerve
C. Auditory nerve
D. Trigeminal nerve

121. In jaundice when there is an unconjugated hyperbilirubinemia is most likely due to:
A. Hepatitis
B. Cirrhosis
C. Obstruction of bite canaliculi
D. Increased breakdown red cells

122. A Patient with grand mal epilepsy would likely be under treatment with:
A. Meprobamate
B. Pentobarbital
C. Trimethadione
D. Phenytoin

123. Admas stokes syndrome is caused due to:
A. Atrial fibrillation
B. Atrial extrasystole
C. Complete AV block
D. Ventilation fibrillain

124. The proper rate of rescue breathing in an adult is:
A. 4 times per minute
B. 12 times per minute
C. 20 times per minute
D. 28 times per minute

125. The rate of injection of intravenous Valium is:
A. 1 ml/min
B. 2.5 ml/min
C. 1 mg/min
D. 2.5 mg/min

126. The term best describes a disease transmitted to man through animals:
A. Communicable
B. Transmissible
C. Zoonotic
D. Vertically transmissible

127. The blood cells responsible for humoral immunity are:
A. T–cell
B. B–cell
C. No cells only antibodies
D. Mostly B cell sometimes T-cells

128. Which of the following is not a method of chlorination of water?
A. Perchloron
B. Ozonation
C. Chroline gas
D. Chloramines

129. Of the following minerals the highest amount found in human body is:
A. Sodium
B. Calcium
C. Phosphorus
D. Iron

130. The Thershold does of fluoride that requires immediate emergency treatment and hospitalization in acute fluoride toxicity is:
A. 4 mg
B. 5 mg
C. 6 mg
D. 7 mg

131. Mouth gourds to prevent accidents to teeth are most practical for
A. All Children
B. All persons engaged in contact sports
C. Automobile passengers
D. Persons on organized athletic team

132. The arch length preservation can be best carried out by:
A. Placing a lingual arch
B. Restoring carious teeth
C. Placing band and loop space maintainer
D. Placing an acrylic removable space maintainer

133. The most common pathogens responsible for nosocomial pneumonias in the ICU are:
A. Gram positive organisms
B. Gram negative organisms
C. Mycoplasma
D. Virus infections

134. Which one of the following drugs has been shown to offer protection from gastric aspiration syndrome in a patient with symptoms of reflux?
A. Ondansetron
B. Metoclopramide
C. Sodium citrate
D. Atropine

135. The following statements comcerning chorda tympani netve are true except that it:
A. Carries secretomor fibers to slubmandibular gland
B. Joins lingual nerve in infratemporal fossa
C. Is a branch of facial nerve
D. Contains postganglionic parasympathetic fibers

136. A women with infertility receives an ovarian transplant f om her sister who is an identical twin. What is the type of gı aft?
A. Xenograft
B. Autograft
C. Allograft
D. Isograft

137. All of the following physiological processes occur during the growth at the epiphyseal plate except:
A. Proliferation and hypertrophy
B. Calcification and ossification
C. Vasculogenesis and erosion
D. Replacement of red bone marrow with yellow marrow

138. Virus mediated transfer of host DNA from one cell to another is known as
A. Transduction
B. Transformation

C. Transcription
D. Integration

139. Barr body is foundin the follwing phase of the cell cycle:
A. Interphase
B. Metaphase
C. \telophase
D. G 1 phase

140. Cellular and flagellar movement is carried out by all of the following except:
A. Intermediate filaments
B. Actin
C. Tubulin
D. Mysoin

141. Heme is converted to bilirubin mainly in
A. Kidney
B. Liver
C. Spleen
D. Bone marrow

142. HIV can be detected and confirmed by
A. Polymerase chain reaction, PCR
B. Reverse transcriptase–PCR
C. Real time PCR
D. Mimic–PCR

143. All of the following hormones have cell surfac receptors except
A. Adrenalin
B. Growth hormone
C. Insulin
D. thyroxin

144. Fluoride, used in the collection of blood Samples for glucose estimation, inhibits the Enzyme.
A. Glucokinase
B. Hexokinase
C. Enolase
D. Glucose-6-Phosphatase

145. Osteoclasts are inhibited by:
A. Parathyroid hormone
B. Clacitonin
C. 1,25-dihydroxycholecaliferol
D. Tumor necrosis factor

146. The protective effects of breast milk are known to be associated with:
A. Igm antibodies
B. Lysozyme
C. Mast cells
D. IgA antibodies

147. A simple bacterial test for mutagenic carcinogens is:
A. Ames test
B. Redox test
C. Bacteriophage
D. Gene splicing

148. Both Vitamin K and C are involved in:
A. The synthesis of clotting factors
B. Post translational modifications
C. Antioxidant mechanisms
D. The microsomal hydroxylation Reactions

149. Enzymes that move a molecular group from one molecule to another are known as:
A. Ligases
B. Oxido-reducatses
C. Transferases
D. Dipeptidases

150. The membrane protein, clathrin Is involved in:
A. Cell Motility
B. Receptor-mediated endocytosis
C. Exocytosis
D. Cell shape

151. The amino acid residue having an imino side chain is:
A. Lysine
B. Histidine

C. Tyrosine
D. Proline

152. CO_2 is primarily transported in the arterial blood as:
A. Dissolved CO_2
B. Carbonic Acid
C. Carbamino-Hemoglobin
D. Bicarbonate

153. 'Endemic Disease' Means that a disease:
A. Occurs clearly in excess of normal expectancy
B. Is constantly present in a given population group
C. Exhibits seasonal pattern
D. Is prevalent among animals

154. Which one of the following statements about influence of smoking on risk of coronary heart disease (CHD) is not true.
A. Influence of smoking is independent of other risk factors for CHD
B. Influence of smoking is only additive to other risk factors for CHD
C. Influence of smoking is synergistic to other risk factors for CHD
D. Influence of smoking is directly related to number of cigarettes smoked per day

155. What is the color-coding of bag in hospitals to dispose off human anatomical wastes such as body parts.
A. Yellow
B. Black
C. Red
D. Blue.

156. WHO Defines adolescent age between:
A. 10–19 Years of age
B. 10–14 Years of age
C. 10–25 Years of age
D. 09–14 Years of age

157. The following tests are used to check the efficiency of pasteurizatioin of milk except.

A. Phosphatase test.
B. Standard plate count.
C. Coliform count
D. Mesthylene blue reduction test.

158. For the treatment of case of class III Dog bite, all of the following are correct except.

A. Give Immunoglobulins for passive immunity
B. Give- ARV
C. Immediately stitch wound under antibiotic coverage
D. Immediately wash wound with soap and water

159. Transplantation of Human organs Act was Passed by Government of India in:

A. 1996
B. 1993
C. 1998
D. 1994

160. Total Cholesterol level=a+b(Caloric intake)+c (Physical activity)+d(Body mass index):Is an Example of.

A. Simple linear regression
B. Simple curvililinear regression
C. Multiple linear regression
D. Multiple logistic regression

161. The Diagonstic power of a test to correctly exclude the disease is reflected by:

A. Sensitivity
B. Specificity
C. Positive predictivity
D. Negative predictivity

162. In Chronic arsenic poisoning the following samples can be sent for laboratory Examination, Except:

A. Nail clippings
B. hair samples
C. Bone biopsy
D. Blood sample

163. The most reliable criteria in Gustafson's method of identification is:

A. Cermentum apposition
B. Transparency of root
C. Attrition.
D. Root resorption

164. The minimum age at which an individual is responsible for his criminal act is :

A. 7 Years
B. 12 Years
C. 16 Years
D. 21 Years

165. The Gold standard for the diagnosis of osteoporosos is

A. Dual energy X-ray Absorptiometry
B. Single energy X-ray Absorptiometry
C. Ultrasound
D. Quantitative computed tomography

166. All of the following can cause Osteoporosis Except:

A. Hyperparathyroidism
B. Steroid use
C. Fluorosis
D. Thyrotoxicosis

167. Hypercalcemia associated with malignancy is most often mediated by:

A. Parathyroid hormone (PTH)
B. Parathyroid Hormone related protein (PTHrP)
C. Interleukin-6(IL-6)
D. Calcitonin

168. 5'-Nucleotidase activity is increased in:

A. Bone diseases
B. Prostate cancer
C. Chronic renal failure
D. Cholestatic disorders

169. Minimal occlusal clearance on centric cusp for cast metal is:

A. 0.5 mm
B. 1 mm
C. 1.5 mm
D. 2 mm

170. Vitamin B12 Deficiency can give rise to all of the following except:

A. Myelopathy
B. Optic atrophy
C. Peripheral neuropathy
D. Myopathy.

171. All of the following organisms are known to surivive intracellularly except:

A. Neisseria meningitides
B. Salmonella Typhi
C. Streptococcus pyogenes
D. Legionella penumophila

172. Viruses can be isolated from clinical samples by cultivation in the following except.

A. Tissue Culture
B. Embryonated eggs
C. Animals
D. Chemicaly defined media

173. It Is true regarding the normal microbial flora present on the skin and mucous membranes that.

A. It cannot be eradicated by antimicrobial agents
B. It is absent in the stomach due to the acidic pH
C. It establishes in the body only after the neonatal period
D. The flora in the small bronchi is similar to that of the trachea

174. The serum concentaration of which of the following human IgG subclass is maximum.

A. IgG1
B. IgG2
C. IgG3
D. IgG4

175. A bacterial disease that has been associated with the 3 "Rs" rats, ricefields, and rainfall is:
A. Leptospirosis
B. Plague
C. Melioidosis
D. Rodent-bite Fever

176. In Radionuclide imaging the most useful radio pharmaceutical for skeletal imaging is:
A. Gallium 67(^{67}GA)
B. Technetium- sulphur-colloid(^{99m}Tc-SC)
C. Technetium-99m (^{99m}TC)
D. Technetium-99m Linked to methylene disphosphonate (^{99m}Tc-MDP)

177. The most common and earliest manifestation of carcinoma of the glottis is:
A. Hoarseness
B. Haemoptysis
C. Cervical Lymph nodes
D. Stridor

178. Abbey-Estlander flap is used in the reconstruction of;
A. Buccal mucosa
B. Lip
C. Tongue
D. Palate

179. Androphonia can be corrected by doing:
A. Type 1 Thyroplasty
B. Type 2 Thyroplasty
C. Type 3 Thyroplasty
D. Type 4 Thyroplasty

180. In which one of the following perineyral Invasion in head and neck cancer is most commonly seen.
A. Adenocarcinoma
B. Adeniod cystic carcinoma
C. Basal cell adenoma
D. Squamous cell carcinoma

181. All of the following are true about manifestations of vitamin E deficiency except:
A. Hemolytic anemia
B. Posterior column abnormalities
C. Cerebllar ataxia
D. Autonomic dysfunction

182. Differential expression of same gene depending on parent of origin is referred to as:
A. Genomic imprinting
B. Mosaicism
C. Anticipation
D. Nonpenetrance

183. All of the following statement are true regarding reversible cell injury, except:
A. Formation of amorphous densities in the mitochondrial matrix
B. Diminished generation of adenosine triphospate (ATP)
C. Formation of blebs in the plasma membrane
D. Detachment of ribosomes from the granular endoplasmic

184. All of the following vascular changes are observed in acute inflammation, Except:
A. Vasodilation
B. Stasis of blood
C. Increased vascular permeability
D. Decreased hydrostatic pressure

185. Which one of the following serum levels would help in distinguishing an acute liver disease from chronic liver disease?
A. Aminotransaminase
B. Alkaline Phosphatase
C. Bilirubin
D. Albumin

186. All of the following are topically used sulphonamides except:
A. Sulphacetamide
B. Sulphadiazine

C. Silver sulphadiazine
D. Mafenide

187. The group of antibiotics which possess additional anti-inflammatory and immunomodulatory activities is:
A. Tetracyclines
B. Polypeptide antibiotics
C. Fluoroquin lones
D. Macrolides

189. S.A. node acts as a pacemaker of the heart because of the fact that it:
A. Is capable of generating impulses spontaneously
B. Has rich sympathetic innervations
C. Has poor cholinergic innervations
D. Generates impulses at the highest rate

190. The first physiological response to high environmental temperature is:
A. Sweating
B. Vasodilatation
C. Decrease heat production
D. Non-shivering thermo genesis

191. Distribution of blood flow is mainly regulated by the:
A. Arteries
B. Arterioles
C. Capillaries
D. Venules

192. In which of the following a reduction in arterial oxygen tension occurs?
A. Anacmia
B. CO poisoning
C. Moderate exercise
D. Hypoventilation

193. A 25 year old female presents with 2 year History of repetitive, irresistible thoughts of Contamination with dirt associated with repetitive hand washing. She reports these thoughts to be her own and distressing: but is not able to

overcome them along with medications. She is most likely to benefit from which of the following therapies.

A. Exposure and response prevention
B. Systematic desensitization
C. Assertiveness training
D. Sensate focusing

195. In which one of the following conditions the sialography is contraindicated?

A. Ductal calculus
B. Chronic parotitis
C. Acute parotitis
D. Recurrent sialadenitis

196. The most common site of leak in CSF rhinorrhoea is:

A. Sphenoid sinus
B. Frontal sinus
C. Cribriform plate
D. Tegmen tympani

197. The technique employed in radiotherapy to counteract the effect of tumour motion due to breathing is known as:

A. Arc Technique
B. Modulation
C. Gating
D. Shunting

198. Gamma Camera in Nuclear medicine is used for:

A. Organ imaging
B. Measuring the radioactivity
C. Monitoring the surface Contamination
D. RIA

199. Type I hypersensitivity is mediated by which of the following immunoglobulin?

A. IgA
B. IgG
C. IgM
D. IgE

200. Lumbar sysmpathectomy is of value in the management of:

A. Intermittent claudication
B. Distal ischaemia affecting the skin of the toes.
C. Arteriovenous Fistula.
D. Back Pain.

Answer Key to MCQs in Self-Assessment Paper

1	C	2	A	3	A	4	B
5	A	6	D	7	C	8	D
9	C	10	B	11	B	12	B
13	C	14	—	15	D	16	A
17	D	18	—	19	—	20	B
21	B	22	C	23	D	24	C
25	C	26	D	27	A	28	B
29	D	30	A	31	A	32	C
33	B	34	C	35	A	36	A
37	A	38	A	39	D	40	D
41	B	42	B	43	B	44	A
45	B	46	C	47	A	48	B
49	B	50	C	51	B	52	B
53	B	54	B	55	A	56	B
57	B	58	D	59	D	60	C
61	B	62	C	63	A	64	A
65	A	66	B	67	B	68	B
69	B	70	A	71	D	72	A
73	D	74	A	75	A	76	B
77	C	78	B	79	B	80	C
81	D	82	D	83	B	84	A
85	B	86	B	87	D	88	C
89	C	90	B	91	C	92	C
93	B	94	C	95	B	96	A
97	B	98	B	99	B	100	B
101	C	102	C	103	B	104	B
105	C	106	B	107	B	108	D
109	A	110	A	111	B	112	A

113	A	114	A	115	A	116	C
117	B	118	B	119	B	120	C
121	C	122	D	123	D	124	B
125	—	126	C	127	B	128	B
129	B	130	B	131	B	132	B
133	A	134	A	135	D	136	D
137	D	138	A	139	A	140	A
141	B	142	B	143	D	144	C
145	C	146	D	147	A	148	D
149	C	150	B	151	D	152	D
153	B	154	A	155	A	156	B
157	D	158	B	159	D	160	C
161	B	162	C	163	B	164	C
165	A	166	D	167	A	168	D
169	B	170	B	171	D	172	D
173	A	174	A	175	B	176	C
177	A	178	B	179	D	180	B
181	A	182	A	183	A	184	B
185	C	186	B	187	D	188	—
189	D	190	B	191	C	192	D
193	B	194	—	195	C	196	C
197	C	198	B	199	D	200	B

Model Test Papers

ORAL SURGERY

1. **The cause of swelling beneath the eye caused by an abscessed maxillary canine is that the**
   A. Lymphatics drain superiorly in this region
   B. Bone is less porous superior to the root apex
   C. Infection has passed into the angular vein which has no valves
   D. The root apex lies superior to the attachment of the caninus and levator labii superioris muscles

2. **A known insulin-dependent diabetic patient feels unwell after the administration of a local anesthetic and becomes pale and sweaty, and does not respond to placing the patient in a supine position. The most likely cause is**
   A. Syncope
   B. Adrenal insufficiency
   C. Hyperglycemia
   D. Hypoglycemia
   E. Carotid sinus reflex

3. **For the cultures from a dental abscess caused by beta hemolytic streptococcus, which of the following is the drug of choice?**
   A. Penicillin
   B. Erythromycin
   C. Tetracycline
   D. Cloxacillin

4. The position of the needle tip during administration of local anesthetic for the inferior alveolar nerve block is?

A. Anterior to the pterygomandibular raphe
B. Superior to the lateral pterygoid muscle
C. Medial to the medial pterygoid muscle
D. Lateral to the sphenomandibular ligament

5. Satisfactory anesthesia in the presence of infection near the injection site cannot be obtained because

A. The swelling causes increased pressure on the nerves
B. Increased blood supply carries the anesthetic solution away too fast
C. Acidity of the infected tissue inhibits action of the anesthetic agent
D. Alkalinity of the infected tissue inhibits action of the anesthetic agent

6. Which muscle is penetrated by the needle during a standard inferior alveolar nerve block?

A. Buccinator
B. Mylohyoid
C. Superior constrictor
D. Masseter
E. Medial (internal) pterygoid

7. After an inferior alveolar nerve block injection, a patient would develop seventh nerve paralysis if the injection was made into the

A. Internal maxillary artery
B. Retroparotid space
C. Internal pterygoid muscle
D. Retromandibular vein
E. Pterygoid plexus of veins

8. In a standard dental cartridge (carpule) containing 1.8 ml 2% lidocaine with epinephrine 1/100,000, the amount of vasoconstrictor is

A. 18.0 mg
B. 0.018 mg

C. 1.8 mg
D. 0.18 mg
E. 180.0 mg

9. A patient suddenly becomes pale and sweaty after an injection of 4 ml of lidocaine 2% with epinephrine 1:100,000. The radial pulse is slow and steady. The respiration is slow. The blood pressure is 80/60. What is the most probable diagnosis?
A. A toxic reaction to lidocaine
B. A toxic reaction to epinephrine
C. An allergic reaction to the local anesthetic
D. Incipient syncope
E. An impending adrenal insufficiency

10. Immediately following a posterior superior alveolar block injection, the patient's face becomes quickly and visibly swollen. The immediate treatment should be to
A. Use pressure followed by cold packs over the swelling
B. Use hot packs over the swelling
C. Refer the patient to a hospital
D. Administer 100 mg hydrocortisone intravenously
E. Administer diphenhydramine hydrochloride (Benadryl®) 50 mg intravenously

11. What is the maximum number of cartridges (1.8 ml) of a 2% local anesthetic solution that can be administered without exceeding a total dose of 300 mg?
A. 2
B. 4
C. 6
D. 8
E. 10

12. For which of the following teeth is the risk of root fracture increased if a rotational force is used during extraction?
A. Upper canine
B. Lower canine
C. Upper first bicuspid
D. Lower first bicuspid
E. Upper lateral incisor

13. In the surgical removal of an impacted mandibular third molar, which of the following would be considered to be the most difficult?

A. Mesio-angular
B. Horizontal
C. Vertical
D. Disto-angular

14. Continued smoking will impair wound healing following a surgical procedure because of

A. Stain development
B. Increased rate of plaque formation
C. Increased rate of calculus formation
D. Contraction of peripheral blood vessels
E. Superficial irritation to tissues by smoke

15. A Le Fort I or Guerin fracture is a

A. Fracture of the zygomatic arch
B. Horizontal fracture of the maxilla
C. Fracture of the malar complex involving the floor of the orbit
D. Pyramidal fracture of the maxilla
E. Craniofacial dysjunction

16. If an odontogenic infection involves the pterygomandi· ular space, the most obvious
clinical sign will be

A. Trismus
B. Facial swelling
C. Swelling in the submandibular area
D. Rise in body temperature above 39°C (102°F)

17. Which of the following will impede healing following the surgical closure of an oroantral fistula?

1. Poor flap design
2. Excessive tissue tension
3. Blowing the nose
4. Sinus infection

A. (1) (2) (3)
B. (1) and (3)
C. (2) and (4)

D. (4) only
E. All of the above

18. Vestibuloplasty is a preprosthetic surgical procedure used to

A. Facilitate reliable impression making
B. Provide adequate posterior inter-arch space
C. Allow placement of teeth over the residual ridge
D. Increase the supporting surface area

19. Bacterial infection may be confirmed by

1. White blood cell count
2. Hemoglobin level
3. Erythrocyte sedimentation rate
4. Platelet count

A. (1) (2) (3)
B. (1) and (3)
C. (2) and (4)
D. (4) only
E. All of the above

20. A surgical flap not repositioned over a bony base will result in

1. Slower healing
2. Foreign body inflammatory reaction
3. Wound dehiscence
4. Necrosis of bone

A. (1) (2) (3)
B. (1) and (3)
C. (2) and (4)
D. (4) only
E. All of the above

21. A periapical infection of a mandibular third molar may spread by direct extension to the

1. Parapharyngeal space
2. Submandibular space
3. Pterygomandibular space
4. Submental space

A. (1) (2) (3)

B. (1) and (3)
C. (2) and (4)
D. (4) only
E. All of the above

22. The washing of hands must be performed before putting on and after removing gloves because it

1. Reduces the number of skin bacteria which multiply and cause irritation
2. Completely eliminates skin bacteria
3. Minimizes the transient bacteria which could contaminate hands through small pinholes
4. Allows gloves to slide on easier when the hands are moist

A. (1) (2) (3)
B. (1) and (3)
C. (2) and (4)
D. (4) only
E. All of the above

23. A patient presenting with diplopia, exophthalmos, nasal bleeding and swelling, may suffer from a fracture of the

A. Neck of the condyle
B. Body of the mandible
C. Zygomatic bone
D. Maxillary tuberosity

24. Ludwig's angina may cause death by

A. Heart failure
B. Asphyxia
C. Convulsions
D. Paralysis of muscles of respiration
E. Pyemia

25. An acute periapical abscess originating from a mandibular third molar generally points and drains in the

A. Submandibular space
B. Pterygomandibular space
C. Buccal vestibule
D. Buccal space

26. When sutures are used to reposition tissue over extraction sites, they should be

1. Placed over firm bone where possible
2. Interrupted, 15 mm apart
3. Firm enough to approximate tissue flaps without blanching
4. Tight enough to produce immediate hemostasis

A. (1) (2) (3)
B. (1) and (3)
C. (2) and (4)
D. (4) only
E. All of the above

27. The design of a mucoperiosteal flap should

1. Provide for visual access
2. Provide for instrument access
3. Permit repositioning over a solid bone base
4. Be semilunar in shape

A. (1) (2) (3)
B. (1) and (3)
C. (2) and (4)
D. (4) only
E. All of the above

28. Which of the following nerves should be anesthetized for extraction of a maxillary lateral incisor?

1. Nasociliary
2. Nasopalatine
3. Sphenopalatine
4. Anterior superior alveolar

A. (1) (2) (3)
B. (1) and (3)
C. (2) and (4)
D. (4) only
E. All of the above

29. The most likely complication associated with the extraction of an isolated maxillary second molar is

A. A dry socket
B. Nerve damage

C. Fracture of the malar ridge
D. Fracture of the tuberosity

30. Trismus is most frequently caused by
A. Tetanus
B. Muscular dystrophy
C. Infection
D. Mandibular fracture

31. An excisional biopsy of a nodule 5 mm in diameter on the lateral border of the tongue was diagnosed as a fibroma. This patient should have
A. Hemisection of the tongue
B. Radiotherapy to site of biopsy
C. No additional therapy
D. Re-excision with wider margins
E. Radium implantation around biopsy site

32. During extraction of a maxillary third molar, the tuberosity is fractured. The tooth with the tuberosity remains attached to the surrounding soft tissue. You should
A. Remove both and suture
B. Leave both and stabilize, if possible
C. Remove both, fill the defect with Gelfoam and suture
D. Reflect the mucoperiosteum, remove the tooth, leaving the tuberosity in place and suture

33. In an acute upper airway obstruction, the entry to the airway on an emergency basis should be made at the
A. Cricoid cartilage
B. Thyroid notch
C. Thyroid membrane
D. Cricothyroid membrane
E. First tracheal ring

34. The most common complication of a venipuncture is
A. Syncope
B. Hematoma
C. Thrombophlebitis
D. Embolus

35. Demineralised bone matrix (DBM) does not have following property?

A. Osteoinductive
B. Osteogenic
C. Osteoconductive
D. All of the above

36. Which of the following is not considered the criteria for the success of the dental implants:

A. There is no evidence of peri-implantitis radioluscency
B. The mean vertical bone loss is less than 0.2 mm per year
C. The individual unattached implant is immobile when clinically checked
D. Slight pain or discomfort is attributable to impant esp to the lateral forces

37. During implant placement, the irreversible bone damage can occur beyond which temprature?

A. 37 C
B. 45 C
C. 55 C
D. 62 C

38. After the removal of impacted mandibular third molar, what is the appropriate time to give analgesics?

A. When pain becomes moderate or severe
B. In the morning of surgery
C. Only after the sensations have returned after effect of L A wears off
D. Before the effect of L A wears off

39. A hemophilic man is having a tooth with periapical radioluscency and putrefied pulp. What is the best Rx for it?

A. Conventional RCT
B. Leaving and waiting till it gives rise to pain
C. Extracting it
D. Sealing formaldehyde to fix the pulp

40. Minimum amount of bone between implant and the inferior alveolar canal is:
A. 1 mm
B. 2 mm
C. 2.5 mm
D. 0.6 mm

41. Which of the following respiratory condition of the patient is most alarming during patient sedation in a dental clinic
A. Apnoea
B. Hyperpnoea
C. Dyspnoea
D. Tachypnoea

42. A thin radiopaque line of bone which outline the root structure is called as:
A. Alveolar crest
B. PDL
C. Nutrient canal
D. Lamina dura
E. Root canal

43. A condition representing with acute gingivitis, punched out papillae and bad taste and breath, low grade fever, poor diet etc point to the condition of
A. ANUG
B. Herpangina
C. Primary herpes
D. Behcet's syndrome

44. A patient with signs of gingival hyperplasia reveals that she on some medicines. Which of the following medicine can be the cause of it?
A. Phenobarbital
B. Phenytoin
C. Diazepam
D. Aspirin

Answer Key to MCQs in Oral Surgery

1	D	2	D	3	A	4	C
5	C	6	C	7	C	8	B
9	D	10	A	11	D	12	C
13	D	14	D	15	B	16	A
17	E	18	D	19	B	20	B
21	A	22	B	23	C	24	B
25	A	26	A	27	A	28	C
29	D	30	C	31	C	32	B
33	D	34	C	35	B	36	D
37	B	38	D	39	A	40	A
41	A	42	D	43	A	44	B

PEDODONTICS

1. A 3 year old requires the extraction of a deciduous maxillary second molar. The local anesthetic technique of choice is
   A. A posterior superior alveolar block
   B. Buccal and palatal infiltration
   C. A tuberosity block plus subperiosteal infiltration of the mesio-buccal root
   D. An infra-orbital block

2. The most appropriate radiographic examination for a 4 year old without visible or clinically detectable caries or anomalies, and with open proximal contacts is
   A. Maxillary and mandibular anterior occlusals
   B. A pair of posterior bite-wings
   C. Maxillary and mandibular posterior periapicals
   D. No radiographic examination

3. A 12 year old child presents with characteristic tetracycline discoloration of the maxillary and mandibular incisors and permanent first molars. The probable age at which this child received tetracycline therapy was
   A. 6 years
   B. 4 years

C. 1 year
D. Before birth

4. The roots of primary molars in the absence of their permanent successors

1. Sometimes are partially resorbed and become ankylosed
2. May remain for years with no significant resorption
3. May remain for years partially resorbed
4. Are always resorbed

A. (1) (2) (3)
B. (1) and (3)
C. (2) and (4)
D. (4) only
E. All of the above

5. A 6 year old patient has a larger than average diastema between the maxillary central incisors.

The radiographic examination shows a mesiodens. In order to manage the diastema, you should extract the mesiodens

A. After its complete eruption
B. Once the patient has reached the age of 12
C. Only if it develops into a cystic lesion
D. As soon as possible

6. In primary molars, radiographic bony changes from an infection are initially seen

A. At the apices
B. In the furcation area
C. At the alveolar crest
D. At the base of the developing tooth

7. In children, the most common cause of a fistula is a/an

A. Acute periradicular abscess
B. Suppurative periradicular periodontitis
C. Acute periodontal abscess
D. Dentigerous cyst

8. An 8 year old patient with all primary molars still present exhibits a cusp-to-cusp relationship of permanent maxillary

and mandibular first molars and good alignment of the lower incisors. The management of this patient should be to

A. Refer for orthodontic consultation
B. Use a cervical headgear to reposition maxillary molars
C. Disk the distal surfaces of primary mandibular second molars
D. Place patient on appropriate recall schedule

9. **The facial and lingual walls of the occlusal portion of a Class II cavity preparation for an amalgam in deciduous teeth should**

A. Be parallel to each other
B. Diverge toward the occlusal surface
C. Converge toward the occlusal surface
D. Not follow the direction of the enamel rods

10. **A large carious exposure occurs on a permanent first molar of a 7 year old. There is no periapical involvement and the tooth is vital. The treatment should be to**

A. Cap the exposure with calcium hydroxide and place zinc-oxide and eugenol
B. Perform a pulpotomy and place calcium hydroxide
C. Perform a pulpectomy
D. Extract the tooth and place a space maintainer

11. **A patient t who has just knocked out his front tooth but that it is still intact. Your instructions should be to**

A. Put the tooth in water and come to your office at the end of the day
B. Wrap the tooth in tissue and come to your office in a week's time
C. Put the tooth in alcohol and come to your office immediately
D. Place tooth under the tongue and come to your office immediately
E. Place the tooth in milk and come to your office immediately

12. **In a 4 year old child, the primary central incisor has discoloured following a traumatic injury. The treatment of choice is**

A. Pulpotomy
B. Pulpectomy

C. Observation
D. Extraction

13. The most appropriate treatment following the extraction of a first primary molar in a 4 year old child is
A. Regular assessment of arch development
B. To perform space analysis
C. Insertion of a space maintainer
D. Extraction of the contra-lateral molar
E. Extraction of the opposing molar

Answer Key to MCQs in Pedodontics

1	B	2	D	3	C	4	A
5	D	6	B	7	A	8	D
9	C	10	B	11	D	12	B
13	C						

CONSERVATIVE

1. Using pins to retain amalgam restorations increases the risk of
1. Cracks in the teeth
2. Pulp exposures
3. Thermal sensitivity
4. Periodontal ligament invasion
   A. (1) (2) (3)
   B. (1) and (3)
   C. (2) and (4)
   D. (4) only
   E. All of the above

2. Sterilization of carious dentin without pulp injury is assured by the application of
A. Phenol
B. 70% ethyl alcohol
C. Chlorhexidine
D. Absolute alcohol
E. None of the above

3. In order to achieve a proper interproximal contact when using a spherical alloy, which of the following is/are essential?

1. A larger sized condenser
2. A thinner matrix band
3. An anatomical wedge
4. Use of mechanical condensation

A. (1) (2) (3)
B. (1) and (3)
C. (2) and (4)
D. (4) only
E. All of the above

4. Endodontic therapy is CONTRAINDICATED in teeth with

A. Inadequate periodontal support
B. Pulp stones
C. Constricted root canals
D. Accessory canals
E. Curved roots

5. What clinical evidence would support a diagnosis of acute dento-alveolar abscess?

1. A negative reaction to the electric vitality tester
2. A positive reaction of short duration to cold
3. A positive reaction to percussion
4. Presence of a draining fistula

A. (1) (2) (3)
B. (1) and (3)
C. (2) and (4)
D. (4) only
E. All of the above

6. The radiographic appearance of internal resorption is

A. Radiolucent enlargement of the pulp cavity
B. Radiolucency around the apex of the root
C. Radiolucency on the surfaces of the root
D. Localized radiopacities in the pulp cavity
E. Radiopacity around the apex of the root

7. Which of the following conditions would NOT require antibiotic premedication before endodontic therapy?

A. Valvular heart disease
B. Cardiac prosthesis
C. Persistent odontogenic fistula
D. Immunosuppressive therapy
E. Organ transplant

8. A 22 year old presents with a fracture of the incisal third of tooth 2.1 exposing a small amount of dentin. The fracture occurred one hour previously. There is no mobility of the tooth but the patient complains that it is rough and sensitive to cold. The most appropriate emergency treatment is to
A. Open the pulp chamber, clean the canal and temporarily close with zinc oxide and eugenol
B. Smooth the surrounding enamel and apply glass ionomer cement
C. Smooth the surrounding enamel and apply a calcium hydroxide cement
D. Place a provisional (temporary) crown.

9. The most important principle dictating location and size of access to the root canal system is
A. Preservation of tooth structure
B. Removal of all caries
C. Straight line access to the canal
D. Removal of all pulp horns

10. Under normal conditions, the most definitive test to confirm the loss of pulp vitality is
A. Applying warm gutta percha to the crown
B. Cutting into the dentin without anesthetic
C. Applying ethyl chloride to the crown
D. Performing a radiographic examination of the tooth
E. Performing an electric pulp test

11. Special attention is given to matrix adaptation for the insertion of amalgam in a MO cavity in a maxillary first premolar because of the
A. Concavity in the cervical third of the mesial surface of the crown
B Restoration being in the esthetic zone
C. Unusual position of the contact area

D. Buccolingual width of the tooth's mesial marginal ridge
E. Size of the interproximal gingival embrasure

12. In pin-retained restorations, the pin holes should be parallel to the
A. Long axis of the tooth
B. Nearest external surface
C. Pulp chamber
D. Axial wall

13. The "smear layer" is an important consideration in
A. Plaque accumulation
B. Caries removal
C. Pulp regeneration
D. Dentin bonding

14. Planing the enamel at the gingival cavosurface of a Class II amalgam preparation on a permanent tooth
A. Should result in a long bevel
B. Is contraindicated because of the low edge strength of amalgam
C. Is unnecessary since the tooth structure in this area is strong
D. Should remove unsupported enamel which may fracture
E. Should result in a sharp gingivoproximal line angle

15. Following root canal therapy, the most desirable form of tissue response at the apical foramen is
A. Cementum deposition
B. Connective tissue capsule formation
C. Epithelium proliferation from the periodontal ligament
D. Dentin deposition

16. In the mandibular first premolar, the occlusal dovetail of an ideal disto-occlusal amalgam preparation is usually not extended into the mesial fossa because of the
A. Small lingual lobe
B. Large buccal cusp
C. Large buccal pulp horn
D. Prominent transverse ridge

17. After initiating preventive management for a 16 year old patient with multiple extensive carious lesions, which of the following restorative treatments is most appropriate?
A. Place amalgam restorations over the next few months
B. Excavate caries and place temporary restorations within the next few weeks
C. Delay any treatment until the hygiene improves
D. Restore all teeth with composite resin over the next few months

18. To ensure maximum marginal strength for an amalgam restoration the cavosurface angle should
A. Approach 45 degrees
B. Approach 90 degrees
C. Be bevelled
D. Be chamfered

19. Generally, glass ionomer cements contain
A. Zinc oxide and distilled water
B. Zinc oxide and polyacrylic acid
C. Fluoroaluminosilicate powder and orthophosphoric acid
D. Fluoroaluminosilicate powder and polyacrylic acid

20. One week after an amalgam restoration is placed in the mandibular first premolar, the patient returns complaining of a sharp pain of short duration when eating or drinking something cold. Teeth respond normally to electric pulp testing and heat and the radiographs are normal. The most likely diagnosis is
A. Hypercementosis
B. Reversible pulpitis
C. Pulpal microabscess
D. Acute periradicular periodontitis

Answer Key to MCQs in Conservative

1	E	2	E	3	E	4	B
5	B	6	A	7	C	8	B
9	C	10	E	11	A	12	B
13	D	14	D	15	D	16	D
17	B	18	B	19	D	20	B

ORTHODONTICS

1. An 8 year old patient with all primary molars still present exhibits a cusp-to-cusp relationship of permanent maxillary and mandibular first molars. The management of this patient should be to

A. Plan serial extractions for more normal adjustment of the occlusion
B. Refer the patient to an orthodontist for consultation
C. Place a cervical headgear to reposition maxillary molars
D. Disk the distal surfaces of primary mandibular second molars to allow normal adjustment of permanent molars
E. Observe

2. A lateral cephalometric radiograph for a patient with a 3 mm anterior functional shift should be taken with the patient in

A. Maximum intercuspation
B. Initial contact
C. Normal rest position
D. Maximum opening
E. Protrusive position

3. If a patient loses a permanent maxillary first molar before the age of 11, the

1. Premolar drifts distally
2. Maxillary second molar erupts and moves mesially
3. Opposing tooth erupts into the space created
4. Overbite increases

A. (1) (2) (3)
B. (1) and (3)
C. (2) and (4)
D. (4) only
E. All of the above

4. Excessive orthodontic force used to move a tooth may

1. Cause hyalinization
2. Cause root resorption
3. Crush the periodontal ligament
4. Impair tooth movement

A. (1) (2) (3)

B. (1) and (3)
C. (2) and (4)
D. (4) only
E. All of the above

5. The angle SNA can be used to evaluate the
A. Maxillary protrusion
B. Overbite
C. Upper incisor inclination
D. Facial height
E. Mandibular angle

6. A single tooth anterior crossbite found in a 9 year old should
A. Self-correct
B. Be treated with a removable appliance
C. Have 2 arch orthodontic treatment
D. Be treated in the complete permanent dentition
E. Be observed and treated when the cuspids have erupted

7. A 7 year old patient has a left unilateral posterior crossbite and a left functional shift of the mandible. The most appropriate treatment for this patient is
A. Bilateral expansion of the maxillary arch
B. Unilateral expansion of maxillary arch
C. Placement of a maxillary repositioning splint
D. Observation until the permanent teeth erupt
E. Bilateral constriction of the mandibular arch

8. The predominant type of movement produced by a finger spring on a removable appliance is
A. Torque
B. Tipping
C. Rotation
D. Translation

9. To prevent mesial drift of a permanent first molar, the ideal time to place a distal extension space maintainer is
A. As soon as the tooth erupts through the gingival tissue
B. After the permanent second molar has erupted
C. Immediately after extraction of the primary second molar
D. As soon as the extraction site of the primary second molar has completely healed

10. The best space maintainer to prevent the lingual collapse that often occurs following the early loss of a mandibular primary canine is a

A. Nance expansion arch
B. Lingual arch
C. Band and loop space maintainer
D. Distal shoe space maintainer

11. A removable orthodontic appliance, producing a light force on the labial of a proclined maxillary central incisor will cause

A. Lingual movement of the crown and lingual movement of the root apex
B. Intrusion of the central incisor and lingual movement of the crown
C. Lingual movement of the crown and labial movement of the root apex
D. Intrusion of the central incisor

12. Recurring tooth rotations occur most frequently after orthodontic correction due to

A. Density of the cortical bone
B. Persistence of tongue and finger habits
C. Free gingival and transseptal fibres
D. Oblique fibres of the periodontal ligament

13. In its classic form, serial extraction is best applied to patients with Class I occlusions with crowding of

A. Less than 10 mm in each of the upper and lower arches and 35% overbite
B. 10 mm or more in each of the upper and lower arches and 35% overbite
C. Less than 10 mm in each of the upper and lower arches and 70% overbite
D. 10 mm or more in each of the upper and lower arches and 70% overbite

14. Following loss of a permanent mandibular first molar at age 8, which of the following changes are likely to occur?

1. Distal drift of second premolar
2. No movement of second premolar

3. Mesial drift of second permanent molar
4. No movement of second permanent molar
   A. (1) (2) (3)
   B. (1) and (3)
   C. (2) and (4)
   D. (4) only
   E. All of the above

15. The most frequent cause of malocclusion is
A. Thumbsucking
B. Mouth breathing
C. Heredity
D. Ectopic eruption

Answer Key to MCQs in Orthodontics

1	E	2	B	3	E	4	E
5	A	6	B	7	A	8	B
9	C	10	B	11	C	12	C
13	B	14	B	15	C		

ORAL PATHOLOGY

1. Caries in older persons is most frequently found on which of the following locations?
A. Pits and fissures
B. Proximal enamel
C. Root surfaces
D. Incisal dentin

2. Benign neoplasms
1. Grow slowly
2. Are generally painless
3. Can be managed conservatively
4. Can metastasize
   A. (1) (2) (3)
   B. (1) and (3)
   C. (2) and (4)

D. (4) only
E. All of the above

3. Which of the following is the LEAST likely primary site for the development of oral squamous cell carcinoma in the elderly?
A. Dorsum of the tongue
B. Floor of the mouth
C. Lateral border of the tongue
D. Tonsillar fossa

4. A radiographic examination of a 10 year old child reveals retention of deciduous teeth and presence of many unerupted supernumerary teeth. This is characteristic of
A. Cleidocranial dysplasia
B. Ectodermal dysplasia
C. Dentinogenesis imperfecta
D. Congenital hypothyroidism

5. A single hypoplastic defect located on the labial surface of a maxillary central incisor is most likely due to a/an
A. Dietary deficiency
B. Endocrine deficiency
C. Tetracycline therapy
D. Trauma to the maxillary primary central incisor
E. High fluoride intake

6. The absence of a pulp chamber in a deciduous maxillary incisor is most likely due to
A. Amelogenesis imperfecta
B. Hypophosphatasia
C. Trauma
D. Ectodermal dysplasia
E. Cleidocranial dysostosis

Answer Key to MCQs in Oral Pathology

1	C	2	A	3	D	4	A
5	D	6	C				

PHARMACOLOGY

1. Acetaminophen in therapeutic doses

1. Retards platelet function
2. Has strong anti-inflammatory properties
3. Produces cns stimulation
4. Has antipyretic properties

A. (1) (2) (3)
B. (1) and (3)
C. (2) and (4)
D. (4) only
E. All of the above

2. In an infection caused by non-penicillinase producing staphylococcus, the drug of choice is

A. Penicillin v
B. Cephalexin
C. Tetracycline
D. Vancomycin

3. Systemic or topical cortisone therapy is used in the treatment of

A. Necrotizing ulcerative gingivitis
B. Erythema multiforme
C. Submaxillary cellulitis
D. Ptyalism (excessive saliva)
E. Herpes simplex

4. Epinephrine should NOT be used as a vasoconstrictor for patients with uncontrolled

A. Hyperthyroidism
B. Hyperparathyroidism
C. Myxedema
D. Asthma

5. Which of the following pharmacokinetic change(s) occur(s) with aging?

A. Absorption is altered by a decrease in the gastric pH
B. Metabolism is decreased by a reduced liver mass
C. Distribution is altered by a decrease in total body fat

D. Excretion is reduced because of lessened renal blood flow
   A. (1) (2) (3)
   B. (1) and (3)
   C. (2) and (4)
   D. (4) only
   E. All of the above

6. Alteration of the intestinal flora by some chemotherapeutic agents can interfere with reabsorption of a contraceptive steroid thus preventing the recirculation of the drug through the enterohepatic circulation. Which of the following can interfere with this mechanism?

1. Codeine
2. Penicillin V
3. Acetaminophen
4. Tetracycline
   A. (1) (2) (3)
   B. (1) and (3)
   C. (2) and (4)
   D. (4) only
   E. All of the above

Answer Key to MCQs in Pharmacology

1	D	2	A	3	B	4	A
5	C	6	C				

MEDICINE

1. A 57 year old man received 10 mg of diazepam intravenously. He becomes unresponsive to verbal stimuli, and his respirations are depressed to 10 per minute. Appropriate treatment is to

A. Administer ephedrine
B. Observe the patient
C. Force the patient to drink coffee
D. Support respiration with oxygen

2. Which of the following would you prescribe for an anxious dental patient with a peptic ulcer?

A. Reserpine
B. Scopolamine
C. Silica gel
D. Diazepam
E. Calcium carbonate

3. A patient who is jaundiced because of liver disease has an increased risk of

A. Post-extraction bleeding
B. Cardiac arrest
C. Postoperative infection
D. Anaphylactic shock
E. Pulmonary embolism

4. Before performing surgery on a patient who is taking warfarin, which of the following should be evaluated?

A. Bleeding time
B. Clotting time
C. Prothrombin time
D. Coagulation time

5. In the treatment of an acute anaphylactic reaction, the first drug that should be administered is

A. Hydroxyzine
B. Epinephrine
C. Hydrocortisone
D. Diphenhydramine

6. Antibiotic prophylaxis is recommended for patients with which of the following?

1. Mitral valve prolapse with regurgitation
2. Cardiac pacemaker
3. Prosthetic heart valves
4. All heart murmurs

A. (1) (2) (3)
B. (1) and (3)
C. (2) and (4)

D. (4) only
E. All of the above

7. Tetracyclines
1. Have no side effects
2. May increase susceptibility to superinfections
3. Are safe to use during pregnancy
4. Have a wide spectrum of antibacterial activity

A. (1) (2) (3)
B. (1) and (3)
C. (2) and (4)
D. (4) only
E. All of the above

8. Which of the following does NOT influence the rate of induction during inhalation anesthesia?
A. Pulmonary ventilation
B. Blood supply to the lungs
C. Hemoglobin content of the blood
D. Concentration of the anesthetic in the inspired mixture
E. Solubility of the anesthetic in blood

9. The usual adult dosage of codeine administered orally is
A. 500–1000 mg
B. 250–500 mg
C. 30–60 mg
D. 2–5 mg

Answer Key to MCQs in Medicine

1	D	2	C	3	A	4	C
5	C	6	A	7	C	8	C
9	C						

PROSTHODONTICS

1. An epinephrine-containing retraction cord has the potential of
A. Interfering with the setting of the impression material

B. Causing tissue necrosis
C. Producing a systemic reaction
D. Discolouring gingival tissue

2. Which of the following is/are (a) useful guide(s) in determining a patient's occlusal vertical dimension?

1. Appearance
2. Phonetics
3. Observation of the rest position
4. Pre-extraction profile records

A. (1) (2) (3)
B. (1) and (3)
C. (2) and (4)
D. (4) only
E. All of the above

3. Upon setting, a mixture of plaster of Paris and water will exhibit

A. Loss in compressive strength
B. Expansion
C. Gain in moisture content
D. Contraction

4. Upon examination of an edentulous patient, it is observed that the tuberosities contact the retromolar pads at the correct occlusal vertical dimension. The treatment of choice is to

A. Reduce the retromolar pads surgically to provide the necessary clearance
B. Reduce the tuberosities surgically to provide the necessary clearance
C. Construct new dentures at an increased occlusal vertical dimension to gain the necessary clearance
D. Proceed with construction of the denture and reduce the posterior extension of the mandibular denture to eliminate interferences

5. A hinge axis facebow records

A. Bennett angle
B. Centric relation
C. Lateral condylar inclination

D. Horizontal condylar inclination
E. Opening and closing axis of the mandible

6. **Following the insertion of complete dentures, a generalized soreness over the entire mandibular alveolar ridge can be caused by**
A. Inadequate interocclusal distance
B. Impingement on the buccal frenum
C. High muscle attachments
D. Excess border thickness

7. **In the design of a removable partial denture, guiding planes are made**
A. Parallel to the long axis of the tooth
B. Parallel to the path of insertion
C. At a right angle to the occlusal plane
D. At a right angle to the major connector

8. **Extreme resorption of an edentulous mandible can bring the alveolar ridge to the level of the attachment of the**
A. Buccinator, styloglossus and geniohyoid muscles
B. Mylohyoid, buccinator and styloglossus muscles
C. Superior constrictor, mylohyoid and buccinator muscles
D. Mylohyoid, buccinator and genioglossus muscles

9. **The location of a crown margin is determined by**
1. Esthetic requirements
2. Clinical crown length
3. Presence of caries
4. Presence of an existing restoration
A. (1) (2) (3)
B. (1) and (3)
C. (2) and (4)
D. (4) only
E. All of the above

10. **A fracture in an all-ceramic crown may be caused by**
1. Inadequate ceramic thickness
2. Sharp line angles in the tooth preparation
3. Excessive occlusal load
4. Use of an inappropriate luting material

A. (1) (2) (3)
B. (1) and (3)
C. (2) and (4)
D. (4) only
E. All of the above

11. The gingival margin of the preparation for a full crown on a posterior tooth, with a clinical crown that satisfies the requirements for retention and resistance, should be placed
A. 0.5 mm subgingivally
B. On the enamel
C. At least 1 mm supragingivally
D. At the cemento-enamel junction
E. At the gingival margin

12. In partial denture design, the major connector should
A. Rigidly connect the bilateral components
B. Act as a stress-breaker
C. Not interfere with lateral forces
D. Dissipate vertical forces

13. A survey of the master cast shows that the 3.5 and 3.7 abutments for a fixed partial denture have different paths of insertion with respect to 3.7. A semi-precision attachment is chosen rather than preparing the teeth again. Where should the male part of the attachment ideally be located?
A. Distal of the 3.5 retainer
B. Distal of the 3.6 pontic
C. Mesial of the 3.7 retainer
D. Mesial of the 3.6 pontic

14. Which of the following should be checked first when a cast gold crown that fits on its die cannot be seated on its abutment?
A. The occlusal contacts
B. The taper of the preparation
C. The proximal contacts
D. The impression used to pour the cast

15. The best way to protect the abutments of a Class I removable partial denture from the negative effects of the additional load applied to them is by

A. Splinting abutments with adjacent teeth
B. Keeping a light occlusion on the distal extensions
C. Placing distal rests on distal abutments
D. Using cast clasps on distal abutments
E. Regular relining of the distal extensions

16. Irreversible hydrocolloid materials are best removed from the mouth by

A. A quick snap
B. A slow teasing motion
C. Twisting and rocking
D. Having the patient create a positive pressure

17. Which of the following structures affects the thickness of the flange of a maxillary complete denture?

A. Malar process
B. Coronoid process
C. Mylohyoid ridge
D. Zygomatic process
E. Genial tubercle

18. During the fabrication of new complete dentures, which of the following can be modified to achieve the desired occlusion?

1. The compensating curve
2. The orientation of the occlusal plane
3. The cusp inclination
4. The condylar inclination

A. (1) (2) (3)
B. (1) and (3)
C. (2) and (4)
D. (4) only
E. All of the above

19. While the teeth are set in wax, dentures are tried in to

A. Verify the maxillomandibular records
B. Verify the vertical dimension of occlusion

C. Evaluate esthetics
D. All of the above

20. A patient with complete dentures complains of clicking. The most common causes are
A. Reduced vertical dimension and improperly balanced occlusion
B. Excessive vertical dimension and poor retention
C. Use of too large a posterior tooth and too little horizontal overlap
D. Improper relation of teeth to the ridge and excessive anterior vertical overlap

21. A maxillary complete denture exhibits more retention and stability than a mandibular one because it
1. Covers a greater area
2. Incorporates a posterior palatal seal
3. Is not subject to as much muscular displacement
4. Is completely surrounded by soft tissue
   A. (1) (2) (3)
   B. (1) and (3)
   C. (2) and (4)
   D. (4) only
   E. All of the above

22. The best means of extending the working time of an irreversible hydrocolloid impression material is to
A. Extend spatulation time
B. Add additional water
C. Use cold water
D. Add a small amount of borax
E. Add potassium sulfate

23. After initial setting, a chemically cured glass ionomer cement restoration should have a coating agent applied to
A. Hasten the final set
B. Protect the cement from moisture
C. Retard the final set
D. Protect the cement from ultraviolet light
E. Create a smooth finish

24. Which of the following cements can chemically bond to enamel?
1. Zinc phosphate cement
2. Polycarboxylate cement
3. Ethoxy benzoic acid cement
4. Glass ionomer cement
   A. (1) (2) (3)
   B. (1) and (3)
   C. (2) and (4)
   D. (4) only
   E. All of the above

25. Compared to unfilled resins, composite resins have
1. Reduced thermal dimensional changes
2. Increased strength
3. Reduced polymerization shrinkage
4. Better polishability
   A. (1) (2) (3)
   B. (1) and (3)
   C. (2) and (4)
   D. (4) only
   E. All of the above

26. The prime advantage of vacuum firing of porcelain is
A. Better colour
B. Less shrinkage
C. More translucency
D. Increased strength

27. In patients wearing complete dentures, the most frequent cause of tooth contact (clicking) during speaking is
A. Nervous tension
B. Incorrect centric relation position
C. Excessive occlusal vertical dimension
D. Lack of vertical overlap
E. Unbalanced occlusion

28. To improve denture stability, mandibular molar teeth should normally be placed
A. Over the crest of the mandibular ridge
B. Buccal to the crest of the mandibular ridge

C. Over the buccal shelf area
D. Lingual to the crest of the mandibular ridge

29. A cast post and core is used to
1. Provide intraradicular venting
2. Strengthen a weakened tooth
3. Redirect the forces of occlusion
4. Provide retention for a cast crown
   A. (1) (2) (3)
   B. (1) and (3)
   C. (2) and (4)
   D. (4) only
   E. All of the above

30. At his first post insertion appointment, a patient with a new removable partial denture complains of a tender abutment tooth. The most likely cause is
A. Overextended borders of the partial
B. Inadequate polishing of the framework
C. Improper path of insertion
D. The occlusion

31. The maxillary cast partial denture major connector design with the greatest potential to cause speech problems is
A. A thick narrow major connector
B. An anterior and a posterior bar
C. A thin broad palatal strap
D. Narrow horseshoe shaped

32. For a cast gold restoration, a gingival bevel is used instead of a shoulder because a bevel
1. Protects the enamel
2. Increases retention
3. Improves marginal adaptation
4. Increases the thickness of gold
   A. (1) (2) (3)
   B. (1) and (3)
   C. (2) and (4)
   D. (4) only
   E. All of the above

33. The anatomical landmarks used to help establish the location of the posterior palatal seal of a maxillary complete denture include the

A. Pterygomaxillary notches and the fovea palatinae
B. Pterygomaxillary notches and the posterior nasal spine
C. Posterior border of the tuberosities and the posterior border of the palatine bone
D. Anterior border of the tuberosities, the palatine raphe and the posterior border of the palatine bone

Answer Key to MCQs in Prosthodontics

1	C	2	E	3	B	4	B
5	E	6	A	7	B	8	D
9	E	10	A	11	C	12	A
13	C	14	D	15	C	16	A
17	B	18	A	19	D	20	B
21	A	22	C	23	B	24	B
25	C	26	A	27	B	28	A
29	C	30	C	31	A	32	B
33	A						

TEST PAPER 1

1. In a Class I occlusion the buccal cusps of maxillary teeth occlude

A. With the lingual surface of the mandibular teeth
B. In the central fossa of the mandibular teeth
C. With the top of the buccal cusp of the mandibular teeth
D. With the buccal surface of the mandibular teeth

2. The most important principle dictating location and size of access to the root canal system is

A. Preservation of tooth structure
B. Removal of all caries
C. Straight line access to the canal
D. Removal of all pulp horns

3. An ideal Class II cavity preparation for an amalgam restoration in a primary molar should have a

A. Proximal box that diverges occlusally
B. Reverse curve
C. Proximal retention grooves
D. Rounded axiopulpal line angle
E. Definite bevel on the gingival cavosurface angle

4. After the crown completion stage, trauma to a developing tooth may be responsible for

A. Enamel hypoplasia
B. Gemination
C. Dilaceration
D. Fusion

5. Radiographic examination of a permanent molar with an acute pulpitis of 24 hour duration would reveal

A. Radiolucency of the bifurcation
B. Normal radiographic appearance
C. Periapical bone rarefaction
D. Altered periodontal ligament space
E. Internal resorption

6. The gingival margin of the preparation for a full crown on a posterior tooth, with a clinical crown that satisfies the requirements for retention and resistance, should be placed

A. 0.5 mm subgingivally
B. On the enamel.
C. Supragingivally
D. At the cemento-enamel junction
E. At the gingival margin

7. To ensure maximum marginal strength for an amalgam restoration the cavosurface angle should

A. Approach 45 degrees
B. Approach 90 degrees
C. Be bevelled
D. Be chamfered

8. In the surgical removal of an impacted mandibular third molar, which of the following would be considered to be the most difficult?

A. Mesio-angular
B. Horizontal
C. Vertical
D. Disto-angular

9. Which articular disease most often accompanies Sjögren's syndrome?

A. Suppurative arthritis
B. Rheumatoid arthritis
C. Degenerative arthrosis
D. Psoriatic arthritis
E. Lupus arthritis

10. Acute osteomyelitis of the mandible differs from malignant neoplasm because it

A. Is asymptomatic
B. Is associated with high fever
C. Has an excellent prognosis
D. Has well defined radiographic margins

11. The maxillary cast partial denture major connector design with the greatest potential to cause speech problems is

A. A thick narrow major connector
B. An anterior and a posterior bar
C. A thin broad palatal strap
D. Narrow horseshoe shaped

12. The principal microorganism in aggressive periodontitis (juvenile periodontitis) is

A. Porphyromonas gingivalis
B. Fusobacterium vincenti
C. Actinobacillus actinomycetemcomitans
D. Prevotella intermedia

13. The objective of scaling and root planing during periodontal therapy is to remove

A. Plaque, calculus, contaminated cementum and junctional epithelium
B. Plaque and calculus exclusively
C. Plaque, calculus and crevicular epithelium
D. Plaque, calculus and contaminated cementum
E. All cementum associated with periodontitis

14. A patient with congestive heart failure may have

1. Epistaxis
2. Shortness of breath
3. Rhinophyma
4. Pitting edema of the ankles

A. (1) (2) (3)
B. (1) and (3)
C. (2) and (4)
D. (4) only
E. All of the above

15. A patient presents with hypodontia, conical teeth, fine, scanty, fair hair, and an intolerance to hot weather. The most likely diagnosis is

A. Achondroplasia
B. Malignant hyperthermia
C. Ectodermal dysplasia
D. Cystic fibrosis

16. The vibrating line of the palate is

1. Always on the hard palate
2. An area which marks the movement of the soft palate
3. Easily located on a cast
4. A useful landmark in complete denture fabrication

A. (1) (2) (3)
B. (1) and (3)
C. (2) and (4)
D. (4) only
E. All of the above

17. In order to achieve a proper interproximal contact when using a spherical alloy, which of the following is/are essential?

1. A larger sized condenser
2. A thinner matrix band
3. A properly placed wedge
4. Use of mechanical condensation

A. (1) (2) (3)
B. (1) and (3)
C. (2) and (4)
D. (4) only
E. All of the above

18. Xerostomia can result from

1. Sjögren's syndrome
2. Radiation therapy for oral cancer
3. Antidepressant drug therapy
4. Anticholinergics (atropine)

A. (1) (2) (3)
B. (1) and (3)
C. (2) and (4)
D. (4) only
E. All of the above

19. The muscles used when closing the jaws to maximum intercuspation include

A. Medial (internal) and lateral pterygoid, masseter, geniohyoid
B. Temporalis, medial pterygoid, masseter, geniohyoid
C. Medial pterygoid, temporalis, masseter

D. Lateral (external) pterygoid, masseter, temporalis, genio-hyoid.

20. Hypothyroidism affects dental development by

A. Causing microdontia
B. Delaying the eruption timetable
C. Causing sclerotic bone to form over the occlusal surface of erupting teeth
D. Accelerating the eruption timetable

21. The lingual nerve contributes sensory fibers to the

1. Tongue
2. Lingual surface of the mandible
3. Floor of the mouth
4. Mandibular posterior teeth

A. (1) (2) (3)
B. (1) and (3)
C. (2) and (4)
D. (4) only
E. All of the above

22. The local anesthetic lidocaine is an

A. Amide
B. Ester
C. Aldehyde
D. Acid

23. Which antibiotic is chiefly bactericidal?

A. Penicillin
B. Erythromycin
C. Tetracycline
D. Chloramphenicol
E. Clindamycin

24. The periodontium is best able to tolerate forces directed to a tooth

A. Horizontally
B. Laterally
C. Obliquely
D. Vertically

25. Abnormalities in blood clotting may be associated with a deficiency of vitamin

A. B_{12}
B. C
C. E
D. K.

26. Molecular attraction between unlike substances is called

A. Adhesion
B. Cohesion
C. Syneresis
D. Absorption

27. Which of the following procedures must be done to ensure acceptable mercury hygiene in a dental office?

A. Use of high volume evacuation when working with amalgam
B. Use of air spray when condensing, polishing or removing amalgam
C. Storage of amalgam scrap in a dry container with a lid
D. A quarterly mercury assessment for office personnel

28. Which of the following is a possible cause for a low density radiograph (light film)?

A. Cold developer
B. Over exposure
C. Improper safety light
D. Excessive developing time

29. After setting, alginate impressions

A. Imbibe water
B. Remain dimensionally stable for 12 hours
C. Have higher tear strength than polyvinylsiloxane impressions
D. Can be poured twice with little effect on accuracy of the resulting cast

30. Cleft lip and palate usually result from

A. Failure of proper union of the median and lateral nasal processes

B. Failure of the union of the median nasal process with the lateral nasal and maxillary processes
C. Anhidrotic ectodermal dysplasia
D. Failure of development of both the lateral nasal and maxillary processes

Answer Key to MCQs in Test Paper 1

1	C	2	C	3	E	4	C
5	D	6	C	7	B	8	D
9	B	10	C	11	A	12	C
13	D	14	C	15	C	16	C
17	E	18	E	19	C	20	B
21	A	22	A	23	A	24	D
25	D	26	A	27	AC	28	A
29	A	30	B				

TEST PAPER 2

1. Sodium content of iontophoresis is:
A. 1%
B. 2%
C. 3%
D. 4%

2. Resistance form of endodontics is:
A. Resists movement of guttapercha in apical area
B. To allow use of spreader in lateral condensation
C. To apply use of plugger in vertical condensation
D. None of the above

3. Appointment for asthmatic patient should be given in:
A. Morning
B. Afternoon
C. Evening
D. Any time

4. **All are true for home bleaching, except:**
   A. Uses 15% carbamide peroxide
   B. In addition to bleaching agent carbapol is used
   C. Vacuum from vinyl trays are used
   D. Both arches bleached simultaneously

5. **Which of the following is true about noise caused by air turbine?**
   A. When above 75 db, it is harmful
   B. Frequency above 1000–8000 cycles/min
   C. Affects elderly individuals more than younger individuals
   D. Its use in younger teeth is contraindicated

6. **I.V. anesthesia is:**
   A. Propofol
   B. Sevoflurane
   C. Flumazanil
   D. Naloxane

7. **About K file all are true, except:**
   A. Has more no. of flutes than reamer
   B. K file is more flexible than reamer
   C. Used to machine the dentin
   D. Made up of triangular/square blank

8. **In class III case to prevent the growth of mandible the force used with chin cup is:**
   A. 0.5 – 1 gm/mm^2 condylar surface area
   B. 6 – 7 gm/mm^2 condylar surface area
   C. 15 – 20 gm/mm^2 condylar surface area
   D. 30 –35 gm/mm^2 condylar surface area

9. **Highest source of vitamin E is:**
   A. Liver
   B. Cod liver oil
   C. Fish
   D. Wheat germ oil

10. **Hypoplasia of enamel caused by deficiency of:**
    A. Vitamin A and D
    B. Vitamin A and B

C. Vitamin B and D
D. Vitamin C and B

11. Pigmentation is caused by all of the following, except:
A. Cushing syndrome
B. Addison's disease
C. Albright's disease
D. Peutz jeghers's syndrome

12. Swollen joint, anemic, loose teeth and dentin dysplasia are because of deficiency of:
A. Vitamin C
B. Vitamin D
C. Vitamin B_{12}
D. Vitamin K

13. All are disadvantage of composite, except:
A. Time consuming procedure
B. Chances of recurrent carries
C. Technique sensitive procedure
D. Causes local abrasion

14. Treatment of dehydrated child patient is:
A. 0.9% Normal saline
B. 5% Dextrose
C. 10% Dextrose
D. 50% Dextrose

15. Culture media of candida is:
A. Methylene blue dextrose agar
B. Sauborad's medium
C. Pingolevin
D. All of the above

16. In saliva bacteria is:
A. 500 million/ml
B. 87 million/ml
C. 45 million/ml
D. 750 million/ml

17. Increased occlusal forces within physiological limit causes:
A Increase width of periodontal ligament

B. Decrease width of periodontal ligament
C. Width remains same
D. Trauma from occlusion

18. Most important content of diet is:
A. Water
B. Proteins
C. Minerals
D. Vitamins

19. High cu content of III generation amalgam is:
A. 12 –32%
B. 2 –12%
C. 1–6%
D. 32 –46%

20. All are true about calcitraumatic line, except:
A. Due to caries
B. Due to death of odontoblastic layer
C. It remains after carries are removed
D. Because of odontoblastic migrate from cell rich zone

21. Motor supply of infrahyoid muscle is:
A. Branches of cervical plexus
B. Vagus nerve
B. Glossopharyngeal nerve
D. Branchial plexus

22. All of the muscles of soft palate supplied by pharyngeal plexus, except:
A. Tensor veli palati
B. Palatoglossus
C. Muscular uvale
D. Palatopharyngeus

23. During preparation of caries vaccine, which is used?
A. IgA
B. IgG
C. IgM
D. IgE

24. **Fluoride in blood carried by:**
    A. Plasma
    B. RBC
    C. Both of the above
    D. WBC

25. **For diagnosis of mouth breathing which is not used?**
    A. Rhinomanometry
    B. Cephalography
    C. Kinesiography
    D. Mouth mirror

26. **What is master apex file?**
    A. Last file selected for obturation
    B. Last file used for removal of soft debris from root canal
    C. File used for determination of length of tooth
    D. File used for master apical preparation

27. **Which of the following immunoglobin shows the maximum amount of immunoglobin after secondary hummoral response?**
    A. IgG
    B. IgM
    C. IgE
    D. IgA

28. **Alkaline phosphate level increase in:**
    A. Hyperparathyroidism
    B. Hypothyroidism
    C. Pernicious anemia
    D. Malnutrition

29. **Chronic non suppurative, low grade infection which leads to localized periosteal reaction is:**
    A. Garre's osteomyelitis
    B. Acute osteomyelitis
    C. Condensing osteitis
    D. Local alveolar osteitis

30. **Regarding pulpal inflammation all are true, except:**
    A. Release of serotonin increases pain

B. There is increase in intrapulpal pressure
C. Platelet aggregation in capillaries causes thrombosis
D. Release of mediators

31. Unattached gingiva:
A. Is interdental gingiva
B. Is below mucogingival fold
C. Cannot be separated by probe
D. Is marginal gingiva

32. Chi square test is:
A. Measures qualitative data
B. Measures both qualitative and quantitative data
C. Measures the qualitative data between two proportions
D. Measures the quantitative data between two proportions

33. All of the following are primary resistance form, except:
A. Rounding of internal line angles
B. Flat pulpal floor
C. Depth at least 1 mm in dentin
D. Include weakened enamel portion

34. Pterygomandibular space contains all, except:
A. Nerve to mylohyoid muscle
B. Long buccal nerve
C. Loose areolar tissue
D. Nerve to medial pterygoid muscle

35. Regarding root caries all are true, except:
A. Caused by actinomycosis viscosis
B. Secondary to gingival recession
C. Remineralization is difficult
D. Slow progress

36. Radiographically lingual developmental groove is seen as:
A. Blurring of root canal
B. Small pulp chamber size and constriction of root canal compare to contralateral tooth
C. Constriction of pulp canal only
D. Large pulp chamber size and constriction of root canal compare to ipsilateral tooth

37. Regarding aesthetics all are true, except:
A. Better when all anterior teeth should be restored simultaneously
B. Better when individual tooth is restored compared to all teeth
C. Crown length can be altered by altering the distance between developmental depressions
D. Crown size can be altered by altering the height of contour

38. Most common malignant tumor in child:
A. Osteosarcoma
B. Ewing sarcoma
C. Metastatic carcinoma
D. Multiple myeloma

39. Multiple punched out lesions seen in:
A. Paget's disease
B. Osteosarcoma
C. Ewing sarcoma
D. Multiple myeloma

40. Folic acid deficiency is precipitated by:
A. Aspirin
B. Ranitidine
C. Cyclosporin
D. Phenytoin

41. All factors are responsible for a normal clotting response, except:
A. Thrombin
B. Plasmin
C. Vitamin K
D. Calcium

42. Incision given within hairline, 45° to zygoma is:
A. Gilli's temporal incisons
B. Alkymat Bramly incision
C. Risdon's incision.
D. Moore's incision.

43. P < .001 is:
A. Highly significant

B. Insignificant
C. Cannot be correlated
D. The probability of significant is not rejected went is true by a magnitude of 1%

44. Darrier's disease is due to deficiency of:
A. Vitamin A
B. Vitamin B_{12}
C. Immune response
D. Glucocorticoids

45. Pain and temperature sensation is carried by:
A. Lateral spinothalamic tract
B. Ventral spinothalamic tract
C. Cortical spinal tract
D. Corticobulbar tract

46. Function of Merkel's cells is:
A. Tactile sensation
B. Melanophage
C. Chemoreceptor
D. Propioception

47. Graft transmitted in same species but not identical is called as:
A. Allograft
B. Isograft.
C. Xenograft
D. Autograft

48. Comparing hatchet and chisel, all are true about hatchet, except:
A. Hatchet blade is heavier and bulkier
B. Hatchet blade is longer
C. Hatchet blade's cutting edge is 90° to long axis
D. Is beveled on one side

49. Impression material of choice in OSMF patient is:
A. Addition silicone
B. Plaster of paris
C. ZnOE
D. Condensation silicone

50. Malunion of fracture of dislocated condyle lead to functional disharmony. This is called as:
A. Ankylosis
B. Dysarthrosis
C. Metaarthrosis
D. Pseudoarthrosis

51. Canine law is used in which classification?
A. Simon's classification
B. Dewey's classification
C. Lischer's classification
D. Bennet's classification

52. Steepest inclined cusp is seen in:
A. Maxillary Ist premolar
B. Maxillary Ist molar
C. Mandibular IInd premolar
D. Mandibular Ist molar

53. After 24 hrs. of setting tensile strength of GIC is:
A. Equal to ZnPO4
B. Greater to ZnPO4
C. Lesser to ZnPO4
D. None of the above

54. Lateral movement of condyle is caused by:
A. Contralateral lateral pterygoid muscle
B. Both lateral and medial pterygoid muscle
C. Epsilateral lateral pterygoid muscle
D. Bilateral contraction of lateral pterygoid muscle

55. Density of radiograph is affected by all, except:
A. mAMP
B. KVP
C. Cone angulation
D. Thickness of object

56. Antirotation effect of post is obtained by:
A. Antirotation notch
B. Antirotation groove in thickest part of root

C. Oval post shape
D. Round cross section post shape

57. About polymerization shrinkage of composite all are true, except:
A. Polymerization shrinkage is greater if bonded surface area is less than unbonded surface area
B. Polymerization shrinkage is high if within 1/3rd enamel margins
C. Acid etching and priming will decrease polymerization shrinkage
D. Microleakage can occur because of polymerization shrinkage

58. Difference between primary and permanent enamel is:
A. In prism arrangement
B. In mineral content
C. No difference in enamel, difference in dentin
D. None of the above

59. WHO 1997 modification of temporary restoration of primary tooth is:
A. Carious
B. Filled with decay
C. Filled without decay
D. Filled tooth

60. All are true about dentin, except:
A. Diameter of dentinal tubules decreases from pulp to dentinoenamel junction
B. No. of dentinal tubules decreases from pulp to dentinoenamel junction
C. 5 –7 μ width of dentinal tubules
D. As depth increases, dentin-bonding strength increases

61. Approximately calcification of root at the time of eruption is:
A. 75%
B. 50%
C. 30%
D. 25%

62. Hypogonadism, developmental delay, loss of taste and smell is due to deficiency of:
A. Cu
B. Zn
C. K
D. Cr

63. Curve passing thru' mandibular buccal and lingual cusp of buccal teeth is:
A. Wilson curve
B. Mansoon curve
C. Curve of Spee
D. Catenary curve

64. Creep rate decreases with:
A. Increase force of condensation
B. Decrease force of condensation
C. Under or overtrituration
D. Delay in time between trituration and condensation

65. Which of the following is untrue regarding exacerbation of phoenix abscess?
A. Tooth is tender on percussion
B. No radiographic change
C. Symptoms are similar to acute alveolar abscess
D. Associated with non vital tooth

66. About guttapercha all are true, except:
A. It contains 60 – 70% guttapercha and 20% ZnO
B. Can be used for lateral condensation
C. With time they become brittle
D. It has two forms α and β on heating

67. All are true about electric pulp test, except:
A. Disintegrated pulp can show normal response
B. Pulp is more sensitive than gingiva
C. Cathode should be placed on tooth
D. Alternating current is best method to illicitate pulp vitality by electric pulp test

68. Adrenal insufficiency causes all, except:
A. Hyponatraemia
B. Hypoglycemia
C. Hypocalcaemia
D. Hypotension

69. Pheochromocytoma is tumor of:
A. Adrenal medulla
B. Adrenal cortex
C. Thyroid gland
D. Parathyroid gland

70. All are true about RVG, except:
A. 80% reduction of patient exposure
B. Instant imaging
C. Easy to storage and retrieval
D. Image is sharper than cause by halogen halide

71. III generation cephalosporin is:
A. Cefadroxil
B. Ceuroxime
C. Cefeperazone
D. Cefaxine

72. Image of superimposition of molar roots on zygoma is avoided by:
A. Paralleling technique
B. Vertical angulation increase by 15°
C. Horizontal angulation is accurate
D. Horizontal angulation of 10° – 20° is best method

73. About bacteriocin produce by bacteria in saliva, all are true, except it:
A. Facilitates growth of other microorganisms
B. Is a peptide
C. Is of therapeutic use in prevention of caries
D. Does not helps in attachment of plaque

74. About acid etching of dentin all are true, except:
A. It removes smear layer
B. It exposes collagen

C. It opens dentinal tubules
D. It increases surface energy

75. Sterilization of hand piece will cause all of the following, except:
A. Loss of torque
B. Wearing of turbine
C. Rusting of body
D. Fibre loss

76. Which of the following is inclusion of cytoplasm?
A. Endoplasmic reticulum
B. Ribosome
C. Golgi body
D. Glycogen

77. Maximum fluoride content is found in:
A. Sea fish
B. Tea
C. Pineapple
D. Coconut water

78. Bond found in GIC is:
A. Covalent bond
B. Ionic bond
C. Hydrogen bond
D. Metallic bond

79. The ratio of no. of death under 1 year of age to total line birth per 1000 live birth per year is:
A. Infant mortality rate
B. Under 5 mortality rate
C. Child mortality rate
D. Life expectancy rate

80. Interradicular bone is:
A. Cancellous
B. Cortical
C. Osteophytic
D. Exophytic

81. All of the following are about efficiency of bur, except:
A. Dianeter of the neck
B. Length and diameter of bur
C. Height of taper of bur
D. Spiral angle and cross-section of bur

82. Gum pads are divide in following section in neonates:
A. 3 in each quadrant
B. 2 in each jaw
C. 5 in each quadrant
D. 2 in each quadrant

83. Outer most covering of nerve fibre is:
A. Perineurium
B. Neurolemma
C. Axolemma
D. Myelin sheath

84. Type or retraction cord used in hypertensive patient is:
A. Plain retraction cord
B. Retraction cord with 8% Alcl3
C. Retraction cord with 2% racemic epinephrine
D. No retraction cord is used

85. Absence of agglutination after mixing patient's blood in Antisera A and Antisera B sample will suggest:
A. Patient's blood group is O Rh (+)
B. Patient's blood group is O Rh (–)
C. Patient's blood group is AB Rh (+)
D. Patient's blood group is AB Rh (–)

86. Engulfment of bacteria is done by:
A. Neutrophilic leukocytes
B. Small lymphocytes
C. Basophilic lymphocytes
D. Large lymphocytes

87. All of the following bacteria are seen in normal periodontium, except;
A. A. viscus
B. Capnocytophaga

C. Vellonella
D. Eubacteria

88. How many no. of scores are found in WHO index for dental fluorosis?
A. 4
B. 5
C. 6
D. 7

89. Axiopulpal line angle should be rounded to:
A. To prevent the fracture of amalgam
B. To prevent the fracture of enamel
C. To remove the unsupported enamel
D. To prevent the fracture of dentin

90. All are true about walking bleach, except:
A. 1 – 3 appointments are required
B. Never be diluted with water and saline
C. Sodium perborate and hydrogen peroxide are mixed
D. Use of eugenol as temporary is contraindicat

Answer Key to MCQs in Test Paper 2

1	B	2	A	3	A	4	A
5	A	6	A	7	D	8	C
9	B	10	A	11	C	12	A
13	D	14	B	15	B	16	D
17	D	18	B	19	A	20	C
21	A	22	B	23	A	24	C
25	C	26	D	27	B	28	A
29	A	30	C	31	B	32	D
33	A	34	A	35	D	36	D
37	A	38	B	39	D	40	D
41	B	42	A	43	A	44	A
45	A	46	A	47	B	48	D
49	A	50	D	51	A	52	B
53	B	54	A	55	C	56	B

57	A	58	A	59	B	60	D
61	A	62	A	63	A	64	A
65	C	66	D	67	A	68	C
69	A	70	A	71	C	72	A
73	A	74	A	75	B	76	D
77	B	78	B	79	A	80	A
81	A	82	C	83	B	84	A
85	B	86	A	87	B	88	B
89	A	90	D				

TEST PAPER 3

1. That the most common contagious disease is the coryza which is:
A. VD
B. Cold
C. Fever
D. Measles

2. US military research shows that an amino acid, tyrosine, boosts brain chemicals that improves motivation and reaction time. Tyrosine is found in:
A. Bananas
B. Chicken
C. Rice
D. Brinjals

3. An Experiment showed that we need sleep to:
A. Rest the body
B. Relax our muscles
C. Dream
D. Reduce brain activity

4. According to Freud, dreams symbolize unconscious desires or anxieties; according to Jung: ideal images. The latest think says:
A. It's recreational
B. It's withdrawal from the real world

C. The brain re-programmers itself in dreams
D. Dreams build up new brain cells

Answer Key to MCQs in Test Paper 3

1 (B) Cold
2. (B) Chicken. Also tuna fish
3. (C) To dream. When a group of sleepers was woken up as their REM-dream stage-began, the showed signs of mental disturbance
4. (C) The brain works on the information it receives in its waking hours and sifts through it during sleep and re-programs itself like a computer

TEST PAPER 4

1. Eating whole-grain bread is said to:
A. Elevate the mood
B. Depress
C. Cause hysteria
D. Improve reflexes

2. Eating bananas helps you combat:
A. Irritability
B. Fatigue
C. Depression
D. Dehydration

3. A tooth which is wholly or party covered by bone gum is called:
A. Buries
B. Non-erupted
C. Sunken
D. Impacted

4. Teeth remain buried in bone and gum due to:
A. Genetic causes
B. Reduction in the size of the human jaw
C. Birth trauma
D. Lack of maturity

5. Chicken pox is infectious 5 days before the rash appears and after that for:

A. 8 days
B. 12 days
C. 10 days
D. 6 days

6. Mumps are infectious 6 days before the glands swell and after that for:

A. 9 days
B. 11 days
C. 13 days
D. 15 days

Answer Key to MCQs in Test Paper 4

1 (A) Elevate the mood. The tryptophan, an amino acid, enters the brain and boots levels of serotonin, the mood-elevating brain chemical
2 (B) Fatigue. Stress drains magnesium from cells resulting in fatigue. Bananas contain magnesium
3 (D) Impacted
4 (B) Gradual reduction in size of human jaw
5 (D) 6 days
6 (A) 9 days

TEST PAPER 5

1. This activity will banish your depression:

A. Wrestling
B. Brisk walking
C. Coffee drinking
D. Sleeping

2. Suffer from insomnia? Exercise:

A. Early in the morning
B. Just before bed-time
C. Four to six hours before bedtime
D. One hour before bedtime

3. Despite a good night's sleep, if your feel very sleepy mid-morning, you could be having

A. Low blood-sugar
B. A brain tumour
C. Low blood pressure
D. A heart problem

4. Mid-morning sleepiness can also be combated by:

A. A 15-minute nap
B. Stretching exercises
C. Pinching yourself
D. Eating chocolate

5. The neuron in the brain is said to look like an insect which is a:

A. Cockroach
B. Mosquito
C. Bee
D. Spider

6. it's called the 'master' because it influences metabolism, growth, second-ary sex characteristics and other hormonal functions. It is the

A. Pituitary land
B. Thyroid gland
C. lymphatic gland
D. nervous system

7. How do you tell if your heart is getting stronger through exercising? Through the:

A. fast pulse rate
B. heavy breathing
C. recovery pulse index
D. the amount you sweat

8. To strengthen your heart while exercising, you must raise your normal heart rate by at least:

A. 50 beats/minute
B. 40 beats/minute
C. 30 beats/minute
D. 20 beats/minute

9. Guess who or what burns the highest number of calories per day?
A. A human being
B. The sun
C. The stars
D. Animals

Answer Key to MCQs in Test Paper 5

1. (B) Brisk walking or any aerobic activity raises nor epinephrine, the natural stimulant that is at a low level in your blood and causes depression
2. (C) Four to six hours before bedtime. When your body temperature is drooping is the best time to nod off into a deep sleep
3. (A) Low blood sugar which arises from skipping meals
4. (B) Stretching exercises. Stand and clasp your hands together and reach as high as you can for 10 seconds. Relax
5. (D) Spider. The cell-body of the neuron has several legs that pick up and pass signals
6. (A) Pituitary gland
7. (C) Recovery pulse index-how much your pulse slows down one minute after you stop exercising. The stronger the heart, the more quickly it recovers
8. (D) 20 beats/minute
9. (B) The sun –at 2000 million million calories per second|

TEST PAPER 6

1. That apart from heart diseases and blood pressure, obesity can also causes
A. Calcium deficiency?
B. Depression?
C. Ageing?
D. Thyroid dysfunction?

2. That the acid-alkaline ratio of our body is:
A. 80% : 20%
B. 70% : 30%

C. 20% : 80%
D. 40% : 50%

3. You should chew your food slowly because it aids digestion and:
A. Cleans your throat
B. Aids teeth maintenance
C. Improves blood circulation
D. Exercises your jaw muscles

4. Sipping a sweet sherbet slowly is:
A. Better than drinking it fast
B. Worse than drinking it fast
C. The some as drinking it fast
D. Recommended for diabetics

5. Khoya made from skimmed buffalo milk has 206 calories in 10 gms. While khoya made from whole cow milk has in 100 gms:
A. 113 calories
B. 213 calories
C. 313 calories
D. 413 calories

6. One glass of buttermilk contains 30 calories. One glass of skimmed milk has:
A. 60 calories
B. 90 calories
C. 120 calories
D. 150 calories

7. If an over the counter drug does not give relief in a certain time-span you must consult your doctor. The time span is:
A. 1 day
B. 2 days
C. 3 days
D. 4 days

8. Pregnant women can ease morning nausea by:
A. Exercising at night
B. Eating a biscuit before rising

C. Sleeping on an empty stomach
D. Taking bed-tea

Answer Key to MCQs in Test Paper 6

1. (A) Calcium deficiency. Excess fat combines with calcium to form an insoluble chemical which penetrate the intestinal wall
2. (C) 20% acid: 80% alkaline
3. (B) Aids teeth maintenance. Chewing secretes more saliva, which prevents bacteria from building up on your teeth
4. (B) Worse that drinking it fast. The sugar dissolves the enamel on your teeth
5. (D) 413 calories
6. (A) 60 calories
7. (B) 2days
8. (B) Eating a biscuit or dry bread before rising

TEST PAPER 7

1. This vegetable is a powerhouse of Vitamin A, which is good for bones, teeth and skin. It is:

A. Spinach
B. Cabbage
C. Carrot
D. Pumpkin

2. Have asthma? Alleviate it which one to two rams of vitamin:

A. A
B. B
C. C
D. D

3. Chemist John Feaerstone of Canada has discovered a new technique that is as effective as brushing your teeth with fluoride. It is:

A. Gargling with alcohol
B. Laser beams shone at the teeth
C. Biting on bark
D. Swallowing fluoride pills

4. Gingivitis is a disease of the:
   A. Gums
   B. Tongue
   C. Inside of lips
   D. Teeth

5. Healthy adults under age 65 should have a physical check-up every:
   A. Year
   B. Two to five year
   C. When they get symptoms
   D. Not required at all

6. Only two to these are professionally qualified to examine eyes and prescribe lens. They are:
   A. Ophthalmologist and optometrist
   B. Optatist and optic neurologist
   C. Optician and optologist
   D. Optimist and opticologist

7. You should take your child for its first dental visit when
   A. The first teeth appears
   B. The first tooth falls
   C. The primary teeth emerge
   D. Any problem occurs

8. If your have disease of gums or bones surrounding the teeth, you should consult a;
   A. Pedodontist
   B. Periodontist
   C. Orthodontist
   D. Prosthodontist

9. About 80 percent of the cholesterol in your blood is produced by your:
   A. Liver
   B. Kidneys
   C. Gall bladder
   D. Heart

Answer Key to MCQs in Test Paper 7

1. (D) Pumpkin
2. (C) Vitamin C. it is a powerful antioxidant and defends the lung against nitrogen oxide
3. (B) Bursts of low-energy laser light beamed at the teeth can prevent cavities says Featherstone
4. (A) Gums is you don't brush your teeth property, bacteria attacks the gums and makes them red
5. (B) Two to Five years
6. (A) Opthalmologist and optometrist
7. (A) When the first primary tooth has emerged
8. (B) Periodontist
9. (A) liver. And 20 percent is influenced by what you eat

TEST QUESTIONS 8

1. The herbs-dried chrysanthemum and gastrodia-are traditional;

A. Headache relievers
B. Blood purifiers
C. Energy givers
D. Digestion aids

2. These herbs were consumed by monks for longevity:

A. Barley
B. Lyceum
C. Ginseng
D. Pine nuts

3. Herbal tea should be drunk:

A. Hot
B. Ice-cold
C. Lukewarm
D. At room temperature

4. Headaches are caused by lowering of:

A. Sugar
B. Serotonin
C. Cholesterol
D. Endorphin

5. Migraine-prone can find relief by taking daily calcium supplements of;
A. 100 mg
B. 200 mg
C. 300 mg
D. 400 mg

6. Plastic surgery has come up with a new laser treatment called surgilase which is for:
A. Facelifts
B. Sagging
C. Crow's feet
D. Fat suctioning

7. Having a problem with spatial intelligence where you feel your ability to view the world accurately is diminishing? Experts say to overcome it, you should:
A. Exercise
B. Weight-train
C. Have a bubble bath
D. Listen to music

8. One cup of the humble pumpkin has 600% of the recommended daily allowance of vitamin a and can prevent certain:
A. Heart diseases
B. Cancers
C. Venereal diseases
D. Skin disorders

9. It's healthier to eat skinned chicken because every 3 ounces of skin has:
A. 4 gms of fat
B. 3 gms of fat
C. 2 gms of fat
D. 1 gms of fat

Answer Key to MCQs in Test Paper 8

1. (A) Headache reliever
2. (D) Pine nuts
3. (D) Room temperature

4. (B) Serotonin-a brain chemical that regulates pain
5. (B) 200 mg
6. (C) Crow's feet around the eyes.
7. (D) Listen to complex music like Mazart's Research has shown that pre-schoolers puzzle building skill improved with music
8. (B) Cancers
9. (A) 4 gms of fat

TEST PAPER 9

1. Osseo-integration is
- A. Structure and functional connection between the bone
- B. Junction between the bone to the overlying mucosa
- C. Structural and functional connection between the ordered living bone and the surface of the load carrying implant or bone
- D. All of the above

2. Implants usually fail due to
- A. Too much heat used fail due to
- B. Improper technique
- C. Improper antiseptic procedure
- D. All of the above

3. the most important aspect for a post implant success is
- A. Type of implant put
- B. Health of the patient
- C. Patients oral hygiene
- D. Position of the implant

4. Medicament used in pulpectomy of deciduous teeth is
- A. Ferric sulphate
- B. Calcium hydroxide
- C. Gluteraldehyde
- D. CCMP

5. The most important step in pulpectomy is
- A. Obturation
- B. Bio-mechanical preparation
- C. Access opening
- D. Extripation

6. Primary teeth have high chances of pulp exposure because

A. Increased blood vessels in the pulp chamber
B. Increased thickness of the dentinal tubules
C. Large pulp chambers with high pulp horns
D. Small pulp chambers with high pulp horns

7. Gingivitis in pregnancy is due to

A. Hormonal changes during pregnancy
B. Gingivitis is not related to pregnancy
C. Pregnancy only accelerates the gingival response to plaque and modifies the existing condition
D. Change in the microbial flora

8. During pregnancy, one should

A. Carry out elective procedure in the 1st or the 3rd trimester only
B. Take drugs whenever required
C. Avoid dental treatment in the 2nd trimester
D. Carry out the dental procedure in the 2nd trimester only with extra care

9. It is important to change your brush every 60 days because

A. Disfigurement of the bristles which could injure your gums
B. Increase in the bacterial flora
C. Old brushes cause systemic and localized diseases
D. All of the above

Answer Key to MCQs in Test Paper 9

1	C	2	D	3	D	4	B
5	C	6	C	7	C	8	D
9	A						

TEST PAPER 10

1. The best X-ray view for maxillary sinus is

A. Water's view
B. Towne's view
C. Submentovertex
D. Occipitomental view

2. In case of an Oro-antral fistula, the fistula has to be excised before surgical closure in

A. Palatal rotation closure in
B. Buccal advancement flap
C. Submucosal pedicle flap
D. All of the above

3. The chain of infection consists of

A. Face makes, puncture resistant gloves and face shield
B. Prophylaxis, immunization and high antibody levels
C. Susceptible host, sufficiently infective pathogen and portal of entry to the host
D. Sanitization, disinfection and sterilization

4. 2% gluteradehyde is used dental infection control procedures for

A. Sanitization only
B. Immersion disinfection
C. Complete sterilization
D. Ultrasonic cleansing agent

5. Hepatitis B viral infection is transmitted through

A. Water
B. Fecal-oral route
C. Air
D. Blood/infectious fluids

6. Extension for prevention in smooth surface caries is

A. Extension to dentino – enamel junction
B. Extension to cavity to areas that are self cleansing
C. Not related to removal of pits and fissures
D. Not related to enamel defects

7. the last primary tooth to be replaced by a permanent tooth is usually the

A. Maxillary second molar
B. Mandibular second molar
C. Maxillary canine
D. Mandibular canine

8. which of the following major physical factors is involve in the use cutting instruments for tooth stricture

A. Heat generated during cutting

B. Vibration developed during cutting

C. Relative effectiveness of efficiency of various cutting instruments

D. All of the above

9. in modern day dentistry the X-ray has become

A. Outlawed due to excessive radiation

B. Unnecessary

C. A foremost aid of diagnosis

D. Inlallible

10. the acceptable radiation limits set by international commission on radiation protection in 1990 is

A. 10 rem per year

B. 2 rem per year

C. 6 rem per year

D. 20 rem per year

11. The interplay between speech pathologist and dental professionals is most vital in management of

A. Cleft lip an palate

B. Soft palate paresis

C. Mandibulectomy and glossectomy due to malignancy

D. All of the above

Answer Key to MCQs in Test Paper 10

1	A	2	D	3	C	4	B
5	D	6	B	7	C	8	D
9	C	10	B	11	A		

TEST PAPER 11

1. The disadvantages of conventional immediate dentures include all except:

A. Inability to plan treatment for failing complete arch fixed prosthesis

B. Inability to correct any prior occlusal discrepancies present in failing prosthesis
C. Multiple visits are required
D. Special laboratory techniques are employed

2. The best type of complete denture patients are:
A. Indifferent
B. Critical
C. Philosophical
D. Skeptical

3. The indications of "the conversion prosthesis" include all except:
A. Failing teeth in an aesthetic area where conventional bridges are not indicated due to span length
B. Extraction sites and immediate placement require an overlying transitional prosthesis
C. Patient cannot wait due to limitation of time
D. Gross occlusal discrepancies requiring immediate correction

4. Exposed vital pulp diagnosed by
A. Radiograph and clinical findings
B. Radiograph only
C. Clinical findings only
D. None of the above

5. In photography, focus refers to:
A. The distance between the nearest and the farthert clearly seen subjects
B. Relationship between the size of the image and size of the subject
C. Degree of clarity of the image on the film
D. Selected period of the time during which light strikes the flims

6. Depth of field is inversely proportional to
A. The shutter speed
B. The area covered in the photograph
C. The size of the aperture
D. The film speed

7. The primary role of a proper access opening is to:
A. Facilitate canal medication
B. Provide good access for irrigation
C. Aid in locating canal orifices
D. Provide straight line access to the apex

8. The solution to combating bad breath of oral origin
A. Tooth brushing and flossing
B. Tongue scraping
C. Mouth fresheners only both a
D. Both a) and b)

9. One characteristic of biofilm is that:
A. It is a homogenous microbial consortia
B. It forms readily over dry surfaces
C. Its development does not have any potential pathogenic effects
D. Its outer layers of microbial-laden material can dislodge into the water stream

10. Microorganisms can enter dental unit waterlines via:
A. Active or passive retraction of patient's oral fluids
B. Municipal water
C. Water bottle or reservoir
D. All of the above

Answer Key to MCQs in Test Paper 11

1	B	2	A	3	D	4	A
5	C	6	C	7	D	8	D
9	D	10	D				

TEST PAPER 12

1. In case of a composite onlay the cusps repuire to be capped if:
A. Caries has greatly undermined the cusps
B. Teeth has been enddontically the cusps
C. The cavity extends more than ½ the cusps width
D. All of the above

2. The degree of the taper in an inlay preparation varies between

A. 5–7 degrees
B. 1–5 degrees
C. 7–10 degrees
D. None of the above

3. In order to establish a satisfactory contact point in an inlay restoration

A. Mark the contact point on the adjacent tooth
B. Fabricate an inlay by an indirect technique
C. Use a split cast model
D. All of the above

4. The major component of the root canal flora are

A. Gram positive aerobes
B. Anaerobic organisms
C. Gram negative aerobes
D. Gram positive and gram negative aerobes

5. which of the following is penicillinase resistant

A. Procaine penicillin
B. Benzyl penicillin
C. Cloxacillin
D. Ampicillin

6. which of the following is the broad - spectrum antibiotic

A. Penicillin
B. Lincomycin
C. Taracycline
D. All of the above

7. The Clarke's rule for the dosage of a drug for a child is

A. Avg. wt of adult x child's wt/adult dose
B. Adult dose x child's wt/avg. wt. of adult
C. Child's wt./avg wt. of adult x adult dose
D. Avg.wt. of adult dose/child' wt

8. Neutral zone is the potential space between

A. The palate and the tongue
B. The tongue and the lingual surfaces of the posterior teeth
C. The cheeks and the buccal surfaces of the posterior teeth
D. Lips and cheeks on one side and tongue on the other

9. A spheroprismatic binocular loupe has primary the following advantage

A. It illuminates the working area brightly
B. Prevents penetration of foreign objects
C. Provides good magnification and relieves eye strain
D. None of the above

10. The interplay between speech pathologist and dental professionals is most vital in management of

A. Cleft lip and palate
B. Soft palate paresis
C. Mandibulectomy and glossectomy due to malignancy
D. All of the above

Answer Key to MCQs in Test Paper 12

1	D	2	A	3	D	4	B
5	C	6	A	7	B	8	D
9	C	10.	A				

TEST PAPER 13

1. As the current adult (Pre-fluoride) generation ages, they are retaining more of their natural dentition and have

A. Greater need for restorative dentistry
B. Less need for restorative dentistry
C. No need for restorative dentistry
D. No need to visit the dentist

2. Evidence-based dentistry is

A. Always using physical diagnostic technique to make decisions about the care of individual patients
B. The conscientious, explicit and judicious use of current best evidence in making decisions about the care of individual patients
C. Providing conscientious, explicit and judicious evidence to individual patients about each dental procedure used in their care
D. None of the above

3. Kay and Locker provided a comprehensive assessment of the literature on the effectiveness of dental health education and concluded that

A. There are no well-designed studies which have shown a decrease in caries through programs aimed at sugar reduction
B. There are many well-designed studies which have shown at decrease in caries through programs aimed at sugar reduction
C. There are no well-designed studies which have shown at decrease in caries through programs aimed at fluoridation
D. None of the above

4. There is strong evidence that supports

A. The role of chewing sugarless gum in the prevention of dental caries
B. The role of aspirin in the prevention of dental caries
C. The role of brushing with fluoride toothpaste in the prevention of dental caries
D. All of the above

5. The 1996 world workshop of periodontics used an evidence-based approach to assess

A. Prevention options for periodontal therapy
B. Diagnostic options for periodontal therapy
C. Treatment options for periodontal therapy
D. All of the above

6. Based on Latin American and Caribbean experience, the prevention of dental disease in lower income developing nations can be best achieved by?

A. Water fluoridation
B. Distributing fluoride tables
C. Promoting brushing
D. Salt fluoridation

7. Organized programs for oral health follow which stages?

A. Assessment, implementation, initial evaluation
B. Assessment, implementation, marketing, long-term evaluation
C. Assessment, implementation, initial evaluation, long-term evaluation
D. Implementation, initial evaluation, long-term evaluation

8. The concentration of fluoride when used in salt fluoridation is:
A. 100–150 ppm
B. 200–250 ppm
C. 150–250 ppm
D. 200–300 ppm

Answer Key to MCQs in Test Paper 13

1	A	2	B	3	A	4	C
5	D	6	D	7	C	8	B

TEST PAPER 14

1. Dental radiographic examinations are:
A. Prescribed after conducting an intraoral examination
B. Indicated based on patient age and history
C. Indicated based on the presence of risk factors
D. All of the above

2. Application of the US FDA guidelines for prescribing radiographic examinations can result in a
A. 43% reduction in periapical radiographs without missing clinically significant disease
B. 25% reduction in periapical radiographs without missing clinically significant disease
C. 43% increase in bitewing radiographs
D. 43% reduction in periapical radiographs: however, clinically significant disease is missed

3. Routine radiographic examinations taken on all patients regardless of clinical indication may
A. Reduce health care costs
B. Substitute for the oral examination
C. Expose the public to unnecessary radiation and costs
D. Contribute to patient care in all cases

4. The US FDA guidelines for prescribing radiographic examinations are designed for
A. Adults
B. Children

C. Pregnant women
D. All of the above

5. The US FDA guidelines for prescribing radiographic examinations
A. Apply to every patient without exception
B. Are subject to clinical judgment
C. Apply to high-risk patients only
D. None of the above

6. What kind of graft promotes osteogenesis?
A. Xenogeneic
B. Autogenous
C. Alloplastic
D. Bioactive glass

7. What is the main disadvantage in the use of barrier membranes in tissue regeneration?
A. They select cell populations occupying the wound
B. They are subject to bacterial colonization
C. They provide space maintenance
D. They are biologically active

8. Periodontal regeneration includes regeneration of the
A. Alveolar bone
B. Periodontal ligament
C. Gingival
D. All of the above

9. In developing countries, oral cancer
A. Is the fifth most common cancer
B. Is the tenth most common cancer
C. Is the third most common cancer
D. Has declined

10. Non-inveasive, early detection of pre-cancerous and cancerous oral lesions can be achieved using a (n)
A. Oral examination
B. Oral epithelium (brush biopsy) screening test
C. Scalpel biopsy
D. None of the above

11. Early stage oral cancers

A. Are often asymptomatic
B. May appear innocuous
C. Are not usually subjected to scalpel biopsy
D. All of the above

12. Preventive dental care must begin before the first tooth erupts

A. In all children
B. In children at high risk
C. In no children
D. None of the above

13. A comprehensive caries management program for children should address

A. Caries
B. Periodontal health
C. Oral function
D. All of the above

14. Periodontal and systemic diseases can occur together without indicating a cause and effect relationship if

A. They have common etiologic factors
B. Periodontal disease is an oral component of the systemic disease
C. The time sequence of occurrence has not been identified
D. All of the above

15. Criteria for assessing relationship from epidemiological studies between periodontal disease and medical inflammatory disease should include

A. Specificity and time sequence
B. Dose-response and strength of the association
C. Biologic credibility and consistency
D. All of the above

Answer Key to MCQs in Test Paper 14

1	A	2	A	3	C	4	D
5	B	6	B	7	B	8	D
9	C	10	B	11	D	12	A
13	D	14	D	15	D		

TEST QUESTIONS 15

1. **Following conditions have been associated with occupational exposure to resin-based restorative materials?**
   A. Rhinitis and conjunctivitis
   B. Parestheria
   C. Dermatitis and urticaria
   D. All of the above

2. **Glass ionomer cement restorations can lead to which of the following adverse reactions?**
   A. Anaphylactic reactions
   B. Mild systemic reactions
   C. Mild pupal irritation
   D. All of the above

3. **Following is the frequency of patients estimated with adverse reactions to dental restorative materials**
   A. More than 1 in 1,000
   B. Between 1 in 1,000 and 1 in 1,00,000
   C. Between 1 in 10,000 and 1 in 1,00,000
   D. Fewer than 1 in 1,00,000

4. **Which compound has been found to have mild mutagenic or carcinogenic potential in mice, but not confirmed in humans?**
   A. Benzoyl peroxide
   B. Methacrylic acid
   C. Camphoroquinone
   D. All of the above

5. **The toxic effects of resin-based dental restorations include**
   A. Cytotoxicity and lichen reactions
   B. Chonic systemic toxicity
   C. Acute systemic toxicity
   D. None of the above

6. **Which of the following contribute(s) to allergic sensitization to resin based dental restorations?**
   A. Degradation of unpolymerized resin
   B. Leaching of unpolymerized resin
   C. Inadequate light curing
   D. All of the above

7. **Which of the following factors is considered to be the most important indicator of high risk for early childhood dental caries?**
   A. Child eats more than three cariogenic snacks per day
   B. Parents do not brush child's teeth regularly
   C. Other family members have caries
   D. Child takes no fluoride supplements

8. **Under what circumstances, Fluoride supplements should be given to young children?**
   A. If they are fed commercial infant formula
   B. If they drink tap water with low fluoride content
   C. If they are less than six months old
   D. All of the above

9. **Strategies aimed at preventing childhood caries should include**
   A. Prenatal treatment of active disease in mothers
   B. Topical fluoride treatment for high-risk children
   C. A series of preventive visits for babies and toddlers
   D. All of the above

10. **Children at high risk for developing caries should**
    A. Receive topical fluoride treatment as soon as teeth emerge
    B. Have the teeth cleaned by dental practitioners
    C. Receive fluoride supplements before six months
    D. All of the above

11. **In children at high risk for dental caries, the topical fluoride treatment begins before the age of**
    A. 6 months
    B. 12 months
    C. 18 months
    D. 24 months

12. **The complication most commonly seen following 3rd molar extractions is**
    A. Dysesthesia
    B. Paresthesia
    C. Alveolitis
    D. Major bacteremia

13. Which of the following are reasonable treatment strategies for unerupted3rd molar?
A. Extraction of some teeth before age 14
B. Extraction of some teeth before age 22
C. Non-intervention and monitoring after age 22
D. All of the above

14. A decision analysis of intervention for unerupted 3rd molar should include
A. Oral hygiene status
B. Risks and benefits of intervention and non-intervention
C. A range of treatment options
D. All of the above

15. Damage to the roots of teeth adjacent to an impacted 3rd molar is
A. Common and easy to seen on x ray
B. Rare and difficult to see on x ray
C. Rare and easy to see on x-ray
D. Common and difficult to see on x-ray

Answer Key to MCQs in Test Paper 15

1	D	2	C	3	B	4	A
5	A	6	D	7	B	8	B
9	D	10	D	11	B	12	C
13	D	14	D	15	B		

TEST PAPER 16

1. Gingival enlargement in Dilantin therapy is an example if:
A. Gingival hypertrophy
B. Gingival hyperplasia
C. Discratr gingival anlargement
D. None of the above

2. Bitewing radiographs are taken to look for:
A. Narrowing of periodontal space
B. Proximal caries
C. Resorption of root
D. Internal resorption

3. Impression material that does Not harden by chemical reaction is:

A. Zinc oxide eugenol
B. Impression compound
C. Alginate
D. Plaster of paris

4. Following metal is most commonly used as an endostral implant

A. Titanium
B. Stainless steel
C. Cobalt-chromium
D. Aluminum

5. The most common clinical sign of trauma to periosontium is:

A. Gingival inflammation
B. Increased attachment loss
C. Increased tooth mobility
D. Pocket formation

6. Which of the following materials should not be used liners or bases under composite restorations?

A. Resin modified Glass lonomers
B. Folwable composite
C. Zinc oxide eugenol
D. Compomer

7. Endodontic implants refer to those:

A. Used to abdurate the canal
B. Used to stabilize periodontally meakened teeth with poor crown root ration
C. Placed between periosteum and cortex of bone
D. Which are embedded in bone

8. Patient complains of losseness of the upper denture while yawning or wide opening, the cause could be

A. III fitting lower denture
B. Posteriorly over extended upper denture
C. Improper occlusion
D. Overextended margins of lower denture

9. The root likely to be pushed into the maxillary sinus during a tooth extraction is

A. Palatal root of maxillary 2nd molar
B. Palatal root of maxillary 1st molar
C. Palatal root of maxillary 1st premolar
D. Mesiobuccal root of maxillary first molar

10. Best treatment for pericoronitis associated with impacted mandibular 3rd molar is:

A. Lrrigating under the operculum
B. Antibiotic and analgesic therapy
C. Extraction of impacted third molar
D. Operculectomy

Answer Key to MCQs in Test Paper 16

1	B	2	B	3	B	4	A
5	C	6	C	7	D	8	B
9	B	10	C				

TEST PAPER 17

1. Borellia Vincenti is a:

A. Mycoplasma
B. Mycobactria
C. Spirochaete
D. Chlamydia

2. Actinomycosis is a:

A. Bacterial infection
B. Viral infection
C. Fungal infection
D. Parasitic infection

3. Techoic acid is present in:

A. Cell wall of Gram-positive organisms
B. Cell wall of Gram-negative organisms
C. Cytoplasm of Gram-positive organisms
D. Cytoplasm of Gram-negative organisms

4. EBV is responsible for all except:
A. Nasopharyngeal carcinoma
B. Burkitt's lymphoma
C. Hepatoma
D. Infectious mononucleosis

5. The most pronounced effect on the oral microflora of a reduction in rate of salivary flow is a:
A. Significant increase in number of oral bacteria
B. Shift towards more acidogenic microflora
C. Significant decrease in number of oral bacteria
D. Shift towards more aerobic microflora

6. Any Principal/dean of recognized Dental College can become a member of Dental Council of India. The maximum members in such category can be:
A. Two
B. Three
C. Four
D. Six

7. The priority program of W.H.O. is:
A. Global eradication of small pox
B. Immunization against common diseases of childhood
C. Surveillance of communicable diseases
D. Child nutrition

8. The headquarter of UNICEF is situated at:
A. Geneva
B. London
C. New York
D. Washington DC

9. The branch of biostatistics which deals with the births, deaths and marriage is called as:
A. Health
B. Medical
C. Demography
D. Vital

10. **When the cry of a child is characterized by a siren like vocabulary, it is called as?**
    A. Compensatory
    B. Frightened
    C. Hurt
    D. Obstinate

11. **Awakening the fundamental desire to learn is known as:**
    A. Motivation
    B. Interest
    C. Learning
    D. Comprehension

12. **"NALGONDA" technique of defluoridation was developed at:**
    A. Chennai
    B. Nagpur
    C. Nalgonda
    D. Banglore

13. **In a path-finder survey, the examination carried out for various age groups in years are:**
    A. 5,10,15,34–45, 65–74
    B. 6,12,15,34–44, 64–75
    C. 5,12,15,34–44,65–74
    D. 5,12,15,30–44,65–74

14. **When a circle is divided into different sector corresponding to the frequencies of the variable in the distribution, the diagram is known as:**
    A. PIE
    B. BAR
    C. HISTOGRAM
    D. PICTOGRAM

15. **In kale water, the highest fluoride value ever recorded is 2800 PPM. In which country this lake is situated?**
    A. Japan
    B. Kenya
    C. Libya
    D. South Africa

16. According to WHO technical series published, CPITN probe is also known as:
A. 611
B. 617
C. 621
D. 625

17. New Zealand type of school dental nurse can perform all of the following clinical duties except:
A. Prophylaxis
B. Pulp capping
C. Root canal treatment
D. Topical fluoride application

18. Sampling which involves grouping the population and then selecting the groups is known as:
A. Cluster
B. Quota
C. Systematic
D. Simple random

19. Dental auxiliaries are not in existence in:
A. America
B. India
C. Saudi-Arabia
D. New Zealand

20. "No Tobacco day " is celebrated every year by the world on:
A. 7th April
A. 31st May
A. 1st August
A. 5th December

21. When making complete denture the occlusal plane should be parallel to the:
A. Frank pert horizontal plane only
B. Inter papillary line only
C. Campers plane only
D. Campers plane and interpupillary line

22. The primary function of the compensatory curve, incorporated in complete dentures is to provide:
A. Stability in centric relation
B. Balanced occlusion, during lateral movements of mandible
C. An esthetically pleasing denture
D. Balancing occlusal contacts, during protrusive movement

23. One of the major disadvantages to immediate denture treatment is:
A. Pain associated with treatment
B. Difficulty in managing occlusions
C. Need foe reline
D. No control over tooth placement and shape

24. Over dentures are indicates over retained roots instead of extracting them and making complete dentures because:
A. To preserve the alveolar bone
B. To allow proprioception from the periodontal ligament of remaining teeth
C. Carrier for patient to adjust
D. All of the above

25. The Gothic arch tracing device is used to record:
A. The vertical dimension of occlusion
B. The centric relation
C. The centric occlusion
D. Vertical dimension at rest

26. "Fluoride sundrome" is a type of:
A. Enamel hypoplasia
B. Dentin hypoplasia
C. Dental caries
D. Fluorosis

27. It is essential that restoration involving the proximal surfaces of deciduous teeth, restore the 2 original mesiodistal dimensions of teeth primarily to:
A. To maintain arch length
B. To maintain esthetics
C. Prevent food impaction
D. Prevent secondary caries

28. Familarization can be the solution of child's behavior problem, in the clinic, if the basis of problem is:
A. Pain
B. Sibling rivarly
C. Fear
D. Parents

29. A mandibular lingual arch with loops mesial to each molar band used in children for:
A. Correction of rotation
B. Regaining the space
C. Space maintenance only
D. Correction of display tilted molar

30. When there is an exposure of the pulp in vital tooth immature apex the treatment of choice is:
A. Apexification
B. Apexogenesis
C. Pulpotomy
D. Pulpectomy

31. When natal teeth are present the most common and preferable approach is to:
A. Extract the teeth
B. Grind the sharp incisal edges
C. Take radiograph and determine the status of adjacent unerupted tooth
D. Retain the teeth if possible

32. The inheritance pattern of dentin genesis imperfecta is:
A. Homozygous
B. Autosomal dominant
C. Recessive
D. X-linked recessive

33. Congenital absence of teeth is most likely to affect the growth of:
A. Palate
B. Maxillary sinus
C. Upper lip
D. Mandibular arch

34. Primary teeth begin to calcify at the age of:
A. 4 to 5 weeks of fetal life
B. Between 4–6 months of fetal life
C. At birth
D. 2–4 months after birth

35. Deviation in which of the following stages of development of dentition result in supernumerary teeth:
A. Apposition
B. Morpho-differenciation
C. Initiation
D. Multiplication

36. The Synder test is designed to:
A. Give a quantitative determination of acidogenic micro-organisms in the oral cavity
B. Predict the acidity of the saliva
C. Estimate the cariogenic potential of dental plague
D. Identify the organisms involved in the carouse process

37. Prolonged use of antibiotics in children can result in:
A. Necrotizing ulcerative gingivitis
B. Candidiasis
C. Actinomycosis
D. Apthous ulcers

38. During mixed dentition stage, which of the following appliance should be used as a space maintain foe missing primary molars in mandibular arch
A. Distal shoe
B. Nances holding arch
C. Passive lingual arch
D. Removable functional acrylic

39. Premature exfoliation of the primary mandibular canine is the most often the sequelae of which the following:
A. Caries
B. Trauma
C. Serial tooth extraction
D. Arch length inadequacy

40. Which of the following provides best guarantee for sterilization in the heat sterilizer?
A. Using chemical indicator strips or pouch
B. Recording a temp/pressure reading from sterilizer gauge
C. Using a bacterial spore test
D. Determining the ability of a sterilizer to kill the Hepatitis B virus

41. Foreign body aspirated during Dental procedures can be retrieved by:
A. Bronchoscopy
B. Gastroscopy
C. Arthroscopy
D. None of above

42. The first brachial arch is called as:
A. Maxillary arch
B. Mandibular arch
C. Hyoid arch
D. None of above

43. Local reaction due to Local Anaesthetic solution:
A. Pain
B. Local irritation
C. Haematoma
D. Dermatitis

44. In Jorqensen technique on IV sedation for dental procedures drugs used are:
A. Pentobardital
B. Mepiridine
C. Scopolamine
D. All above

45. Pick out odd drugs for anaesthetic emergencies are:
A. Aminophylline
B. Epinephrine
C. Atropine sulphate
D. Amoxicillin

46. Nerves anaesthetized in incisive nerve block are:
A. Incisive nerve only
B. Incisive and mental nerve
C. Incisive and inferior alveolar nerve
D. Mental and inferior alveolar nerve

47. Masticator space infection usually result from:
A. Infections of the last two lower molars
B. Non aseptic technique in local anacsthesia
C. External or internal trauma to the mandibular angle region
D. All of above

48. The horizontal fracture of Maxilla is called as:
A. Lefort I fracture
B. Floating jaw fracture of Maxilla
C. Both of above
D. None of above

49. Pre auricular pain, grating sensation and parial trismus are the symptoms of:
A. T.M. joint fibrous ankylosis
B. T.M. joint bony ankylosis
C. T.M. joint pain dysfunction syndrome
D. Ear infection

50. Which of the following is not a surgery for anterior open bite:
A. Thomas trapezoid
B. Thomas corticotomy
C. Thomas Y osteotomy
D. Limberg's osteotomy

51. Apoptosis is:
A. Single cell necrosis
B. Intracytoplasmic accumulation
C. Degenerative change
D. Neoplastic change in the cell

52. Type II collagen is present in:
A. Skin
B. Bone

C. Cartilage
D. Basement membrane

53. Caission disease refers to:
A. Aminiotic fluid ambolism
B. Fat embolism
C. Arterial embolism
D. Gas embolism

54. All of the following malignancies metastasize except:
A. Basal cell carcinoma
B. Adenocarcinoma
C. Squamous cell carcinoma
D. Melanoma

55. Kaposi's sarcoma is more commonly seen in patient with:
A. AIDS
B. Amyloidosis
C. Leukemia
D. HSV infection

56. All of the following lab tests can be used to distinguish streptococci mutans from other oral streptococci, except
A. Gram staining
B. Fermentation of mannitol and sorbital
C. Production of intracellular and extracellular adherent polysaccharide
D. Colony morphology on saliva agar

57. Which of the following is not a characteristics of exotoxins?
A. Produced in minute amounts
B. Released from bacterial cell wall
C. Destroyed by proteolytic enzymes
D. Weakly antigenic

58. Which of the following are correctly matched?
A. Transfer of antibody from mother to child is through colostrums and acquired passive immunity naturally
B. Injection of antibody (hepatitis) is artificially acquired passive immunity

C. Antigenic stimulus given by vaccine(Polio) is artificial active immunity
D. All of the above

59. The common site in oral cavity for lesions of lymphogranuloma venerum
A. Gingiva
B. Tongue
C. Lips
D. Palate

60. Chronic sinus tract present at the angle of lower jaw, yellow purulent granular
A. Tuberculosis
B. Staphyloccal infection
C. Actinomyces
D. Histoplasmosis

61. The crown formation of all permanent teeth except third molar is completed between:
A. Birth to 6 years
B. Birth to 8 years
C. Birth to 12 years
D. 6 years to 12 years

62. The formation of which of the following does not represent normal phyciogical process of dentin formation:
A. Primary and secondary dentin
B. Secondary dentin and circumpulpal dentin
C. Tertiary dentin and sclerotic dentin
D. All of the above

63. Basal lamina consists of:
A. Type I collagen fibres
B. Type II collagen fibres
C. Type IV collagen fibres
D. Type III collagen fibres

64. Secretion of salivary gland is:
A. Apocrine
B. Holocrine

C. Merocrine
D. Endocrine

65. Which of the following has a nonfunctional cusp?
A. Mandibular canine
B. Maxillary second premolar
C. Mandibular first premolar
D. None of the above

66. Buprenorphine acts by following mechanism:
A. Mu receptor antagonist
B. Kappa receptor antagonist
C. Mu receptor partial agonist
D. Kappa receptor partial agonist

67. Which of the following drugs undergoes "Hoffmann elimination"?
A. D-tubocurarine
B. Acetylcholine
C. Atracurium
D. Atropine

68. Mention the drugs causing gynecomastia, hirsuitism, menstrual disturbance on long-term use:
A. Hydrochlorthiazide
B. Amiloride
C. Sporionolactone
D. Acetazolamide

69. Magnesium trisilicate should not be combined with
A. Aluminium hydroxide gel
B. Oxithiazaine
C. Sucralfate
D. Ranitidine

70. I.N.H. induced neuropathy is treated with:
A. Thiamine
B. Pyridoxine
C. Niacin
D. Riboflavin

71. Which of the following conditions causes transudative pleural effusion?
A. Cirrhosis of liver
B. Tuberculosis
C. Bronchogenic
D. Rheumatoid arthritis

72. Hepatitis B infection spreads through all of the following routes except:
A. Blood transfusion
B. Sexual contact
C. Faeco oral route
D. Perinatal transmission

73. Treatment of choice for pneumocystis carinii pneumonia is
A. Trimethoprim/sulgamethoxazole
B. Erythromycin
C. Ofloxacin
D. Tetracycline

74. All of the following are becteriocidal drugs against Mycobacterium tuberculosis except
A. Rifampicin
B. Lsoniazid
C. Pyrezubamide
D. Tetracycline

75. What are the symptoms of diabetes mellitus?
A. Polydipsia
B. Poliuria
C. Poliphagia
D. All of the above

76. Which type of R.P.D. can best resist the forces, to which it is subjected?
A. Class I
B. Class II
C. Class III
D. Class IV

77. How far should be the border of a maxillary major connector be far from the gingival crevices of the teeth?

A. 1 cm
B. 4–6 cm
C. 1–2 mm
D. 0 mm

78. When a large unoperable palatal torus is present major connector of choice is the?

A. Palatal strap
B. Antero-posterior palatal strap
C. Antero-posterior palatal bar
D. Complete palatal plate

79. Compared to resin base the main disadvantage of a metallic denture base in distal extension situation is that, metal bases:

A. Are difficult to keep clean
B. Transfer thermal changes quickly to mucosa
C. Cannot be relined in event of ridge resorption
D. Are subjected to distortion and breakage

80. In Distal extension base partial dentures the impression is recorded in:

A. Pressure impression technique
B. Microstatic impression technique
C. Physiologic impression technique
D. Minimum pressure impression technique

81. Ante's law concerns the:

A. Degree of tipping allowable in the abutment tooth
B. Amount of increase in retentive factor with a full crown verses a 3/4th crown
C. Crown: root ratio
D. Ratio of combined pericemental root surface area of the abutment teeth and the pericemental root surface areas of the teeth to be replaced

82. Extra retention in abutment teeth is obtained by:

A. Dovetail
B. Slots, pins and grooves

C. Outline from
D. Increasing tooth reduction

83. Predictable compliment of optimum tooth preparation should satisfy

A. Biological requirement
B. Esthetic requirement
C. Combination of compromises among the prevalence biological and mechanical considerations
D. Biological mechanical and esthetic requirement

84. Tissue displacement commonly need to obtain

A. Adequate assess to prepared tooth
B. To expose all necessary surfaces, both prepared and not prepared
C. Both of the above(A-B)
D. None of the above

85. Post and core is indicated for:

A. Vital tooth with primary caries
B. Badly damaged non-vital endodontically treated tooth
C. Badly damaged vital tooth
D. Tooth with fractured incisal third

86. A cyst can be differentiated from granuloma rediographically by injecting

A. Radio opaque dyes
B. Poliacrylamide gel
C. Sodium morrhuate
D. Corticosteroids

87. In a pin retained amalgam restoration use of pins

A. Do not reinforces the tooth
B. Weakens the tooth
C. Reinforces the amalgam structure
D. Improves retention of restoration

88. Mercury rich condition in a slow setting amalgam alloy system in a restoration result in

A. Accelerated corrosion
B. Fracture of the restoration

C. Marginal damage
D. All of the above

89. Ethoxy benzoic acid increases the strength and solubility of the cement:
A. Zinc oxide eugenol
B. Polycarboxylate cement
C. Zinc phosphate cement
D. Silicate cement

90. A15% solution of EDTAC has a pH:
A. 5.5
B. 7.3
C. 7.9
D. 7

91. Percussion is a dental diagnostic procedure used in determining whether:
A. The tooth is vital
B. A pulp is metaplastic
C. A periodontitis exist
D. The pulp is metaplastic

92. Glass bead endodontic sterilizer is operated at temperature range:
A. 425–475° F
B. 550–760° F
C. 285–330° F
D. 218–246° F

93. Average length of maxillary cuspid is:
A. 26 mm
B. 33 mm
C. 21 mm
D. 18 mm

94. Internal resorption is characterised by:
A. Pain on percussion
B. Slow dull continuous pain
C. No charaterstic feature symptom free
D. Increased pulpal pain when lying down

95. Uerthane dimethacrylate based composite resin is cured by:
A. Ultraviolet light
B. Visible light
C. Chemical means
D. None of the above

96. A giromatic hand piece for endodontic instrumentation operates by:
A. Rotating motion
B. Oscillating motion
C. Zig-zag motion
D. All of the above

97. Which of the following restorative material is the most biocompatible to the pulp?
A. Silver amalgam
B. Composite resin
C. Glass ionomer cement type II
D. Silicate cement

98. The rate of tarnish and corrosion of class II cast material having VHN 200 is:
A. 0%
B. 2 to 3%
C. 5 to 10%
D. Less than 1%

99. Effective conditioning of the tooth enamel for retention purpose prior insertion of tooth coloured resin-restoration using aqueous solution of phosphoric acid has the concentration
A. 8 to 85%
B. As low as 15%
C. 35 to 50%
D. None of the above

100. A dental bur cuts the tooth structure more effectively when rake angle of bur is:
A. Positive
B. Negative

C. Radial
D. None of the above

101. Which of the following tests will be abnormal in a patient with haemophilia?
A. Bleeding time
B. PTT (Partial Thromboplastin Time)
C. PT (Prothrombin Time)
D. Platelet count

102. Confirmatory test for HIV infection is:
A. ELISA
B. Western blot
C. RIA
D. None of the above

103. The most important investigation done in infective endocarditis is:
A. 2-D ECHO cardiography
B. ECG
C. Serial blood cultures
D. ASO titer

104. Which of the following is not correct about nephrot c syndrome?
A. Proteinuria
B. Hypoalbuminemia
C. Hypolipidemia
D. Lipiduria

105. Which of the following represents the serologic evidence of recent hepatitis B virus infection during "window" period?
A. HBs Ag
B. IgM anti-HBc
C. Anti HBs
D. None of the above

106. Cryoprecipitate is a rich source of:
A. Factor V
B. Factor VII
C. Factor VIII
D. Factor XII

107. Essential granulation tissue constituents include all except:
A. Fibroblast
B. Macrophages
C. Polymorphs
D. Budding blood vessels

108. Toxic effect of local anesthetic includes:
A. Convelsions
B. Asystole
C. Methemoglobinemia
D. All of the above

109. Punched out edge is a characteristic of which type of ulcer:
A. Tuberculous
B. Rodent ulcer
C. Syphilitic
D. Non specific

110. Cystic Hygroma is:
A. Lymphangiectasia
B. Canernous haemangioma
C. Sebaceoua cyst
D. Non specific

111. Early post-operative complications of tracheostomy are all, expect
A. Apnoea
B. Haemorrhage
C. Pneumomedisatinum
D. Tracheal stenosis

112. Treatment strategy in ludwigs angina includes:
A. Amoxycilline plus metronidazole
B. Decompression of both submandibual triangles
C. Tracheostomy
D. All of the above

113. Symptoms of hyperthyroidism are the following except:
A. Emotional lability
B. Heat intolerance

C. Weight gain
D. Excessive appetite

114. Eighty per cent of the salivary stones occur in:
A. Parotid
B. Submandibular
C. Sublingual
D. Minor salivary glands

115. The weakest part of mandible where fracture occurs is:
A. Neck of condyle
B. Angle of mandible
C. Canine fossa
D. All of the above

116. The swollen degenerating epithelial cell due to acantholysis is:
A. Anitschow cell
B. Tzank cell
C. Ghost cell
D. Prickle cell

117. The rate of malignant transformation is highest in:
A. Leukoplakia
B. Oral submucous fibrosis
C. Oral lichen plans
D. Erythroplakia

118. ackerman's tumor is a acronym for:
A. Fibrous dysplasia
B. Epithelial dysplasia
C. Verrucous carcinoma
D. Epithelial dysplaisa
e) Basal cell carcinoma

119. Nikolsky's sign is positive in:
A. Herpes labialis
B. Pemphigoid
C. Pemphigus
D. Herpes zoster

120. Ghost cells are seen in:
A. Ghost teeth
B. Pindborg's tumour
C. Odontogenic keratocyst
D. Calcifying odontogenic cyst

121. Oral hairy leukoplakia is a feature of:
A. White sponge neavus
B. Hairy cell leukemia
C. Speckeled leukoplakia
D. None of the above

122. Liquefaction degeneration of basal cell layer is a histological feature of:
A. Hairy leukoplakia
B. White sponge neavus
C. Oral lichen planus
D. Recurrent apthous ulceration

123. Arecanut chewing is aetiological factor in
A. Leukoedema
B. Oral submucous fibrosis
C. Erythema multiformae
D. Oral lichen planus

124. Oral co-carinogenesis concept is suggested by:
A. Thoma
B. Golbhaber
C. Shafer
D. Pindborg

125. Which of following is not a Oral pre-cancer:
A. Leukoplakia
B. Leukoedema
C. Verrucous hyberplasia
D. Erythroplakia

126. What is the most common skeletal finding in cephalometric radiographs in a patient with a history of cleft palate and anterior cross-bite?
A. Maxillary retrusion

B. Mandilbular protrusion
C. Mandibular retrusion
D. Maxillary protrusion

127. Orthodontics brackets attached directly to the tooth are retained by a:
A. Compressive force
B. Hydrostatic force
C. Mechanical bond
D. Chemical bond

128. Eruption of the permanent maxillary second molar prior to the maxillary second premolar is:
A. Normal and desirable
B. Abnormal and undesirable
C. Abnormal and desirable
D. Normal and undesirable

129. Frankfort horizontal plane is drawn from:
A. Sella to Nasion
B. Orbitale to Nasion
C. Orbitale to Porion
D. Subnasion to Nasion

130. Head gear applied to maxillary molars can improve anteroposterior skeletal dysplasia by:
A. Maxillary growth redirection
B. Bilateral expansion of the palate
C. Anterior repositioning of the maxillary teeth
D. Stimulating growth of the mandible

131. The type of resorption seen when light continous orthodontic forces are applied:
A. Apical
B. Frontal or direct
C. Indirect or undermining
D. No resorption is seen

132. After 6 year of ago, the lengthening of mandible occurs mainly:
A. At the symphysis

B. Between the canines
C. Distal to first permanent molar
D. Along the lower border

133. An early prepubertal growth spurt indicates:
A. Metabolic disturbance
B. Fast maturing child
C. Endocrine dysfunction
D. Slow maturing child

134. "Growth spurt" means:
A. Period of uniform growth
B. Period of sudden acceleration of growth
C. Axis of increased growth extending from head towards the feet
D. None of the above

135. Mechanism of bone growth is by:
A. Bone deposition and resorption
B. Cortical drift
C. Displacement
D. All of the above

136. Grinspan syndrome is associated with:
A. Leukoplakia
B. Lichenplanus
C. Apthous ulcer
D. Oral submucous fibrosis

137. in hemophilia A there is deficiency of:
A. Factor VIII
B. Factor V
C. Factor VI
D. Factor X

138. Ibuprofen is contraindicated in:
A. Patient's having fever
B. Patient's having asthma
C. Patient's having Amoebic dysentery
D. Patient's having Bronchitis

139. Putez-jegher syndrome is characterized by:
A. Deafness
B. Multiple supernumerary teeth
C. Multiple intestinal polyps
D. Scleroderma

140. Cyst that has high recurrence rate is:
A. Incisive canal cyst
B. Periapical cyst
C. Dentigerous cyst
D. Odontogenic keratocyst

141. Routine assessment of Jaw function does not consists of:
A. Palpation of T.M. joint
B. Determination of maximum opening
C. Observation of lateral devastation
D. Arthrography

142. Which is the best for diagnosis of primary herpes simplex infection?
A. Smear stained with Giemsa stain
B. Smear stained with Write's stain
C. Fluourescent staininf of cytology smear
D. Routine cytology

143. Normal bleeding time is:
A. 1 to 6 minutes (modified lvy's method)
B. 8 to 10 minutes
C. 30 to 40 seconds
D. 40 to 50 seconds

144. Most common tumour associated with ADS is:
A. Carcinoma
B. Kaposis sarcoma
C. Melanoma
D. Eving's sarcoma

145. In sickle cell anaemia there is:
A. 75% to 100% Haemoglobin S
B. 10% to 20% Haemoglobin S
C. 20% to 30% Haemoglobin S
D. 50% to 60% Haemoglobin S

146. Why an increased target-film distance is required in the paralleling techniques:
A. To avoid image magnification
B. To avoid distortion
C. To reduce scattered radiation
D. To improve film placement

147. Which of the following is not a type of particulate radiation?
A. Alpha particles
B. Beta particles
C. Protons
D. Nucleons

148. Thyroid dose from panoramic radiography is about:
A. 22 μGY
B. 34 μGY
C. 51 μGY
D. 74 μGY

149. Of the following which is the best projection to study the fracture of zygomatic arch
A. Lateral oblique
B. P.A. Caldwell view
C. Submentovertex view
D. Lateral cephalmetric view

150. Most commonly used colour of the filter used in dark room safelight is:
A. Blue
B. Red
C. Green
D. Yellow

151. When the jaw is opened
A. Condyles move upwards
B. Anticular disc moves posteriorly
C. Lateral ptergoids contract
D. Moves around vertical axis

152. When a patient is asked to say "ah", if the uvula is drawn upwards to the left the cranial nerve likely to be damages is:
A. Vagus

B. Right accessory
C. Left accessory
D. Hypoglossal

153. All of the following are examples of fibrous joint except:
A. Symphysis
B. Gomphosis
C. Sutural
D. Syndesmosis

154. Regarding teeth which statement is wrong?
A. Enamel is harder than dentine
B. Enamel has no cells
C. Ameloblast secrete enamel and dentine
D. Odontoblast produce dentine

155. First pharyngeal arch derivatives includes which of the following structures?
A. Hyoid bone
B. Maxillary process
C. Stapes
D. Styloid process

156. Following are the features of Cretinism, except:
A. Pot-belly
B. Idiotic look
C. Normal intelligence
D. Stunted growth

157. The part of Nephron, "least permeable to water" is:
A. Proximal tubule
B. Descending limb of loop of henle
C. Ascending limb of loop henle
D. Collecting tubule

158. Haemphilia is due to deficiency of:
A. Factor V
B. Factor VII
C. Ca ions
D. Prothrombin

159. At neuromuscular junction following neurotransmitter is released.:
A. Nor-adrenaline
B. Glycine
C. Serotonin
D. Acetylcholine

160. Following are extrapyramidal tracts except:
A. Reticulospinal
B. Corticospinal
C. Rubrospinal
D. Vestibulospinal

161. Liver cells cannot utilize ketone bodies as source of energy due to deficiency of:
A. Glucose 6 phosphatase:
B. Thiophorase
C. Thiolase
D. Thiokinase

162. The hormone which exerts hypoglycemic effect is:
A. Insulin
B. Glucagon
C. Growth hormone
D. Epinephrine

163. Scurvy is a deficiency disease of:
A. Pyridoxine
B. Niacin
C. Riboflavin
D. Ascorbic acid

164. Urea synthesis takes place mainly in:
A. Muscle
B. Liver
C. Kidney
D. Adipose tissue

165. Normal serum calcium level is:
A. 5 to 7 mg%
B. 7 to 9 mg%

C. 9 to 11 mg%
D. 11 to 13 mg%

166. If two elements form an intermetallic compound the mechanical properties of this compound:
A. Are higher then those of either element
B. Are lower than those of either element
C. Fall between those of either element
D. Can not be predicated

167. The term "chroma" aspect in selection of artificial teeth refers to:
A. Degree of saturation of hue
B. Intensity of value
C. Both value and hue
D. None of the above

168. Advantages of minimum mercury technique or Eames technique is all except:
A. High strength
B. Sets quickly
C. Needs no squeezing of excess mercury
D. Greater plasticity and adapts well to cavity walls

169. Gold with highest strength and can be used in stress bearing areas:
A. Gold foil
B. Mat gold
C. Spherical gold
D. Electroply

170. When selecting a dental wire for is ability to withstand a certain stress without experiencing permanent deformation one should consult data tables for the property known as:
A. Elastic limit
B. Fracture strength
C. Modulus if elasticity
D. Precent elongation

171. Inorganic phase of the composites aid in:
A. Increasing the mechanical strength

B. Decrasing the coefficient of thermal expansion
C. Reducing the polymerisation shrinkage
D. All of the above

172. The solder used for soldering two metal alloy parts should have:

A. Fusion temperature below the fusion temperature of both the alloys
B. Fusion temperature above the fusion temperature of both the alloys
C. Fusion temperature equal to the either of the alloys
D. None of the above

173. The main advantage exhibited by the porcelain compared to the tooth coloured restorations:

A. Good marginal integrity
B. High tensile strength
C. Better colour harmony
D. Highly insoluble

174. knoop hardness number of the enamel is :

A. 68
B. 110
C. 343
D. 450

175. Suck back porosity in the casting can be eliminated by:

A. Increasing the mould metal temperature differential
B. Increasing the flow of molten metal
C. Flaring the point of the sprue attachment
D. None of the above

176. There stages in progression of acute odontogenic infection are:

A. Periapical osteitis-Cellulitis - Abcess
B. Abcess-Cellulitis-preiapical osteitis
C. Cellulites-abcess-preiapical osteitis
D. Periapical osteitis-abcess-cellulities

177. Which one of the following is not a sign of recurrence of injured inferior alveolar nerve?

A. Prikling sensation

B. Hyperesthesia
C. Anaesthesia
D. Partial return of sensation

178. Which of the following are known for recurrence?
A. Keratocyst
B. Amaeloblastoma
C. Both of them
D. None of them

179. A lesion composed of microscopic vessels is called as:
A. Haemangioma
B. Angioma
C. None of haemangioma and angioma
D. Haemangioma and angioma

180. Spontaneous closure can be expected in
A. Chronic oroantral fistula
B. Acute oroantral fistula
C. Both chronic and acute oroantral fistula
D. None of above

181. Dendritic cell located among keratinocytes at all suprabasal levels and belonging to reticulo-endothelial system derived from bone marrow are:
A. Melanocytes
B. Langerhans cells
C. Lymphocytes
D. Merkel cell

182. One of the following systemic diseases involving periodontal tissues is not a disorder of neutrophil function
A. Agranulocytosis
B. Chediak-Higashi syndrome
C. Leukemia
D. Cyclin neutropenia

183. The predominant fibre groups affected in the early lesion of gingivitis are:
A. Circular and dentogingival
B. Circular and horizontal

C. Circular and alveolar crest
D. Circular and transseptal

184. All of the following are biologic properties of IgG except:
A. Passes the placental barriers
B. Neutralizes bacterial toxins
C. Binds with organisms enhancing phagocytosis
D. Most efficient activator of complement system

185. The distance between the bottom of calculus and alveolar crest in human periodontal pocket is constant having an approximate length of.
A. 0.97 mm
B. 1.97 mm
C. 2.97 mm
D. 3.97 mm

186. Which of the following is not an instrument grasp during scaling procedure?
A. Pen grasp
B. Thumb grasp
C. Modified pen grasp
D. Palm and thumb grasp

187. Gracey curettes have an offset blade placed to the shank of the instrument at an angle if:
A. 180 degree
B. 100 degree
C. 70 degree
D. 50 degree

188. The concept of calculus formation in which seeding agents induce small foci of calcification which enlarge coalesce to form a calcified mass is termed as:
A. Mineral precipitation
B. Calculus adaptation
C. Heterogenous nucleation
D. None of the above

189. Patients exaggerated concept that something is mechanically wrong in his/her occlusion or jaw is termed as:
A. Bruxism

B. Skeletal malocclusion
C. Phantom bite
D. Jubenile occlusal disharmony

190. The inorganic component of sub gingival plague is derived from:
A. Saliva
B. Gingival cravicular fluid
C. Inorganic matter of tooth
D. Food debries

191. Gingival fluid from diabetics contain a reduced luvel of cuclic adenosine monophosphate which may lead to:
A. Increased severity of gingival inflammation
B. Decreased severity of gingival inflammation
C. No response on gingiva
D. Epithelial desquamation

192. The overall effect of HIV is to gradually impair the immune system by interference with:
A. Helper T Lymphocytes
B. Natural killer cells
C. Plasma cells
D. Macrophages

193. The region in which cementum formation is most rapid is:
A. Middle
B. Coronal
C. Apical
D. Interradicular

194. Alveolar bone proper is also known as:
A. Lamina lucida
B. Lamina densa
C. Lamina propria
D. Lamina dura

195. One of the following drug can slow the loss of alveolar bone in periodontics.
A. Dexamethasone
B. Ibuprofen

C. Penicillin
D. Calcium channel blockers

196. Which of the following is a feature of class I type 3 malocclusion?
A. Posterior cross bite
B. Anterior cross bite
C. Mesial drifting of molars
D. Protrusion of mandibular incisors

197. In occlusion the teeth have:
A. Cusp to cusp contact
B. Edge to edge contact
C. Marginal contact
D. Surface to surface contact

198. The condition in which the occlusal plane of the teeth lies nearer the frank plane than it dose in normal occlusion is term:
A. Distraction
B. Contraction
C. Attraction
D. Retraction

199. All of the following are dental characteristics of a skeletal class III malocclusion, expect:
A. Anterior cross bite
B. Distocclusion
C. Linguoversion of the mandibular molars
D. Posterior cross bite

200. In orthodontics treatment, in order to avoid injuries to the tissues, the forces applied should not exceed the.
A. Arterial blood pressure
B. Capillary blood pressure
C. Masticatory forces
D. Muscular forces of facial muscles

Answer Key to MCQs in Test Paper 17

1	C	2	A	3	A	4	C
5	B	6	C	7	B	8	C
9	D	10	D	11	A	12	B
13	C	14	A	15	B	16	C
17	C	18	A	19	C	20	B
21	D	22	D	23	C	24	D
25	B	26	C	27	A	28	C
29	B	30	B	31	D	32	B
33	D	34	B	35	C	36	A
37	B	38	C	39	D	40	C
41	A	42	B	43	B	44	D
45	D	46	B	47	D	48	D
49	C	50	B	51	A	52	C
53	D	54	A	55	A	56	A
57	D	58	D	59	B	60	C
61	B	62	C	63	C	64	C
65	C	66	C	67	C	68	C
69	C	70	B	71	A	72	C
73	A	74	D	75	D	76	C
77	B	78	C	79	C	80	C
81	D	82	B	83	D	84	C
85	B	86	B	87	D	88	D
89	A	90	B	91	C	92	A
93	A	94	C	95	B	96	B
97	C	98	B	99	B	100	A
101	B	102	B	103	C	104	C
105	B	106	C	107	C	108	D
109	C	110	A	111	D	112	D
113	C	114	B	115	A	116	B
117	D	118	C	119	C	120	D
121	D	122	C	123	B	124	B
125	B	126	A	127	C	128	B
129	C	130	A	131	B	132	D
133	B	134	B	135	D	136	B
137	A	138	B	139	C	140	D
141	D	142	C	143	A	144	B

145	A	146	A	147	D	148	D
149	C	150	B	151	B	152	A
153	A	154	C	155	B	156	C
157	C	158	B	159	D	160	B
161	B	162	A	163	D	164	B
165	C	166	D	167	A	168	D
169	B	170	A	171	D	172	A
173	D	174	C	175	C	176	A
177	C	178	C	179	D	180	B
181	B	182	C	183	A	184	D
185	B	186	B	187	C	188	C
189	C	190	B	191	A	192	A
193	C	194	D	195	B	196	B
197	D	198	C	199	B	200	B

Reader's Notes

Reader's Notes

Reader's Notes

Reader's Notes